HEALTH, ETHNICITY, AND WELL-BEING

AN AFRICAN AMERICAN PERSPECTIVE

Edited by:

Penelope J. Kinsey, PhD
Consulting Psychologist
The Lincoln University, Pennsylvania

Delroy M. Louden, PhD, FRSPH
President
Anguilla Community College
Anguilla, British West Indies

i

Library of Congress Control Number:		2013911869
ISBN:	Hardcover	978-1-4836-5391-4
	Softcover	978-1-4836-5390-7
	eBook	978-1-4836-5392-1

Rev. date: 02/15/2014

To order additional copies of this book, contact:
Xlibris LLC
1-888-795-4274
www.Xlibris.com
Orders@Xlibris.com
590051

ii

This book is dedicated to the mother of Dr. Kinsey,
and
countless other women who died before their time.

The design for this book was done by Dameshe Hardy, a 2013 graduate of Lincoln University with a BS in Graphic Design. Dameshe is currently a freelance graphic designer. Her immediate plans are to pursue a Master of Arts degree at The Academy of Art University in San Francisco.

Acknowledgments

This book is not the result of one person; and, we thank those colleagues who believed in the worth and significance of this book in the form of their contributions. We also gratefully acknowledge the support of The Lincoln University (PA) in making this publication possible. We sincerely thank the staff at Anguilla Community College, especially Ms Suzanna Proctor, for their invaluable assistance. We also thank Ms Allison Kinsey for her editorial skills in the final preparation of this book. We appreciate the research skills of our scholar-students, Gervon Anderson, Morgan Heath, Chelsea Small, and Emmanuel Woodson, who helped to bring this project to completion.

Finally, we are eternally grateful to our spouses, Bradshaw and Jonice, who not only understood and appreciated our deep commitment in writing this book, but who also provided us with love, encouragement, and the time and space needed to complete this labor of love

Penelope Kinsey
Delroy Louden

Preface

This book is the third in a series of anthologies by noted faculty members from historically black colleges and universities (HBCUs) who are trained health care researchers and professionals, and, by distinguished researchers and health care practitioners dedicated to developing more culturally competent strategies to eliminate disparities in health care outcomes for African Americans. A main theme of the book is that current models and practices of health care present many practitioners with challenges for which their training does not prepare them. With the prediction of a rapid, increase in the size of the African American population in major cities across America, the implications for client knowledge and training of health care professionals lacking sufficient cultural competence are extremely important, relevant, and timely. Although training for improving interactions with African Americans has received much attention in the last decade, it has been inadequate, stemming from misinterpretation of culturally based behaviors, misdiagnosis, misuse of health care procedures, and "unintentional racism." Consequently, lack of training means that many health care professionals are deficient in the skills, attitudes, and sensitivities needed to effectively deliver health care to African Americans.

Health care professionals are becoming increasingly aware of the need to respond to the enormous challenges posed by a culturally diverse population. Other practitioners recognize the inadequacy of the models used to conceptualize and strategize health care for African Americans. Various attempts to develop research strategies aimed at targeting reasons for the disparities in health care outcomes have yielded discouragingly low success and high dropout rates, Other problems stem from the lack of knowledge and skills necessary to engage African Americans in health care delivery, and the lack of effective, culturally significant, tools of assessments. In spite of great, technological advances in medicine and health care delivery, there is strong evidence of the inadequacy of practitioners' knowledge base to deliver culturally appropriate services to African Americans.

A central argument posed in this book is that the primary purpose of culturally competent health care is the alleviation of disparities in health care outcomes. The search for solutions to the problem of disparities is of crucial significance. This book is an attempt to address the problem by giving voice to a diverse, interdisciplinary group of researchers and practitioners in twelve chapters segmented into four parts. Part I presents some critical issues that impact African Americans with respect to the historical barriers that have prevented access to health care, epidemiological challenges, issues relating to gender and age, the role that economics plays in the neglect of health in the African American community, and the specific, health concerns of the youth culture. Part II focuses on two, significant factors impacting health care delivery—self-assessments and educational approaches. Part III presents examples of culturally competent strategies which have been instituted in African American communities throughout the country. Part IV examines future directions and challenges for the twenty-first century related to cultural competency.

CONTENTS

Virginia J. Smith, PhD, MSW
    The Lincoln University, Pennsylvania
Frank P. Worts, MSW, MA
    The Lincoln University, Pennsylvania
Jennifer Smith, DMD
    University of Pennsylvania School of Medicine

William K. Dadson, PhD, MBA
    The Lincoln University, Pennsylvania

Charles Pinckney, PhD
    University of North Carolina at Charlotte
Elizabeth Alston-Pinckney, MA
    Livingstone College

II. CULTURE IN EFFECTIVE HEALTH CARE DELIVERY:
     ASSESSMENT AND EDUCATIONAL ISSUES

Tawara D Goode, MA
    Georgetown University
Sonja Harris Haywood, MD, MS
    Case Western Reserve U. School of Medicine
Suzanne Bronheim, PhD
    Georgetown University School of Medicine

Kristyn Smith, BA
Emory University at Washington DC
Laurie Murphy, MBA, MPH
Case Western Reserve U. School of Medicine

Linda Fleisher, PhD, MPH
Children's Hospital of Philadelphia
Sarah Bauerie Bass, PhD, MPH
Temple University
Evelyn Gonzalez, MA
Fox Chase Cancer Center
Stacy N Davis, PhD, MPH
H. Lee Moffitt Cancer Center
Rachael Slamon, MSc
American Diabetes Association, Philadelphia
Stephanie Ravitch, BA
Fox Chase Cancer Center
Maria Jibaja-Weiss, EdD
Baylor College of Medicine
Luis O Rustveld, PhD
Baylor College of Medicine
Venkata Kandadai, MPH
Children's Hospital of Philadelphia
Michael C. Gibbons, MD, MPH
Johns Hopkins Medical Institutions

III. PREVENTION AND INTERVENTION STRATEGIES IN AFRICAN AMERICAN COMMUNITIES: SELECTED EXAMPLES

Domenica F Mcbride, PhD
Help Institute, Inc.

About the Editors: Dr. Kinsey

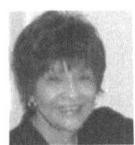

Dr. Penelope Kinsey is a Clinical Psychologist who recently retired from The Lincoln University, Pennsylvania, the nation's oldest historically black university. During her long tenure at the University, Dr. Kinsey was a Professor and Past Chair in the Department of Psychology. She is currently developing a consulting service that will provide consultation for the development and use of test protocols in the assessment of chronic pain, and for the use of culturally sensitive instruments in the evaluation of health care effectiveness for underserved populations.

In addition to her long tenure as an academician at Lincoln, Dr. Kinsey worked as a psychologist in private practice. In addition to her clinical work with Margolis and Associates, LLC, a practice located in Philadelphia, PA, Dr Kinsey served as Research Coordinator for the group. She was primarily responsible for coordinating research activities that focused on the development of reliable and valid instruments for assessing pain and the therapeutic effectiveness of the procedures used by the group to reduce pain in chronic diseases.

In her role as Consulting Psychologist, Dr. Kinsey has been, and continues to be, involved in the development of program evaluations for primary, medical care/outpatient, medical services, and formulation of protocols that focus on the role of spirituality/religiosity in the assessment and treatment of African Americans. One notable example was her work on a grant from the Pew Foundation that focused on the development of culturally competent assessment procedures and tools for health care staff serving minority patients with HIV/AIDS in three, major, Philadelphia area hospitals. Her collaboration with Dr. Delroy Louden, a co-editor and contributor for this book, and two previous ones, attest to her commitment toward easing health disparities among historically underserved populations.

Dr. Kinsey is the recipient of three Woodrow Wilson Fellowships, the Charles Lindback Award for Distinguished Teaching, and the

Lincoln University Faculty Award for Distinguished Teaching. She has been noted in the Who's Who Executive and Professional Registry, Directory of American Scholars, and Who's Who among American Teachers. Dr. Kinsey received her PhD in Clinical Psychology from the University of Delaware.

About the Editors: Dr. Louden

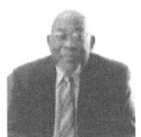

Dr. Louden is the first President of Anguilla Community College (ACC), British West Indies. Prior to this, Dr. Louden was a Professor and Past Chair in the Department of Psychology at The Lincoln University, Pennsylvania, and, while at Lincoln, served as Principal Investigator on several funded research projects in collaboration with major research institutions, most notably those focusing on adolescent obesity with Children's Hospital of Philadelphia, colorectal cancer with Penn State College of Medicine and the North East Cancer Center; and, on the elimination of cancer health disparities via research and training with Fox Chase Cancer Center of Philadelphia.

Dr. Louden's international experience includes the development of peer health educator training to combat HIV/AIDS in Nigeria, the investigation of the prevalence and incidence of drug abuse in Toronto, service as a member of the Jamaican government's task force on work attitudes, and service as a member of the Organization of American States to investigate family planning attitudes in adolescent parents within the English speaking Caribbean. He has provided consultation in a variety of settings, more recently with the Substance Abuse and Mental Health Administration (SAMSHA), and as Track Co-Chair at the CDC 2002 HIV/AIDS Prevention Conference.

Dr. Louden brings a distinguished record of research, teaching, and scholarship, having held senior appointments in academic and in the non-profit world, most notably in Nigeria, UWI-Mona, Canada, and the United States. He also served as Director of Epidemiology and Surveillance-Bureau of Tuberculosis for the New York City Department of Health, and, later as Vice President for Research at the National League for Nursing in New York. He is the recipient of several awards, notably a Fulbright Scholarship, the US Bureau of Primary Health Care Policy Fellowship, and a fellowship from the Royal Society of Public Health. He is a Fellow in the Royal Society of Public Health, United Kingdom. Dr. Louden received his PhD in the Department of Mental Health from the University of Bristol, England, and post-doctoral training in Epidemiology and Public Health from the Johns Hopkins University.

About the Contributors: Professional Highlights

Professor Elizabeth Alston-Pinckney

Mrs. Alston-Pinckney is the Director of Counseling Services at Livingstone College. She is also an Instructor in the Department of Psychology. Prior to joining Livingstone College in 2007, Ms. Alston-Pinckney served as the Vice President of the Palmetto Group, an educational non-profit organization in Columbia, South Carolina. She is a freelance writer and producer with over ten years of experience as a social worker. Mrs. Alston-Pinckney received her MA in Counseling from Webster University. Currently, she is pursuing her PhD in Counseling at Liberty University

Dr. Sarah B. Bass

Dr. Bass is an Associate Professor of Public Health and Undergraduate Program Director in the Department of Public Health at Temple University. Dr. Bass has almost twenty years of experience and training in communication message development, public health research and teaching at both the undergraduate and graduate levels. As Co-Director of Temple's Risk Communication Laboratory, Dr. Bass' research focuses on health and risk communication and how public health messages are crafted for all audiences. She also has researched the use of new technologies such as the Internet and their impact on patient/public self-efficacy and behavior intention. She has widely published in the area of health communication and recently authored a guide on Health Literacy. In addition, she has developed and implemented a number of community based health education programs, including interventions in the areas of HIV/AIDS, Drug Abuse Prevention and Child Care Education. Dr. Bass received her Ph.D. in Health Education from Temple University and a MPH in Community Health from Temple University.

Dr. Lula Beatty

Dr. Beatty is the Senior Director, Health Disparities, American Psychological Association. She is responsible for the development and implementation of APA's strategic initiative on health disparities, including the conceptualization of initiatives, goals, and translation into programs and activities, and the development of resources and collaborations. Until 2012, Dr. Beatty was the Director of the Special Populations Office, Office of the Director, National Institute on Drug Abuse, National Institutes of Health. She was responsible for the overall development and execution of diversity and health disparities programs for NIDA. In addition to administering continuing programs (e.g., the Diversity Supplement Program), she developed special initiatives on South Africa, African Americans and criminal justice, and health disparities in boys and men. Before joining NIDA, she was Director of Research at the Institute for Urban Affairs at Howard University, where she was involved in training and research programs, child abuse and neglect, Black family strengths, and mental health in the Black community. She has published in the areas of health disparities, drug abuse and addiction, diversity in science, health disparities in boys and men, and racial/ethnic, health concerns. She is a Fellow in the Society of Women in Psychology and the Society for the Psychological Study of Ethnic Minority Issues, American Psychological Association (APA). She has served as President of the Section of the Psychology of Black Women, APA, and is a founding faculty member of the Leadership Institute for Women in Psychology. Dr. Beatty received her Ph.D. in Developmental Psychology from Howard University.

Dr. J. Robert Beck

Dr. Beck holds several executive positions at Fox Chase Cancer Center. He is the Senior Vice President, Chief Academic Officer, Chief Medical Officer, and is the H.O. West and J. R. Wike Chair in Cancer Research. As Chief Academic Officer, Dr. Beck supervises the Office of Academic Programs, the Office of Corporate Partnerships, the Office of Health Communications and Health Disparities, and the Institutional Review Board, as well as a number of core research facilities and information technology. As the Chief Medical Officer, he works with physicians and nurses to improve the delivery of clinical care in both the inpatient and outpatient departments, and senior administrative leaders to improve processes, quality, and safety in all patient-related areas. Dr. Beck also helps foster academic collaborations with a wide variety of national and international universities, research institutions and oncologists. One notable example of these linkages is his collaboration with colleagues at Lincoln University. Dr. Beck led the joint Fox

Chase-Lincoln effort to obtain a NCI P20 award which has provided many Lincoln faculty and senior students with opportunities to partner with colleagues at Fox Chase for the purpose of developing faculty research projects and mentoring experiences. He previously served as Fox Chase's Deputy Director of the Population Science Division, and, as Vice President for Information Services and Chief Information Officer. Before joining Fox Chase in 2001, Dr. Beck was Vice President for Information, Research and Planning at Baylor College of Medicine in Houston, Texas. He was also a Professor of Pathology and Professor of Family and Community Medicine. In the recent past, he has served as Editor-in-Chief of *Medical Decision Making*. Dr. Beck served on the editorial boards of *Disease Management* and the *Journal of Biomedical Informatics* until last year. Dr. Beck received his MD from Johns Hopkins University with a specialization in Clinical Decision Making.

Ms. Theresa E. Berger

Ms. Berger has twenty-five years of experience in health care and research administration and regulation. Currently, she is the Director of the Office of Academic Affairs at Fox Chase Cancer Center. Her work involves the development, facilitation, and maintenance of academic partnerships, student training and professional development, and the dissemination of career information, program development, and bioethics training for STEMM (Science, Technology, Engineering, Mathematics, and Medicine) careers to decrease workforce disparities among underrepresented student populations. Ms. Berger received a MBE in Bioethics from the University of Pennsylvania, completed the certification to become a Nationally Certified Bioethics Trainer at Tuskegee University's Center for Bioethics in Research and Health Care, and is working toward the PhD in Health Policy at the University of the Sciences in Philadelphia.

Mr. William Brokaw

Mr. Brokaw is currently an Adjunct Professor of Psychology at Norfolk State University. He is also working toward becoming licensed as a professional counselor. Mr. Brokaw earned a BA in Psychology from the University of Arizona, and a MA in Community and Clinical Psychology from Norfolk State University.

Dr. Suzanne Bronheim

Dr. Bronheim is a Senior Policy Associate at the National Center for Cultural Competence and Associate Professor of Pediatrics at the Georgetown University Medical School. In addition to her work on cultural and linguistic competence, Dr. Bronchium's research and clinical interests focus on services for individuals with disabilities and chronic health conditions, with a particular emphasis on children, youth and families. She is currently Principle Investigator of Maternal and Child Health Bureau funded research to address the demonstrated racial and ethnic disparities in families' access information they need to obtain services for their children. She has co-authored several organizational cultural and linguistic competence self-assessment tools and conducted policy research on requirements for cultural and linguistic competence for health care providers. She provides training and technical assistance to providers and organizations on implementing cultural and linguistic competence. She has written several book chapters and published numerous research findings. Dr. Bronheim received her PhD in Clinical Psychology from the Catholic University of America.

Ms. Dayna Campbell

Ms. Campbell currently serves as a Research Associate/ Coordinator for the Institute for Partnerships to Eliminate Health Disparities (IPEHD) at the University of South Carolina, and is a research consultant for the South Carolina Primary Health Care Association (SC), and Frazier-Anderson Research and Evaluation, LLC in Norwalk, Connecticut. Her research interests are diverse, but are primarily focused on the assessment of disparities in health status and outcomes across multiple conditions/illnesses, and the social, economic and environmental exposures that influence health. Ms. Campbell received her MS degree in Health Education, Promotion, and Behavior, and is completing her Ph.D. in Health Services, Policy and Management from the University of South Carolina.

Dr. Dionne Smith Coker-Appiah

Dr. Coker-Appiah, an Assistant Professor in the Department of Psychiatry at Georgetown University School of Medicine. She is a licensed psychologist and has expertise in adolescent health and community-based participatory research (CBPR) approaches.

Her research program focuses on adolescent dating violence prevention, adolescent mental health, and adolescent sexual health. She has conducted both quantitative and qualitative research among African Americans in both rural and urban settings. Recently, Dr. Coker-Appiah received training in adolescent neuropsychology at the National Institutes of Health. She plans to use fMRI research to expand her dating violence research program. Dr. Coker-Appiah continues to present her research at local, national, and international conferences, and has won numerous awards for her scholarship, including a Kellogg Health Scholarship. Dr. Coker-Appiah received her Ph.D. from the University of Tennessee, Knoxville and completed postdoctoral training at Johns Hopkins University of Public Health.

Dr. William Dadson

Dr. Dadson is currently a Professor of Economics and Finance in the Department of Business and Entrepreneurship Studies at The Lincoln University, Pennsylvania. He was a past Chair for the Department and spearheaded its development. He is a Fulbright/ Hays Scholar; for which he went to Togo, Benin, and Sierra Leone for the purpose of investigating the impact of privatization on the economies of Togo and Sierra Leone. Dr. Dadson received a MBA in Finance from Texas Tech University, and, a PhD in International Studies with a major concentration in International Economics and a second concentration in Finance from the University of Denver.

Dr. Dawnavan Davis

Dr. Davis is a medical psychologist and obesity researcher with nearly twenty years of experience in community health education, obesity prevention and treatment research. She currently serves as the Director of Health Promotions at BlueCross BlueShield of Kansas City (BlueKC), where she is charged with the development and implementation of evidence-based health promotion programs in the areas of childhood obesity prevention and treatment. Prior to joining BlueKC, Dr. Davis was a Research Assistant Professor of Medicine and the Director of the Community-Based Participatory Research Program at the University of Chicago School of Medicine. Additionally, Dr. Davis is the founder of A.C.T.S of F.A.I.T.H—Actions Connected To Spirituality—Forming Alliances In Transforming Health—a faith-based health equity non-profit organization serving the Chicago area. Dr. Davis received her Ph.D. in Medical Psychology from the Uniformed Services University of the Health Sciences.

Dr. Stacy N. Davis

Dr. Davis is currently a postdoctoral fellow in the Health Outcomes and Behavior Group at the H. Lee Moffitt Cancer Center. Her research interests are focused on understanding the impact of behavior, culture, and the role of genetics on cancer health disparities, factors involved informed decision making and community-based participatory research among immigrant populations. Her past research experience has included investigating the impact of culturally targeted interventions on cancer screening in African American men, understanding early detection and informed decision making related to prostate cancer and breast cancer in immigrant populations, and the implementation of a health and wellness program in African American church congregations. Dr. Davis received her Ph.D. in Public Health, with a specialization in Social and Behavioral Health Sciences from Temple University and a MPH with a specialization in Epidemiology from the University of Medicine and Dentistry of New Jersey.

Dr. Ernestine Duncan

Dr. Duncan is an Associate Professor of Psychology and Acting Department Chair for the Department of Psychology at Norfolk State University. Dr. Duncan's research interests include issues related to student learning and faculty success in higher education. Additionally, she has conducted health psychology research focusing on HIV/AIDS prevention in African Americans. Dr. Duncan received her Ph.D. in Clinical Psychology from Georgia State University.

Dr. Linda Fleisher

Dr. Fleisher is the Senior Scientist for the Center for Injury Research and Prevention at The Children's Hospital of Philadelphia. She recently accepted this position after serving as Assistant Research Professor and Vice President of the Office of Health Communications and Health Disparities (OHCHD) including Community Outreach, Cancer Screening, the Resource and Education Center and other health communications research projects at Fox Chase Cancer Center. Dr. Fleisher has over twenty-five years of experience in cancer control, health communications, program planning, management and evaluation, as well as intervention research. She has developed numerous health education materials and resources, co-authored health communication tools (print and new media), technical guides and peer-reviewed publications. As a researcher, she has led multiple community-based and health disparities research projects and built many cancer education and navigation programs and initiatives. She has directed a number of successful cancer control efforts focusing on tailoring health communications materials to underserved audiences and on the use of formative evaluation and community participation in developing cancer-related programs with special interest in health literacy, health disparities and informed consent. Dr. Fleisher received her PhD in Health Studies/Health Communication from Temple University, and a MPH in Community Health Education from Temple University.

Dr. Pamela Frazier-Anderson

Dr. Anderson is the Principal Investigator for Frazier-Anderson Research and Evaluation, LLC in Atlanta, GA. She has over twelve years of experience in education, including the academic, behavioral, and cognitive assessment of children in grades Pre-K through twelfth, serving special populations including children with autism and children from at-risk populations and settings. Her experience in charter school settings, as well as the development and implementation of educational programs for non-profit and private organizations have addressed the needs of individuals from historically underserved populations. She has provided evaluation assistance to private and public organizations, and to individuals in the areas of survey development, project development/ implementation and program evaluation. Dr. Frazier-Anderson received her Ph.D. in Educational Psychology from Arizona State University.

Professor Denise Gaither-Hardy

Professor Gaither-Hardy is an Assistant Professor and Interim Chair in the Department of Psychology at The Lincoln University, Pennsylvania. She has held several positions during her tenure at the University, most notably as Assistant to the President, Assistant to the Vice President for Academic Affairs, Director of the Industrial/ Organizational Psychology Program, and Director of the University Student Enhancement Fund. Her research experience includes investigating the impact of culturally targeted interventions focusing on obesity, colorectal cancer, and HIV/AIDS for African and African American communities. She is a statistician with extensive experience and has worked on grants funded by the Department of Defense, the US Naval Health Research Center, the National Institutes of Health, and the Pennsylvania Department of Health. In addition to her university appointments, she has been a Kellogg Fellow, a Phelps-Stokes Fund Recipient, and has served as a member of the National Advisory Group for SAT development at the Educational Testing Services. Professor Gaither-Hardy received her MA in Social Psychology from the University of Delaware.

Dr. Michael C. Gibbons

Dr. Gibbons is an Associate Director of the Johns Hopkins Urban Health Institute and an Assistant Professor of Medicine, Public Health and Health Informatics at the Johns Hopkins Medical Institutions. Dr. Gibbons' is a Physician Informatician, Healthcare Disparities and Urban Health Expert whose research focuses on the use of technology and Consumer Health informatics to improve healthcare disparities. He has been named a Health Disparities Scholar by the National Center for Minority Health and Health Disparities at the National Institutes of Health and has authored/edited several books such as *eHealth Solutions for Healthcare Disparities.* He is an advisor and expert consultant to several state and federal agencies and policymakers in the areas of urban health, ehealth, minority health and healthcare disparities. Dr. Gibbons received his MD from the University of Alabama School of Medicine, and a MPH with a specialization in health promotion among urban and disadvantaged populations from Johns Hopkins University.

Ms. Evelyn Gonzalez

Ms. Gonzalez is the Senior Director for Community Programs in the Office of Health Communications and Health Disparities at Fox Chase Cancer Center. Ms. González has over twenty-five years experience as a public health advocate and educator focused on health disparities and health equity. She currently oversees the implementation of community cancer education and outreach programs focused on improving health outcomes. Nationally, Ms González serves as a mentor to junior researchers in NCI's *Research to Reality* program, guiding others in the adaptation and translation of research into practice at the community level. She has co-authored a book, *Managing a Public Speaker Bureau*, a manual that provides hands-on experiences and tools to assist organizations with establishing, maintaining, and evaluating the impact and outcome of a speaker's bureau. Her professional career includes work in reproductive healthcare, maternal and child health, genetics, cardiovascular disease, oncology and community health workers. Ms. Gonzalez received her MA in Health Advocacy from Sarah Lawrence College.

Professor Tawara Goode

Ms. Goode is the Director of the National Center for Cultural Competence and an Assistant Professor in the Department of Pediatrics, Georgetown University Medical Center. She is nationally recognized as a thought leader in the area of cultural and linguistic competence and had a primary role in developing curricula, assessment tools, professional development series, and other resources to advance and sustain cultural and linguistic competence for individuals, organizations, and systems. Ms. Goode is actively involved in the development and implementation of programs and initiatives in the area of cultural and linguistic competence at local, national, and international levels which focus on diverse audiences including health care, mental health, social services, professional societies, and institution of higher education. She conducts research on cultural and linguistic competence and its role in addressing health care disparities and is currently involved in a collaborative effort to create validated measures of cultural and linguistic competence in health care settings. She is the author of numerous publications. Ms. Goode received a MA in Education and Human Development from George Washington University.

Dr. Sonja Harris-Haywood

Dr. Harris-Haywood is currently an Assistant Professor in the Research Division, Department of Family Medicine, at the Case University School of Medicine. In this position, she has been

Principal Investigator of NIH funded grants focusing on cultural competence in primary care and cancer health disparities. In addition to her research activities, Dr. Harris-Haywood is a Family Medicine physician at the University Hospital Medical Center. In that capacity, she is the Director of the Department of Family Medicine and the Representative from Case Western Reserve University School of Medicine. Her research interest in the use of cultural competency as an intervention to reduce health disparities evolved from fellowships and a residency she received from the University of North Carolina at Chapel Hill, from the Robert Wood Johnson Medical School in New Brunswick, NJ, and, as a Medical Director for a federally qualified health center in rural North Carolina. Dr. Harris-Haywood received her MD from the University of Medicine and Dentistry (UMDNJ), New Jersey Medical School and a MS in Science Education from New York University

Dr. Karen Holmes

Dr. Holmes is an Associate Professor of Psychology at Norfolk State University. Her professional interests are varied and include the examination of the mental health consequences of the "Strong Black Woman," the issues related to the mental health outcomes of African Americans, and, psychology pedagogy and the scholarship of teaching and learning. Dr. Holmes is the author of many peer-reviewed manuscripts and has presented at numerous local, regional and national conferences. Her honors include an Instructional Research Award from the Society for the Teaching of Psychology (APA Division 2). Dr. Holmes received her PhD in Social Psychology from Wayne State University.

Dr. Maria Jibaja-Weiss

Dr. Jibaja-Weiss is Associate Professor in the School of Allied Health Sciences and the Department of Family and Community, Baylor College of Medicine and the Director of the Office of Outreach and Health Disparities for the Dan L. Duncan Cancer Center. She has been involved in health promotion and cancer prevention and control research among low-income and minority populations for over two decades, including the development and evaluation of novel, multilingual educational interventions designed to motivate lower-literate, underserved populations to learn about various health topics, including management skills for type 2 diabetes, cancer screening, breast health, cancer treatment patient decision-making, and breast cancer risk reduction. As a lead investigator she has been supported by such federal agencies as the Agency for Healthcare Research and Quality, the National Cancer Institute, Department of Defense, Susan G. Komen for the Cure, the Cancer Prevention and Research Institute of Texas (CPRIT), as well as by private donors. Dr. Jibaja-Weiss received the EdD in Health and Physical Education from the University of Houston.

Dr. Dionne J. Jones

Dr. Jones is an Adjunct Professor in the Department of Psychology in the Department of Social, Behavioral, Natural, and Mathematical Sciences, University of Maryland University College (UMUC). She previously managed a research grant portfolio that focused on women, HIV/AIDS, criminal justice, and health disparities. Dr. Jones has held administrative and research positions at nonprofit and for profit organizations, including the National Urban League, Howarad University, The Lewin Group, and the Pacific Institute for Research and Evaluation. She was also Managing Editor of *The Urban League Review*, a policy research journal of the National Urban League, and, was Guest Editor for supplemental issues of *Public Health Reports* and the *Journal of Urban Health*. She has published journal articles, book chapters and a monograph on drug abuse and addiction, HIV/AIDS, women's issues in HIV, and health disparities research. Dr. Jones received her Ph.D. in Educational Psychology from Howard University.

Mr. Venk Kandadai

Mr. Kandadai is currently a Senior Research Associate for the Center for Injury Research and Prevention at The Children's Hospital of Philadelphia (CHOP). Prior to working at CHOP, Mr. Kandadai was the Research Manager in for the Office of Health Communications and Health Disparities at Fox Chase Cancer Center. He has over six years of experience in public health research methods, database development and analysis, and project management. He has developed databases for a prostate cancer study and has performed all the data analysis related to the project. He also has performed similar work for numerous other studies, including one on patient navigation. Mr. Kandadai received his MPH in Community Health from Temple University.

Dr. Dominica McBride

Dr. McBride is Co-Founder and Co-President of the Help Institute, Inc in Chicago, Ill. She has conducted domestic and international program development and evaluation projects with marginalized communities, including rural communities in Tanzania, East Africa, African American communities, Hispanic communities, urban Native American communities, and women. She has also provided clinical psychotherapeutic services to individuals, couples, families, and groups. Dr. McBride has led myriad, multicultural projects, with a focus on community involvement and participatory approaches. She has designed and implemented workshops nationally focusing on such topics as cultural competence, wellness, social and emotional intelligence, coalition building, program evaluation, and logic modeling for a variety of clients (e.g., Goodwill Industries International, prevention specialists, lawyers, mental health professionals, substance abuse professionals, municipal governments, and community organizations). She is widely published on culturally responsive evaluation, cultural competence, prevention and human rights, and health disparities. Dr. McBride received her Ph.D. in Counseling Psychology with a Specialization in Consultation from Arizona State University.

Ms. Laurie Murphy

Ms. Murphy is a doctoral student in the Department of Epidemiology and Biostatistics at Case Western Reserve University School of Medicine with a concentration in Health Care Organization, Outcomes, and Policy. She received a MBA from the William E. Simon Graduate School of Business at the University of Rochester with a concentration in Marketing, and a MPH from Cleveland State University.

Dr. George Myers

Dr. Myers, an administrator at The University of Michigan, Ann Arbor, has held several positions at the University for over twenty years. During this time, he has had the opportunity to teach and conduct research in the area of health with an emphasis on the use of such qualitative methods as the oral histories of prospective members of underserved cultural and ethnic groups. One specific instance of this newly emerging methodology is his work as the Principal Investigator/Project Director of an oral history investigation sponsored by the W.K. Kellogg Foundation and the University of Michigan Medical School. An important finding of this project is the living evidence from the recorded histories of African Americans that attest to the many ways in which members of that cultural group have persisted despite the actual and perceived barriers to their access to, and usage of, health care in the United States. Dr. Myers received his Ph.D. in Urban, Technological, and Environmental Planning from the Taubman College of Architecture and Urban Planning at The University of Michigan.

Dr. Charles Pinckney

Dr. Pinckney is a lecturer, speaker, consultant, and educator. He is Co-Founder and President of the Educational Research Group, a public health educational research—based consulting firm whose mission is to provide innovative research, communication strategies, logistical marketing solutions and program development aimed at advancing human health and knowledge. Dr. Pinckney is faculty member in the African-Studies Department at the University of North Carolina at Charlotte. He is noted for his expertise on Hip-Hop culture, both nationally and globally, and is a pioneer in the investigation of the relationships between social policy, mental health research, and the Hip-Hop culture. He received his Ph.D. in Psychology from Walden University.

Ms. Stephanie Raivitch

Ms. Raivitch is the Director of Health Communication Programs in the Office of Health Communications and Health Disparities (OHCHD) at Fox Chase Cancer Center. Ms. Raivitch oversees operations and staff of the Resource and Education Center (REC), a multi-media learning center which provides educational services to Fox Chase patients, their families and those at risk through both in-person encounters and a web-based service. Previously Ms. Raivitch had six years of experience working for the National Cancer Institute's Atlantic Region Cancer Information Service as an Information Specialist, then as the Resource Coordinator for the service, and finally as a Special Projects Coordinator managing several grant-funded programs and contracts. Currently, she also chairs Fox Chase's Health Literacy Committee, oversees the institution's Health Literacy Assessment Team and manages the health communication services of the OHCHD including the provision of readability and plain language evaluation services for research interventions, administrative and clinical areas. Ms. Raivitch received her BA in Psychology from Temple University.

Dr. Luis Rustveld

Dr. Rustveld is an Epidemiologist and Assistant Professor in the Department of Family and Community Medicine at Baylor College of Medicine. He completed an NIH post-doctoral fellowship (National Research Service Award T32) in the same department. His research interests include interventions for the prevention, and management of chronic diseases such as diabetes, obesity, cardiovascular disease, and cancer. Dr. Rustveld is Program Coordinator for the *Collaborative Network for Cancer Prevention (CNCP)*, funded by the Cancer Prevention Research Institute of Texas (CPRIT). This network engages the Harris County community in building an infrastructure to enhance colorectal and cervical cancer screening services for the medically underserved, and improve delivery of colorectal and cervical cancer services in the Harris County Hospital District and other partner organizations. He is also Program Analyst and Project Co-Director for the Sugar, Heart, and Life diabetes education program. He is also a Registered and Licensed Dietician. Dr. Rustveld received his PhD in Epidemiology from the University of Pittsburgh.

Ms. Rachel Slamon

Ms. Slamon is the Youth Outreach Manager for the American Diabetes Association in Philadelphia. Her responsibilities include planning and implementing an overnight camp for children with type 1 diabetes, developing a type 2 diabetes prevention program for at-risk youth, and managing the *Safe at School* program. She is also responsible for local advocacy and outreach efforts with an emphasis on youth and at-risk populations. Prior to her current position she served as a Health Educator at Fox Chase Cancer Center. While there, she managed the *Pennsylvania Patient Navigator Network*, working on health literacy research projects and managing internal and external communications for the Office of Health Communications and Health Disparities. Her work has contributed to a number of research publications and presentations related to health disparities, genetic literacy, and health communication. She received her MSc degree in Health Communication from Boston University.

Dr. Jennifer Smith

Dr. Smith is an Orthodontic Resident at the University of Pennsylvania, School of Dental Medicine. She has worked on several research projects involving medical issues relating to older adults, with an emphasis on health outcomes for underserved populations. Dr. Smith received a DMD in General Dentistry from the University of Pennsylvania, School of Dental Medicine. She is licensed to practice dentistry in the states of Pennsylvania and Maryland.

Ms. Kristyn Smith

Ms. Smith is currently a Research Project Coordinator at the Institute for Health and Productivity Studies at Emory University, which is located in Washington, DC. Prior to this position, she was a Research Assistant in the Family Medicine Research Division of Case Western Reserve University's School of Medicine where she contributed to several studies devoted to assessing health care provider cultural and linguistic competence, evaluating physician-patient communication, and reducing healthcare disparities. Ms. Smith obtained her BA in Sociology (with a concentration in Health & Aging) and minored in Chemistry. She has just completed the necessary pre-medical requirements needed for admission to medical school from Case Western University.

Dr. Virginia Smith

Dr. Smith is an Associate Professor in the Master of Human Services Program in the Graduate School at The Lincoln University, Pennsylvania. Her area of expertise is in social analysis and planning for the elderly and their families. Dr. Smith has been involved in the development of research strategies designed to decrease poor health outcomes for African American older adults.

Her work has contributed to a number of scholarly presentations at regional and national conferences related to health disparities among African Americans and other underserved populations. She is a member of the Academy of Certified Social Workers of the National Association of Social Workers and is a Licensed Social Worker in the state of Pennsylvania. Dr. Smith has a PhD. in City and Regional Planning from the University of Pennsylvania, and a MSW from the University of Pennsylvania.

Dr. Tiffany Townsend

Dr. Townsend is the Senior Director of the Office of Ethnic Minority Affairs for the American Psychological Association (APA). Before joining APA, Dr. Townsend served as a full time faculty member in the Department of Psychiatry at Georgetown University Medical Center. Her work has involved the implementation of community based research and prevention programs to decrease health and mental health disparities among ethnic minority women, children, and families. She has received most of her funding to support HIV prevention research among youth populations of color. In particular, she served as the Principal Investigator on three federally funded grants and was the co-investigator on two other grants. Currently, she serves as the Associate Editor of the *Journal of Black Psychology* and has authored numerous peer-reviewed journal articles and book chapters. Dr. Townsend received her doctorate in Clinical Psychology from George Washington University,

Professor Frank Worts

Mr. Worts is an Assistant Professor in the Master of Human Services Program in the Graduate School at The Lincoln University, Pennsylvania. His area of specialization is Systems Theory in Sociology. For much of his career, he has been involved in research, planning, and training in areas relating to older adults. Mr. Worts received a MSW from the University of Pennsylvania and a MA from Gregorian University, Rome, Italy. He is completing his work for the PhD in Education with a specialization in Technology at Walden University.

Foreword

J. Robert Beck, MD
Senior Vice President
Chief Academic and Medical Officer
H.O. West & J.R. Wike Chair in Cancer Research
Fox Chase Cancer Center
Philadelphia, Pennsylvania USA

The historical experience of African Americans has been characterized by slavery, exclusion, and persistent overt and institutionalized racism. Although much progress in civil rights has been made since the 1950s, the effects across sectors of society have been variable. Disparities in access and poor relative outcomes testify to the persistence of inequities in healthcare in the 21st Century (Watts, 2003). Healthcare policymakers and providers must make specific efforts to overcome unconscious biases in the allocation of resources to effect change the health and well being of African Americans.

Cultural competence refers to the ability to interact effectively with persons from different sociological or ethnic backgrounds. According to Martin and Vaughn (2007), the culturally competent professional possesses four attributes: (a) awareness of one's own cultural worldview, (b) an open attitude towards cultural differences, (c) knowledge of different cultural practices and worldviews, and (d) cross-cultural skills. Close interaction with people from different cultures engages the healthcare worker in activities that can promote cultural competence, but a comprehensive approach necessitates study.

Therefore I am honored to recommend this compendium to those who influence or provide the delivery of health services to African Americans, especially policymakers, administrators, legislators and clinicians whose attitudes and beliefs affect the scope of services in our communities. Over the past six years I have worked with Drs. Louden and Kinsey, initially on the Lincoln-Fox Chase Partnership in Cancer Research and Training supported by the U.S. National Cancer Institute, and subsequently on developing cancer registries and educational programs in America and the Caribbean. From having no specific background in health disparities research and education I have been tutored by the editors and several of the chapter authors, to the point where I may have reached "conscious competence" within the four stages of learning (Gordon Training International, 2011).

Among many excellent chapters in this book, for the student or practitioner, I would specifically identify Goode, et al's article on the role of self-assessment in achieving cultural and linguistic competence. This chapter provides a comprehensive examination of the evidence on recent attempts to determine the usefulness of the self-assessment process in achieving cultural and linguistic competence. A noteworthy element is the introduction of a new, validated measure of cultural and linguistic competence for health care providers. Fleisher et al's contribution highlights some of the best practices used in health education and health communications aimed at targeting the role of the community and the integration of cultural and linguistic factors.

For the investigator, the theoretical framework discussed in Kinsey, Gaither-Hardy, and Berger's chapter on gender and race offers a more effective model for developing scholarship in cultural competence as applied to the African American community. Specifically, they advocate for a more culturally competent way of conceptualizing the lives of African American women in terms of their shared history and cultural values. Louden's chapter vividly illustrates how the demographic landscape is changing, and the need for professionals in health, education, and elsewhere to deal effectively with this reality in their practice. Additionally, he illustrates, with several examples taken from research being conducted at the Agency for Health Care Research and Quality (AHRQ), the usefulness of Community Based Participatory Research (CBPR) as a more effective strategy than the current research designs in use. He indicates that such an approach can contribute, not just to better outcomes, but to a stance in which researchers become less rigid in their selection of research designs to address the cultural needs of America's increasingly, diverse population. Taken as a whole, the take home message of this book is clear; it is not the color of your skin that defines you; it is geography, culture, history, and religion!

It is the editors' and my hope that this book will empower all professionals who provide education, healthcare, and social services for African Americans, and will stimulate increased cultural competence among those who develop laws, policies and programs that support inclusive and healthy communities.

Riverton, NJ
March, 2012

References

http://www.gordontraining.com/free-workplace-articles/learning-a-new-skill-is-easier-said-than-done/ Accessed 3/10/2012.

Martin, M. and Vaughn, B. (2007). *Strategic Diversity & Inclusion Management Magazine*. San Francisco, CA: DTUI Publications Division, 31-36.

Watts, R. (2003). Race consciousness and the health of African Americans. *Online Journal of Issues in Nursing. Vol. 8* No. 1, Manuscript 3.
Available: www.nursingworld.org//MainMenuCategories/ANAMarketplace/ANAPeriodicals/OJIN/TableofContents/Volume82003/No1Jan2003/RaceandHealth.aspx. Accessed 3/9/2012.

Part I

**Foundations and Selected Critical Issues:
Challenges for Culturally Competent Health Care**

CHAPTER ONE

The Spirit of Advocacy: How the Past Impacts Today and the Future in Health Care Delivery for African Americans

George Myers III
The University of Michigan

Abstract

This chapter provides some answers to questions of health disparities through the exploration of unethical research and systemic inequities leading to a climate of distrust for many minorities. This climate can be abated through education, advocacy, increased cultural competencies, and more racial representation in health care professions. Real-life examples of what African American practitioners encountered in their effort to reduce health care disparities through hospital reform of the segregated health care system in Detroit are used as a primary source throughout the chapter. These excerpts illustrate counteractions and social activism at the local and national level that changed the racial landscape of the hospital system. In summary, minorities must remain vigilant activists against health care injustice by monitoring the government in the enforcement of the laws governing the ethical conduct of research. By delving into the past, insights can be gained when addressing inequality and inadequate access to health care.

Introduction

In conversations surrounding the disparities of health care between African Americans and White Americans, one of the focal points of these conversations, whether it's among professional colleagues or the local barbershop, is lack of access due to the high costs of medical care. Statistically, however, this argument does not hold. The National Center of Health Statistics (2010) published data that reported for those who did not get or delayed medical care due to cost in 1997, 10.8% of the White American population and 10.8% of the African American population fell into this category. In 2009, the percentages are 15.2 and 16.7, respectively. The report also surveyed the number of health care visits in a 12-month period. The largest percentage of responders made between 1-3 visits in the past 12 months. Of this group, in 1997, 46.1% of White Americans and 46.1% of African Americans equally reported making 1-3 visits in the past 12 months. For 2009, these percentages are 46.5 and 46.8, respectively. If one were to graph these statistics, the lines would practically superimpose each other. But we are inundated with study after study that highlights the disparities in health and mortality rates between these two races. If African Americans do not delay medical care due to economic factors and visit doctor's offices, emergency rooms, or have home visits at the same rate, why does the disparity exist?

To answer this question and explore this anomaly, we need to follow-up our original question with three key questions. First, although African Americans do not delay medical care due to cost, is there another reason that medical care is delayed? Secondly, although African Americans make the same number of medical visitations on average as White Americans; does the delay when African Americans conduct medical visits result in more acute stages of illness and disease? Lastly, when African Americans are diagnosed, are they receiving the same level of competent care and treatment modalities?

This chapter will provide some answers to these crucial questions through the exploration of unethical medical research and systemic medical inequities toward the African American community that has led to a climate of distrust and reluctance to access medical professionals. This distrust is directly attributed to the disparities in the African American health status and can be abated through education, advocacy, an increase in cultural competencies, and more racial representation in the American health care professions.

The National Institute on Minority Health and Health Disparities defines health disparities as differences in the incidence, prevalence, mortality, burden of diseases, and other adverse health conditions that exist among specific population groups in the United States (US Department of Health and Human Services, NIH News, 2010). African Americans continue to have poorer health (i.e. higher rates of morbidity and mortality) and receive lower quality of care than whites when factors such as insurance status and income are controlled. Despite several decades of health care reform legislation, limited impact on the elimination of health and health care disparities for minority groups has occurred. Most statistics focus on the end result of these disparities and do not get at the root causes of the complex problems caused by barriers that contribute to health disparities between racial groups. Many of the systemic barriers are from institutional and governmental policies, administration, and delivery of appropriate treatment models and stem from the complexity of social factors of institutional racism and discrimination toward African Americans (David and Collins, 1991; Massey, 1990).

During the late nineties, I had the most professionally rewarding experience directing an African American Health Care Oral History Project. My education in urban and regional planning, experience in public health, and interest in medical history enabled me to establish a highly effective community participatory model necessary for successfully conducting this type of academic research. The project represents a tremendous collaboration with the University of Michigan Medical School, various Detroit institutions, and several African American residents in Detroit, Michigan.

A portion of this chapter is built on the inspirational stories of lesser-known African Americans in Southeast Michigan who overcame adversity stemming from inadequate access, availability, and quality of care under a segregated health care system. The study time period of 1940-1969 represents three decades in which significant historical events transpired, both known and unknown, that facilitated the transformation of the segregated health care system. Lead Principal Investigator Norman L. Foster, states "the research is based on stories of unsuspected and unsung innovation and entrepreneurship as energetic and talented individuals tried to overcome adversity to achieve their own personal goals. Also, many of their personal testimonies are living evidence of their ability to overcome structural societal barriers to provide the best health care available for African Americans during the time period". Foster further states "these stories are inspirational and deserve to be told" (*The Archive*, 2000). This chapter is written with that same spirit in mind.

The project originated in the Historical Center for the Health Sciences in the University of Michigan Medical School. Nicholas Steneck, Professor of History provided the initial leadership during the early stages of the project. Norman L. Foster, M.D., Professor of Neurology and Senior Research Scientist at the

Institute of Gerontology and Harold W. Neighbors, Ph.D., Professor in the School of Public Health lead the research team. This multidisciplinary research work assembled the most comprehensive information, highlighted by 41 oral histories, about African American health care in Southeast Michigan. Secondary resource materials were also compiled, interpreted, and disseminated as part of the research process. The extensive oral history collection consists of five linear feet of written material.

The W.K. Kellogg Foundation and The University of Michigan Medical School funded the research project. The overall goal of project was to document, collect, and preserve information on historical experiences of African Americans in Southeast Michigan with regard to the legally segregated health care system during the period of 1940-1969. Specifically, the research team conducted oral histories of African American physicians, nurses, non-traditional health care providers, and community residents with regard to health care, the health professions, and the health sciences.

Excerpts from the oral interviews are interspersed throughout the chapter as a primary source. These excerpts represent invaluable and irreplaceable permanent testimony reflecting the nuances of the spoken word and emotional zeitgeist of those with personal knowledge of past unethical practices in health care and medicine. Furthermore, this historical perspective conveys the groundwork for exploring past unethical medical events and the lingering negative effects that these events have on treatment-seeking and health care behavior of African Americans today.

This chapter is divided into three sections. The first section highlights unethical medical research that has fostered African Americans' distrust of the medical establishment. The second section focuses on a discussion of unequal treatment of African Americans by the Detroit medical establishment. The final section will discuss the role of advocacy in reducing health care disparities for African Americans.

Unethical Research Practices: A History

The Tuskegee Study. The infamous *Tuskegee Study of Untreated Syphilis in the Negro Male* also known as "The Tuskegee Syphilis Study" is the focus of this section because it is one of the most well-known and salient examples of past medical atrocities in the United States. Gamble (1997) describes the Tuskegee Syphilis Study as being a major source behind African American distrust of medical institutions. Please note it is not my intent to ignore or make light of other past medical abuses in this country, because they have had equally deleterious and lingering effects on the psyche of African Americans, but for the sake of brevity this most known study will receive focused attention.

Numerous books and articles have been written about this infamous study (Jones, 1981; Washington, 2006; Reverby, 2009). Even though the details of the study have been well documented by researchers, academics, and the media the study is often the source of misinformation. For the purpose of this section, the following brief overview of the Tuskegee Syphilis Study serves as a backdrop for the latter discussion of the importance of accurately reporting the facts of the study.

The Tuskegee Experiment conducted from 1930-1972 involved six hundred (600) African American men in a government sponsored study to research the effects of untreated syphilis in African Americans. Three hundred and ninety-nine (399) of the men were in the degenerate or late stages of tertiary syphilis. The remaining men (201) who did not have the disease served as the control group. All of the men were from low socioeconomic backgrounds, were illiterate, or had limited educational backgrounds (Jones, 1981). The major issue centered on the deception and outright fabrication used by the U.S. Public Health Service informing the men in the study that they were being treated, when in actuality, the men were being studied to track the progression of symptoms associated with the disease and subjected to invasive procedures associated with the disease, and subjected to other invasive procedures that would not lead to treatment. It is also important to note that the men were not made aware of the seriousness of the disease and were only informed they were being treated for "bad blood", a local term describing several ailments (Jones, 1981).

As diabolical as it may sound, even when the cure for syphilis was discovered in 1947, the study participants were deliberately denied the medication (penicillin). A reliable internet database educational site reports that despite the fact that 250 of the men also registered to serve in the armed services, the United States

Public Health Service exempted them from receiving treatment. The study still continued and the men went untreated even after the enactment of the Henderson Act in 1943, requiring testing and treatment for venereal disease. In 1964, there was still another opportunity to end the study with the passing of the World Health Organization's Declaration of Helsinki (1964), in which "informed consent" was required for experimentation involving human beings (InformationPlease, 2007).

Because of this malfeasance, many of the men and their families by the end of the forty-two year period suffered unnecessarily. Twenty-eight (28) of the subjects died directly of syphilis, 100 were dead of related complications, 40 of their spouses had been infected, and 19 of their children had been born with congenital syphilis (Brandt, 1978; James 1993; Freimuth et al, 2001; Thomas, 2008).

The aforementioned overview of the study provides concrete evidence that the study was unethical despite any rationalization that might have been introduced by the medical community over the years. Some researchers have stated that ethical standards at the time were not as stringent as a rationale for alleviating some of the major criticism associated with the unethical nature of the study (Wasserman 2006). In an article written by the Associated Press (2011), many felt that medical research was different then because of the high mortality rate from infectious diseases. Therefore, many doctors felt professionally committed to testing and discovering cures sometimes at the risk of greater harm to research participants. Furthermore, many felt it was legitimate to experiment on people who did not have full rights in society (i.e., prisoners, mental patients, minority groups, and impoverished people (*Associated Press*, 2011).

According to the Final Report of the Tuskegee Syphilis Study from an Ad Hoc Advisory Panel of the U.S. Department of Health, Education, and Welfare (1974), "this study was ethically wrong based on the fundamental rule that a person should not be subject to avoidable risk of death or physical harm unless he or she freely and intelligently consents". The panel found no evidence that such consent was obtained from the participants in this study. Furthermore, the panel also reported that this was a scientifically unsound experiment as the results are disproportionately meager compared with the known risks to the human subjects involved.

However, one can take exception with the panel's possible rationale on how the study might have been justifiable. It is possible that a scientific study in 1932 of untreated syphilis, properly conceived with a clear protocol and conducted with suitable subjects who fully understood the implications of their involvement, might have been justified in the pre-penicillin era. This is especially true when one considers the uncertain nature of the results of treatment of late latent syphilis and the highly toxic nature of therapeutic agents then available. Most research subjects are often unable to provide informed and voluntary consent. Many individuals that participate in research studies have impoverished backgrounds and often are mentally ill or substance abusers, and have limited educational backgrounds. There is no justification for this type of study that was designed to cause harm and undue suffering to unwilling research subjects. Logically, who would consent to participate in the study knowing the negative repercussions? Often individuals from institutionalized and impoverished groups are coerced into consenting to participate in medical research by their institutions and governments (P. Wright: *USA Today*, August 21, 2006).

The Impact of Prison Studies. Prison studies provide a prime example of this point. The United State penal system has an extensive history of allowing prisoners to be abused by medical establishments, research institutions, governmental agencies, and major pharmaceutical and biotech companies. The following overview of the studies conducted in the early 20th century using prisoners as research participants provide concrete evidence of the exploitation of this population for the sake of medical research. Mike Stobbe (2011) in an AP review of past research reported that:

In 1915, the U.S. government's Dr. Joseph Goldberger recruited Mississippi inmates who were offered pardons for their participation to go on special rations to prove his theory that the painful illness pellagra was caused by a dietary deficiency. Even today, many consider him a public health hero despite his unethical behavior. Five years later, another study conducted by Dr. L. L. Stanley at San Quentin prison in California attempted to treat older, 'devitalized men' by implanting in them testicles from livestock and from recently executed convicts (AP Press, 2011, p. 13).

To further support this history of victimization, Wright's review of the Holmesburg prison study provides another example of medical abuse and exploitation of prisoners from 1951 to 1974. In his review, Wright notes that the study conducted by Hornblum (1998) documents how prisoners were exposed to carcinogenic agents over a 23-year period. The majority of prisoners used in these experiments were from impoverished backgrounds and in poor health, which further compromised their decision-making ability to provide voluntary consent. Wright (2006) commented:

> Many prisoners were often coerced into thinking that they were receiving better health care or consented to participation because of fear of retaliation from prison officials. Prisons have been a vast laboratory for researchers representing major corporations, and biotech and pharmaceutical companies. Some researchers have had a moral indifference to using this population as research subjects and have subjected others to risks outside the prison population. Until the early 1990's, private companies used prisoners in Arkansas and Arizona as plasma donors which dramatically increased the contamination of the US blood supply with hepatitis and HIV (Wright, 2006, p. 10).

This moral indifference can be likened to the Tuskegee Syphilis Study in which several of the wives and the offspring of the men were unknowingly exposed and infected with the disease. The above-mentioned studies, along with what occurred in Tuskegee, Alabama; serve to reinforce the African Americans' belief and distrust of the medical system. The lingering effects of the Tuskegee Study are dangerous because it causes cultural transmission of African American myths from one generation to another that have led to conspiracy theories of genocide (Gamble, 1997). For example, during testimony to the National Commission on AIDS, a health educator stated: "So many African American people that I work with do not trust hospitals or any of the other community health care service providers because of the Tuskegee experiment. It is like if they did it then, they will do it again" (Thomas & Quinn, 1991).

Wasserman (2006) reports that the Tuskegee Syphilis Study is probably one of the most inaccurately reported medical experiments in terms of misconception and misinformation about the exact nature of the study. He further summarizes that ignoring context and producing inaccurate information has real impact on health care, particularly for African Americans. Failure to do so often produces mythic knowledge, which is transmitted from one generation to another in the African American community. The inaccuracies and often embellishment of past and present medical events such as the Tuskegee Syphilis Study have real implications on the health seeking and health care behavior for African Americans (Wasserman, 2006). For example, knowledge of this study is often associated with the conspiracy theory existing among many African Americans that HIV/AIDS is a government-induced genocide against the African American community (Corbie-Smith, Thomas, Williams, Moody-Ayers, 1999).

The Role of Inaccurate Reporting. Educators, researchers, health care practitioners, academicians, the media, the African American community, and the public at large share in the responsibility for accurate reporting of past unethical or questionable health care events and practices. Wasserman (2006) lists several examples in which academicians and the media have reported either inaccurate or ambiguous information that has often led to misconceptions about the Tuskegee Syphilis Study. The following are two examples reported in the Wasserman article. Tom Brokaw, on April 8, 1997, reported on the NBC Nightly News that the government had infected the men in the study with syphilis. The other example is of a Philadelphia newspaper headline that stated hundreds of men "were infected with syphilis and denied treatment . . ." As Wasserman points out, at the start of the study, the men did have the disease but the ambiguous term "were infected" could be misconstrued that the researchers purposely infected the men.

Many sources that have been produced over the years inaccurately report the number of men that actually had the disease in the study. A summary of James Jones's book, *Bad Blood*, describes the non-therapeutic experiment as involving "over" 400 black male sharecroppers infected with syphilis. Another published source in a major journal reported that 600 men had been infected with syphilis (Calloway, 1995). In actuality, according to the final report of the Tuskegee Syphilis Study produced in 1973 by the U.S. Department of Health, Education, and Welfare, only 399 men had the disease and the other 201 were in the control group (i.e., men without the disease). This study has often been depicted as a secret experiment conducted by the Government of the United States. In actuality, the study was anything other than secret, because several articles were published in professional journals about the study. Some of the articles focused on the increased mortality and a reduction in life expectancy of the subjects (Tuskegee Syphilis Study Ad Hoc Advisory Panel Report, 1973). However, the nature of the secrecy theory could be somewhat supported by the fact that information about the study was not disseminated to the public at large until July 1972 in an Associated Press story.

An interesting study focused on African Americans' views on research and the Tuskegee Syphilis Study. Investigators found that the accuracy of their knowledge about the study was limited, which is a contributing factor in the lack of recruitment of African Americans in medical trials and research studies (Frimuth, Quinn, Thomas, Cole, Zook, and Duncan, 2001). Their study involved seven focus groups with 60 African Americans in five major cities to examine the participants' knowledge of the Tuskegee Study and reaction to 1997 film of *Miss Ever's Boys* created by the Home Box Office Productions. The researchers report that the majority of the participants were familiar with the study but lacked specific knowledge about the details of the experiment. A significant number of the participants believed that the research participants were purposely injected with syphilis. Many of the focus group participants expressed sentiment that the Tuskegee experiment was typical based on their overall perceptions that African Americans are not valued as much as whites.

Other Unethical Practices. A more in-depth review of unethical practices that have taken place in the United States would be unreasonable for the chapter because the literature is voluminous.

Therefore, the general overview of one of the most well known documented unethical medical practices provides contextual background for the discussion regarding the lingering effects that unethical practices have had on health seeking and health behavior of African Americans. Past research has illustrated that knowledge of these injustices are correlated with African Americans unwillingness to participate in medical research and often promote distrust of medical researchers and practitioners (Shavers, Lynch, Burmeister, & Toner, 1997).

Numerous researchers have been able to document the systematic mistreatment of African Americans by the medical establishment since the enslavement of Africans in the United States (Randall 1993; Savitt 1998; Gamble 1997; Bryd and Clayton 2000; Washington 2006). Author and scholar Harriet Washington's (2006) book, *Medical Apartheid: The Dark History of Medical Experimentation on Black Americans from Colonial Times to the Present,* provides the most comprehensive chronological account of overwhelming miscarriages of justice pertaining to the medical exploitation of African Americans in this country. The book reveals that private individuals as well as governmental institutions and agencies in the United States have conducted many unethical medical experimentations and practices. Washington provides a strong account of the infamous Tuskegee Syphilis Study as well as other lesser-known medical abuses that have occurred in this country since the 17th century. One of the most poignant points of her work in documenting a history of medical malfeasance in the United States is that, despite past history, she strongly encourages African Americans to participate in the health care system. But, at the same time, she encourages African Americans to remain vigilant through advocacy and education of potential abuse in health care practices.

Inequality: Detroit

Of all forms of inequality, injustice in health is the most shocking and the most inhumane (Rev. Dr. Martin Luther King, Jr.).

The first section provided a selective history of major medical atrocities, which showed the inhumane side of health care for

African Americans. This section will explore the injustice side by examining real-life examples of what African American medical practitioners encountered during the time period of 1940-1969. This period represents the era that facilitated the transformation of the United States from a segregated to a more integrated society. During this time period, many African Americans advocated for change in the health care system in Detroit, Michigan. Individual counteractions, as well as social activism at the local and national level, changed the racial landscape of the hospital system. At a national meeting in August 2002, Dr. L. Natalie Carroll, President-Elect of the National Medical Association, commented, "Dr. King's declaration is a powerful statement telling us that health care equality is an essential component of the civil rights struggle. It also tells us that the gap between the health status of blacks and whites has been with us for a long time." Therefore, it is imperative that the struggle for civil rights in health care and medicine remain a priority on the national health care agenda in the fight to eradicate health disparities for African Americans. To this end, the African American, Oral History Health Care Project sponsored by the Kellogg Foundation provides an excellent example of how African American medical practitioners, who worked during the crucial years from 1940 to 1969, viewed the Tuskegee Syphilis Study. An excerpt from the project is presented below to show how the Tuskegee study can be used as an educational platform for increased advocacy for equality in health care for African Americans.

> You may have read in recent months . . . it's been published . . . a national study showing that blacks in America do not receive health care on the basis that is equal to white people. And, we're not now talking about the problem of segregation per se, we talking about (and the study demonstrates that) the problem that develops because black people do not receive as aggressive medical attention as do white people on average. Now why is that? A White doctor at Columbia Presbyterian, who was being interviewed on this matter, said he was sorry to say, but he could not think of anything but race that determined that difference. That you know, this is

kind of an extension of the Tuskegee experience and different waters on different land. The question is if you are going to see a doctor complaining, is he going to send you to the best specialist he knows about, and is that specialist going to order all the tests when you get to see him, that could be ordered, to determine what is the nature of your problem? And will he call in the best resources to treat you? And the record shows that in general white people get better treatment Arthur Johnson, Ph.D. (Oral History Interview, June 6, 1997.)

The above excerpt from Dr. Arthur Johnson provides an excellent example of the saliency of the Tuskegee Syphilis Study and how the memory of this unethical study can be used as an impetus for advocacy in the fight for health care equality. His reasoning for health care disparity is two-fold. First, the inequality in health care today is an extension of the Tuskegee Syphilis Study, and, secondly, Africans Americans are treated differently in terms of medical treatment; hence his statement *"different waters on different land"*. Medical Historian, Vanessa Gamble, assertion "that African Americans' beliefs are undervalued by white society and influence their relationships with the medical establishment, further supports Johnson's insight. They perceive, at times correctly, that they are treated differently in the health care system solely because of their race, and such perceptions fuel mistrust of the medical profession." (Gamble, 1997).

Dr. Johnson's assertion about unequal treatment based on race is further supported by numerous studies. For example in 1999, a study conducted with one-hundred and sixty-four medical students found that a patient's race and gender could significantly influence treatment recommendations. This particular study using actors as patients found that African American males, along with white and black females, were substantially less likely than white males to be recommended for cardiac surgery (Ratnore, Lenert, Weinfurt, Tinoco, Taleghani, Harless, Schulman, 2000). In June 2007, the *Science Daily* reported the results of one study indicated that African American Medicare patients received less lifesaving medical procedures such as angioplasty following a heart attack than whites. The same is true whether they were admitted to hospitals that provided or did not provide these procedures. As recent as June 2011, a study conducted by the University of Michigan Health System, found that:

> Black patients having a heart attack wait longer in hospitals as white patients to receive revascularization medical procedures that will restore blood flow to their hearts. Researchers found the difference in care is explained more by hospital quality rather than the race of the patient. Black patients were more likely to go to less responsive hospitals than whites which resulted in longer waiting times to receive lifesaving medical procedures. Even though researchers found race may play less of a role in the difference in care, the end result is still driven by race. Hospitals that most blacks often have to go are inferior because they often lack the staff and capacity to perform angioplasty or revascularization medical procedures. The lack of resources and poor organization of many of these hospitals that serve black populations must be improved to standards of white hospitals" (*Science Daily*, 2011, p. 1).

Societal structural contexts of poverty, racism, and segregation resulting from being disadvantaged which disproportionately affect African Americans remain a major factor in the unequal medical treatment for this group. Equally astonishing, Dr. Johnson's recollection of the Tuskegee Syphilis Study actually served as a precursor to his general mistrust of white medical doctors in terms of providing unequal medical treatment based on race. For many African Americans, the memory of these events contributes to attitude and belief systems that have detrimental consequences for African Americans (Wasserman 2006). Whether these reconstructions are real or perceived, they are still prominent barriers that foster distrust in African Americans about the medical establishment. The Tuskegee Study has far reaching impact in that it is, for many African Americans, a "symbol of their mistreatment by the medical establishment, a metaphor for deceit, conspiracy, malpractice, and neglect, if outright racial genocide" (Jones, 1992 p.38).

Dr. Rachel Keith, another participant in the Oral History Project supports the above-mentioned statements. In her interview, Dr. Keith indicates that publicity about the Tuskegee Syphilis Study has had detrimental consequences, often resulting in the reluctance of African Americans to participate in research studies. She furthermore elaborated that African Americans tend to gravitate toward black physicians because they are more comfortable with a health care professional that is familiar with their cultural background and heritage.

> Blacks feel they are being treated as guinea pigs and they don't want to be experimental guinea pigs. They want the attention from their own private physician and they like the fact that they can communicate a little easier with people who understand their culture. For that reason, they tend to gravitate toward black physicians (Rachel B. Keith, MD (oral history interview, July 16, 1998).

The Kellogg African American Health Care Project presents many real life examples of how individual counteractions and social activism helped to create a more just (i.e., free of discriminatory practices) medical system for African Americans in Detroit, Michigan. Several excerpts from the Kellogg Oral History Project are integrated in this section to support the idea that equality in health care is worth fighting for as a civil right granted to all Americans. These excerpts represent a spirit of mentorship and social activism as demonstrated by African Americans through individual and highly organized counteractions.

Historically, during the period from 1940 to 1969, African American doctors were not admitted to residency programs and were denied hospital appointments and staff privileges at the white hospitals in Detroit. As a result, African American practitioners were not able to provide the necessary care for their patients (mainly, African Americans) in the hospitals. They were also denied admission to the major medical societies such as the American Medical Association (AMA). These injustices set the political platform to protest the discriminatory practices of hospitals and the AMA. Individual African American physicians pressured the hospitals through civil rights organizations and the National Medical

Association (NMA—the black counterpart to the AMA) via political and social activism at both the local and national levels. These actions forced hospitals to change their segregation policies and discriminatory practices.

Dr. Johnson, in the excerpt below, discusses the effect of institutional racism and discrimination in health care in Detroit.

> The major hospitals in Detroit in 1950 operated with patterns of racial segregation in placement of patients. They didn't want a black and a white person in a semi-private room, and they consistently worked to avoid that. I mean this was it. This [was] commonplace. And everybody . . . black people could sense this, and black doctors who had graduated from medical school here and elsewhere, working on the assumption that they would become doctors, soon discovered that they were to be "black doctors" in the sense that they would not be treated equally, fairly, with white doctors in the privileges they were [granted] in these hospitals in Detroit. The major hospitals in many cases did not even respond to [the] letters [from black doctors] requesting appointment. And it was because of these racial segregation conditions in health care that we began to think about ways of how we could break that pattern, and it finally came with the legislation passed by Congress that sought to bar discrimination based on race. Arthur Johnson, Ph.D. (Oral History Interview, June 6, 1997.)

The integration of the hospital staff originated with the acceptance of African American nurses. Overall, hospital nursing staffs were well integrated before most medical institutions in America; however, the nurses still faced the challenges of overcoming institutionalized discrimination and racism that were prevalent at many of the hospital across the nation as well as in Detroit (*Blecher*, 2002). Researcher and author, Darlene Clark Hines states, "It should be recognized that black nurses were in many ways the most important providers of health care for the black community. Indeed, the community would hardly have survived without them".

Hines, the author of *Black Women in White: Racial Conflict in the Nursing Profession* (1993), states, "If you want to gauge how well blacks did at achieving certain liberties, the experience of black nurses is a good indicator."

To further support Hines's assertion, the following excerpt is an example of an individual counteraction that was courageously made by Registered Nurse Oretta Todd against racial segregation.

> When I got through with that experience and I actually started working on staff at Hutzel [Hospital] while I was waiting for students to come, I decided that I was going to put blacks and whites wherever they had to be—I wasn't going to keep them upstairs in labor and delivery—I mean in the recovery room. So, I assigned them a room as long as . . . you'd have what rooms are available. I just pulled them and sent them down there. I made the mistake . . . Dr. S. had this very, very important lady from Grosse Pointe. I put her in a room and then when the next patient came in and they had "semi-private", I put her in the same room. Dr. S. happened to come in that evening and he said, "Who did this? I don't mix my patients with blacks!" So he came flying up to labor and delivery. I said, "I did Dr. S." I said, "The two patients got along real well and I saw no reason to let your patient be alone when she was associating with this other patient up in recovery." Oh, he was furious with me! But, because I was black, he didn't do anything, but I think he said something to somebody else. So when Dr. [Charles] Wright came up I said, "You know Dr. Wright, I don't think Dr. S. is happy with me, I mixed the patients." He said, "Good!" That was the first time they had actually mixed racial groups there. (Oretta Todd, RN, PhD (oral history interview, May 1, 1997).

Similar counteractions were made by other nurses to combat segregated wards in white hospitals in an effort to provide African American patients with care equal to whites. "Overall, African American nurses were some of the most vigilant whistleblowers against health care facilities that were receiving federal funds but ignoring orders to integrate" (*Blecher, 2002*). Nurses were also politically involved as change agents working diligently with local civil rights organizations in the reform of the discriminatory practices in the hospital system in Detroit, Michigan.

African American physicians also played an instrumental leadership role in hospital reform as well as in the Civil Rights Movement. Dr. Lionel Swan, as Past President of the National Medical Society, spearheaded the Hospital Reform Movement at both the local and national levels. This distinguished warrior of hospital reform worked with the National Association for the Advancement of Colored People (NAACP) and local and national government officials to place health care for African Americans on the national agenda. In 1964, he met with President Lyndon B. Johnson to discuss the health care needs of African American physicians and their inability to provide quality health care for their patients due to discriminatory practices at medical institutions.

The following excerpt demonstrates Dr. Swan's commitment to hospital reform in the United States. In the excerpt, he talks about leaving the South only to find the same policies of segregation in place in the North. The major difference in the North is that there was a place to practice because of the existence of the black proprietary (i.e., black owned and operated) hospitals.

> I became president of the National Medical [Association] . . . somewhere by [19]67, But, before that I still remember that one of the things we had lacking was hospitalization for our patients. [One of the disadvantages of practicing in Birmingham was the lack of hospital privileges for black doctors. If one of my patients needed hospital care, I had to refer that patient to a white doctor. I had such a patient and my doctor friend had secured her a hospital bed. But when she reached the hospital her husband was asked who his doctor was. When he said "Dr. Swan", he was told that Dr. Swan was not on the staff. So, the patient was not admitted. She died shortly after. And I called Governor Fulsome and the TV stations. The TV stations jumped on it. The hospital said they didn't have a bed, and that's

the reason they didn't admit the woman. The mayor of the city and the governor condemned the action of the hospital. One of the women that worked there said they did have beds because she made the bed up for this woman. The woman's husband was grief stricken, but he had no desire to sue anyone. And, so, nothing came of that. This incident confirmed my desire to leave Birmingham.

When I arrived in Detroit in 1951, this situation with non-hospital privilege was similar to Birmingham], except that we had the black hospitals. [For example, Burton Mercy Hospital, Trinity Hospital, Edyth K. Thomas Hospital, Dr. Samuel B. Milton's hospital [Sumby Memorial] in River Rouge, the Drs. Daisy and David Northcross' Mercy General, the new Southwest Detroit Hospital, and others where both patients and doctors were treated with dignity. And they were doing some very good work. As a matter of fact, they trained some people. Dr. Charlie Green trained here in surgery. Dr. Arrington trained here. They were doing some good work, but obviously, they couldn't get on the staff of the major hospitals.

In the major hospitals, very few black doctors were admitted. The effort for hospital privileges was continuous, especially after board certified black specialists appeared on the scene. The fight to secure hospital privilege was led by several doctors. Dr. Lawrence Lackey, Sr, who was in River Rouge and followed me as President of the Detroit Medical Society, was among them. I think Dr. Charlie [Charles H.] Wright was trying to get in and several others. So he and I wondered what we were going to do, Then he moved somewhat on his own. I remember him saying, "What have they offered you?" Once, I think, he said, "I think we're going to make it." And precisely when and what was done I don't know, because I didn't have anything to do with that, but I do know that he called me to say they would take four doctors. (Lionel F. Swan, MD (oral history interview, June 18, 1999).

The struggle for equality in health care was the plight of many health care practitioners and not just a few individuals. Many had leadership roles in the political fight to desegregate the hospital system in Detroit. Dr. Charles Wright provides another illustration of an individual counteraction made against segregation in "white" institutions.

> I went to Hutzel . . . it was called Woman's Hospital then, that was a very prominent women's hospital, and it was a white hospital, it still is—anyway it was very prominent, and it was prominent for me as an obstetrician because I was . . . this is what I did—OB-GYN. What happened though, in 1956, three years after I got started, a senator from Michigan wrote in the *Detroit Free Press* that the government had appropriated $600,000, I think, in renovation money for Hutzel (that's the name of it—Hutzel Hospital) to alter its operating room, delivery room, and this kind of thing, and this was their participation in the medical center development.

> So his name was Hart, Phil Hart was his name, senator, and so that afternoon (and this was the morning paper) I sent him a letter telling him, "Don't give them a dime." I said, "They discriminate against my patients." They wouldn't allow my patient to come into the hospital if there was not a vacancy in a room where another black patient was. And they didn't accept black interns and residents. And they took me largely because I had been recommended by [the same doctor at Sinai Hospital], and I knew that was no way to do it. So I wrote him and told him, "Don't send them a dime," and I said, "now you don't have to come at any time, any particular time to check on it, come any time and see for yourself." And he sat down and sent copies of everything I said to him to the chairman of the board of trustees at Hutzel. He said,

"Dr. Wright is accusing you of this. Is it true?" Well, he made such a noise until he might come and look. And did you know the next day they were integrated.

They never forgave me for whistling. I was a whistle-blower. But that didn't matter. You take your lumps, and then you go ahead. But the community knew what we were doing, and so rather than lose that money, they came along. That was just part of our fight. We used to go into the board rooms in Grace [Hospital] and other places, and meet with the superintendent of the hospital. We wanted to know, "Why aren't you integrating? What are your plans? Do you have any long-term plan?" And they would hem and haw and promise and stuff, but nothing much happened until we threatened to shut it down, and then they got the message. (Charles Wright, MD, oral history interview, April 15, 1997).

The City of Detroit has a rich and extensive history in health care and was considered by many to be the capital of African American-owned and operated hospitals in the United States during the era of racial segregation (Wright, 1995). These institutions provided a place to practice and train while providing medical care for African Americans. Even though African American doctors did the best that they could in providing health care for the city residents, they still faced deficits due to inadequate training after medical school and working in technologically inferior hospitals. Many of these hospitals had insufficient staffing, inadequate and outdated equipment, poor standards of cleanliness, and overcrowding. Therefore, discrimination against African American physicians by the white medical institutions seriously affected patient care. The integration of the hospital system, and the fact that these smaller institutions could not compete with the major majority hospitals, led to their demise. Norm Foster states, "On the one hand there is the tragedy of this loss of grass roots health systems among the African American community. On the other hand, its demise was, in part, because of improved access to health care, which was the ultimate goal of all of these pioneers to begin with. So they succeeded in achieving their ultimate goal and they also demonstrated the ability to overcome obstacles to provide good health care" (University of Michigan Press Release, October 25, 2000).

Unfortunately, based on the information already presented in this chapter and in the next section with regard to the health disparities confronting African Americans, the health care system is still not adequately meeting the needs of the African American population. However, as we have learned from the past, advocacy at both the local and national level can be instrumental in creating another platform in which to continue to address issues of diversity and cultural competency in the medical professions as a means of reducing health care disparities and unequal treatment for African Americans.

Solutions: Advocacy, Cultural Competency, and Diversity in the Medical Profession

Those who fail to learn from history are doomed to repeat it (Sir Winston Churchill).

This quote represents the dichotomy for African Americans. What African Americans have learned from past medical practice history, and the attitudes and efforts African Americans display in order to avoid repeating past medical atrocities, is actually leading to doom as evidenced by the health statistics and disparities. Has history taught us anything that could possibly be used in the effort to eliminate racial health care disparities for minority groups, especially African Americans?

This section reintroduces some valuable lessons from the past that could help to increase African Americans' trust in the medical establishment. Many researchers have reached conclusions that awareness of past injustices in medicine correlate with African Americans reluctance to fully participate in the health care system. Non-participation in the health care system has detrimental effects on health care seeking behaviors. The causes of health care disparities are extremely complex because they can stem from numerous sources such as poverty, education levels, access to health care, cultural differences and biases, societal constructs of racism and discrimination, etc.

As mentioned in the first part of this chapter, the saliency of the Tuskegee Syphilis Study continues to have long term and serious consequences on health behaviors and equality for African Americans. Many African Americans simply do not trust the medical establishment because of this unethical experiment (Freimuth et al, 2001). It is a major source of suspicion and lack of trust in the medical profession for many African Americans. Misconceptions and misinformation about this study as well as lesser-known abuses can be counterproductive for reestablishing trust among African Americans in the medical establishment. Many of the concerns and fears are justified, but must be handled in such a manner as that it is still in the best interest of the community to have a more trusting relationship with the medical establishment.

Past research shows the knowledge or belief in past unethical medical events, whether perceived or factual, can act as impediments to African American participation in the health care system in terms of low participation rates in clinical trials and medical research. The book, *The Immortal Life of Henrietta Lacks* (Skloot, 2010); focuses on the ethical debate of using a black woman's cells without her consent. Her cells have been bought and sold around the world and launched a multibillion dollar industry. Unfortunately, none of the proceeds were shared with her surviving family members. An excerpt in the book supports the suspicion that many African Americans have of the medical establishment.

A relative of Henrietta Lacks shares his opinion with family members about his belief regarding the frightening nature of John Hopkins Hospital.

> Well what you expect from Hopkins. I wouldn't go there to get my toe nails cut. Back then they did things, especially to black folks. John Hopkins was known for experimentation on black folks. They'd snatch em off the street . . . experimentin' on them (Skloot, 2010, p.165).

The previous review of the Tuskegee Study, coupled with other documented abuses, serves as icons of distrust and suspicion for many African Americans. In order to change the paradigm of non-participation in the medical establishment, advocacy based on accurate information within the African American community should be undertaken as illustrated in the oral history excerpts integrated throughout this chapter. As we have learned, individual counteractions and large-scale social activism proved to be the impetus for hospital reform during the period of segregation. The importance of the excerpts is that they demonstrate how past experiences can powerfully affect attitudes and belief about health care system. Through a social activism and advocacy movement, changes to the health system in the United States can be made that would not be detrimental to the health status of African Americans.

Health care practitioners and medical researchers must have knowledge of past misuse of African Americans in research and be prepared and willing to discuss these issues with patients and during the recruitment of African Americans in medical research and clinical trials. Their discussion should cover their commitment to ethical research and safeguards in place to protect participants' rights, and perceived benefit to the patients, and, if applicable, to the African American community. Taking time to discuss these issues with patients and potential study participants can promote better trust between African Americans and the health care profession. In addition, this enhanced communication could also combat rumors often associated with folklore similar to the above belief that hospitals and health care providers should be avoided unless it is necessary. Therefore, trust and education of a patient's/participant's rights are important factors in promoting better health-seeking behaviors in African Americans.

One of the major barriers that have been problematic in the reduction of racial health care disparities is the lack of cultural competency in the health care profession and the disproportionate numbers of African American practitioners. Cultural competency training has been included in medical school curricula for some time focusing on awareness, attitudes toward cultural differences, cross-cultural skills communication skills between medical practitioners, patients, families, and other health care providers. There is sometimes a thin line in drawing the distinction between racism and cultural insensitivity of health care providers for many African Americans. The excerpt below from an interview with Dr. William Anderson provides additional insight on the subject matter that may be beneficial to medical students as well as practicing health care professionals.

> I happen to believe that there is a direct correlation between the cultural sensitivity of the providing physician and the patient. There is a direct correlation. So much so, that in a recent report of the Council on Graduate Medical Education that advises the [U.S.] Congress on health care related matters, one of its recommendations was to meet the needs of the underserved populations. I'm talking about blacks. One of the means that they are recommending to do that is to culturally sensitize and educate white doctors, Needless to say, I went ballistic when they said that. I believe that white doctors [are] not sufficiently sensitized to the needs of black folks, as well intentioned as they may be.

> I look upon racism as being an overt, conscious act. There are a lot of white people that are culturally insensitive, but they don't have any negative feelings or negative thoughts about a black. It is as though it has never come into their thought process that here's a black that has the same need, same sensitivities, same desires as whites. It has never been a part of the thought process. They're not anti-anything, but they have not had the occasion to have to get into that thought process that [says] black people want that, too. It has never been an issue, they've been so isolated. So, I just think that a lot of those white people, even today, fall into that category. They are not "anti." They have just not had the occasion to deal with a black. (William G. Anderson, D.O., Oral History Interview, June 24, 1998).

Through health care reform, government sponsored and funded programs are needed to continue to support initiatives that focus on introducing minorities at the K-12 grade levels to the health professions. Additional government funding should be provided to researchers that would encourage continued research in the area of health care disparities and cultural competency. Funding should also be provided to support physicians working in underserved and poor communities. Hopefully, employing these strategies will increase the number of African Americans in the medical profession.

It is paramount that the past and the present are not linked in such a way that African American participation in medical research and personal health care is hampered too much today. Accurate knowledge of past and present unethical medical practices is important to share with the African American community. The African American community must approach this health crisis with the same veracity and fearlessness used in securing civil rights in this country during the period of segregation. This time the new civil rights movement focuses on equality in health. We must be vigilant activists and whistleblowers against health care injustice by monitoring the government in the enforcement of the laws that govern the ethical conduct of the research activities of private and public institutions.

The intent of this chapter was to provide a richer understanding of what took place in the past with respect to the possible causes of racial health care disparities and unequal medical treatment for African Americans. By delving into the past, lessons can be learned and insights gained to help facilitate future discussions that could possibly lead to solutions and strategies in addressing inequality and inadequate access to health care for African Americans.

References

Aetna.com. (n.d.). (2002). *African American History Calendar: Introduction*. Retrieved from http://www.aetna.com/diversity/aahcalendar/2002/intro.html.

Anderson, William (1998, June 24).Interviewed by George Myers and Ron Amos [Transcript and tape recording].Kellogg African American Health Care Project, University of Michigan Bentley Historical Library, Ann Arbor, Michigan.

Berry, Winbush, G. (1996). African-American health care: Beliefs, practices, and service issues. In M. Julia (Ed.), *Multicultural awareness in health care professionals*. Boston, MA: Houghton Mifflin, 18.

Boulware, L. e., Cooper, L. A., Ratner, L. E., LaVeist, T. A., & Powe, N. R. (2003). Race and trust in the health care system. *Public Health Reports*, *118*, 358-364.

Calloway, K. T. (1995). Bioethical issues confronting the African American community. *Bioethics Forum*, Summer, 31-34.

Carmichael, M. (2010). The great divide: Why racial disparities in health care persist. *Newsweek Web Exclusive.* Retrieved from http://www.newsweek.com/id/233629.

Centers for Disease Control and Prevention. (n. d.). *The Tuskegee Timeline*. Retrieved from http://www.cdc.gov/tuskegee/timeline.htm.

Clayton, L. A., & Byrd, W. M. (2000). Race: A major health status and outcome variable 1980-1999. *Journal of the National Medical Association, 93*(3), 125-135.

Corbie-Smith, G., Thomas, S. B., Williams, M. V., & Moody-Ayers, S. (1999) Attitudes and beliefs of African Americans: Toward participation in medical research. *Journal of General Internal Medicine, 14*(9), 537-546. doi:10.1046/j.1525-1497.1999.07048.x.

Freimuth, V. S., Quinn, S. C., Thomas, S. B., Cole, G., Zook, E., & Duncan, T. (2001). African Americans' views on research and the Tuskegee syphilis study. *Social Science & Medicine, 52*, 797-808.

Foster, N., Neighbors, H., & Myers, G. (2000). *University of Michigan Kellogg African American Health Care Project.* Retrieved from http://www.med.umich.edu/haahc/

Gamble, V. N. (1997). Under the shadow of Tuskegee: African Americans and health care. *American Journal of Public Health, 87*(11), 1773-1778.

Hine, D, (1993). Black women in white: racial conflict and cooperation in the nursing profession, 1890-1950. *Medical Anthropology Quarterly, Volume 7*, Issue 4, 403-405.

JAMA and Archives Journals (2007, June 14). Black patients less likely to receive certain coronary procedures following heart attack. (2007). *ScienceDaily.* Retrieved from http://www.sciencedaily.com/releases/2011/06/110620103939.htm

Johnson, Arthur (1997, June 6).Interviewed by George Myers and Ron Amos [Transcript and tape recording].Kellogg African American Health Care Project, University of Michigan Bentley Historical Library, Ann Arbor, Michigan.

Jones, J. H. (1993). *Bad blood: The Tuskegee syphilis experiment.* New York, NY: The Free Press.

Keith, Rachel (1998, June 16).Interviewed by George Myers and Ron Amos [Transcript and tape recording].Kellogg African American Health Care Project, University of Michigan Bentley Historical Library, Ann Arbor, Michigan.

National Center for Health Statistics. (2011). *Health, United States, 2010: With special feature on death and dying,* Hyattsville, MD. 2011. Retrieved from http://www.cdc.gov.nchs/data/hus/black. htm#access.

Randall, V. R. (1996). *The basis for African American distrust.* Retrieved from http://academic.udayton.edu/health/05bioethics/ slavery02.htm.

Ratnore, S., Lenert, L., Weinfurt, K., Tinoco, A., Taleghani, K., Harless, W., & Schulman, K. (2000). *The effects of patient sex and race on medical students' ratings of quality of life.* Accessed from www.sciencedirect.com/science/journal/00029343, Pages 561-566.

Reverend Dr. Martin Luther King Jr. (1966, March). In a speech presented at the Second National Convention of the Medical Committee for Human Rights, Chicago, Illinois.

Reverby, S. M. (2009). *Examining Tuskegee: The infamous syphilis study and its legacy.* Chapel Hill, NC: The University of North Carolina Press,

Rich, W. C., & Wright, R. H., (1999). In B. K. Hughes Smith (Ed.), *The Wright man: A biography.* Detroit/Southfield, MI: Charro Books,

Samuels, A. (2010) Health-care injustice. *Newsweek Web Exclusive.* Retrieved from http://www.newsweek.com/id/233671.

Shavers-Hornaday, V., Lynch, C., Burmeister, L., & Torner, J. (1997). Why are African Americans under-represented in medical research studies? Impediments to participation. *Ethnicity and Health, 2,* 31-45.

Savitt, T. L. (1988). Slave health and southern distinctiveness. In T. L. Savitt & J. H. Young (Eds.), *Disease and distinctiveness in the American south.* Knoxville, TN: University of Tennessee Press, 120-121.

Skloot, R. (2010). *The immortal life of Henrietta Lacks.* New York, NY: Crown Publishers,

Stobbe, M. (2011, February 27). Past medical testing on humans revealed. *The Washington Post.* Retrieved from http://www.washingtonpost.com/wp-dyn/content/article/2011/02/27/AR2011022700988.html.

Sussman, D. (1999). Separate but unequal: Black nurses waited decades for place at bedside. *NurseWeek.com.* Retrieved from http://www.nurseweek.com/features/99-12/blacks.html.

Swan, Lionel (1999, June 18).Interviewed by George Myers and Ron Amos [Transcript and tape recording].Kellogg African American Health Care Project, University of Michigan Bentley Historical Library, Ann Arbor, Michigan.

The Tuskegee Syphilis Experiment. (n.d.). *Infoplease.com.* Retrieved from http://www.infoplease.com/ipa/A0762136.html.

Todd, Oretta (1997, May 1).Interviewed by George Myers and Ron Amos [Transcript and tape recording].Kellogg African American Health Care Project, University of Michigan Bentley Historical Library, Ann Arbor, Michigan.

United States Department of Health, Education, and Welfare. (1973). *Final report of the Tuskegee syphilis study ad hoc advisory panel.*

University of Michigan Health System (2011, June 20). Black heart attack patients wait longer for advanced treatment, study shows. *Science Daily.* Retrieved from http://www.sciencedaily.com/releases/2011/06/110620103939.htm.

Washington, H. A. (2006). *Medical apartheid: The dark history of medical experimentation of black Americans from colonial times to present.* New York, NY: Doubleday.

Wasserman, J., Flannery, M. A., & Clair, J. M. (2007). Raising the ivory tower: the production of knowledge and distrust of medicine among African Americans. *Journal of Medical Ethics, 33*(3), 177-180.

Wright, Charles (1997, April 15).Interviewed by George Myers [Transcript and tape recording].Kellogg African American Health Care Project, University of Michigan Bentley Historical Library, Ann Arbor, Michigan.

Wright, P. (2006, August 22). Looking elsewhere for subjects; Rules rightly protect vulnerable population in coercive setting. *USA Today.* Retrieved from https://pqarchiver.com/USAToday/access/1103746101.

CHAPTER TWO

Epidemiological Issues: Critical Factors in Culturally Competent Health Care

Delroy M. Louden
Anguilla Community College
British West Indies

Abstract

This chapter examines the demographic features that are the driving forces toward acceptance of culturally competent care as an acceptable feature of modern professional practice, whether in industry, commerce, education or health care. No longer can cultural competency be seen as a warm and fuzzy idea or feeling lacking any empirical basis, but as an essential ingredient of health service delivery in an increasingly diverse, multi-ethnic, and multicultural population. It is argued that there is a need for more evidence based practices, among these diverse groups who live, work, and play amongst us. This requires that health service delivery practitioners engage in a multidisciplinary approach in understanding the relationship between attitudes, behaviors, cultural practices, health seeking behaviors and health outcomes. There must be no assumption that one size fits all and once we have understood any one group we can then extrapolate to other diverse populations. The lessons from health disparity research clearly illustrates that we missed the boat when we focused on one group to the detriment of others. Community Based Participatory Based Research (CBPR) provides us with a paradigm shift and its utility in addressing cultural competency is outlined. The utility and versatility of this approach is illustrated by the variety of studies and settings in which it has been used through the Agency for Health Care Research and Quality in particular its multidisciplinary characteristics as well as its usefulness in translational research and population based research. Successful cultural competence practices must be guided by evidence based outcomes so that individuals seeking professional services, employers, and purchasers of services whether it be managed care organizations or accreditation bodies can subscribe to it. Notions of targeting literacy, offering patients navigation facility and broadening or redefining our understanding of health and wellbeing in the broadest possible sense must become central to academic discourse.

Introduction

The movement of populations from city to city and from country to country has been a constant feature of human existence from time immemorial. What is different today is that the configuration of groups that constitute the majority of this transition has changed dramatically. More specifically, the new groups in our midst share a different history, geography, ethnicity and cultural practices.

These new and emerging groups demand that we address their health, education and social needs in a manner that is ethical and culturally appropriate, as well as meeting all the requirements pertaining to human rights and citizenry. For the practitioner the question is not whether these groups should remain distinct; the fact is their needs must be addressed in culturally appropriate ways, otherwise such practices are clearly inadequate in professional terms. In short, the demography that once shaped North America, and in particular the United States, has changed dramatically for those who provide services and also for those who receive services due to this new population. As a result, the cultural competence of all providers of care has become critically important in ensuring positive health outcomes. Equally important is our need to comprehend more fully the attitudes, risk, and vulnerability factors associated with these changing demographics and their impacts on service delivery.

Paradoxically, this new diverse population has forced many practitioners to finally recognize that a diverse population has existed in our midst for a long time, but their needs have never been addressed adequately. In the US, it has taken a long time to recognize that culturally competent health care does not mean simply recruiting personnel who look like the patient /client population to staff many of these organizations. As a consequence, health disparities exist and health systems have very little evidence that cultural competency techniques or evidenced based practice has been part of their service delivery model.

U.S. Census Bureau Projections Show a Slower Growing, Older, More Diverse Nation a Half Century from Now

The U.S. population will be considerably older and more racially and ethnically diverse by 2060, according to *projections* released by the U.S. Census Bureau, December 2012. "The next half century marks key points in continuing trends—the U.S. will become a plurality nation, where the non-Hispanic white population remains the largest single group, but, no group is in the majority," said Acting Director Thomas L. Mesenbourg. (US Census Bureau, 2012). Furthermore, the population is projected to grow much more slowly over the next several decades, compared with the last set of projections released in 2008 and 2009. That is because the projected levels of births and net international migration are lower in the projections released today, reflecting more recent trends in fertility and international migration.

According to the projections, the population, ages 65 and older, are expected to more than double between 2012 and 2060, increasing from 43.1 million to 92.0 million. The older population would represent just over one in five U.S. residents by the end of the period, up from one in seven today. The increase in the number of the "elderly" would be even more dramatic—those 85 and older are projected to more than triple from 5.9 million to 18.2 million, reaching 4.3 percent of the total population.

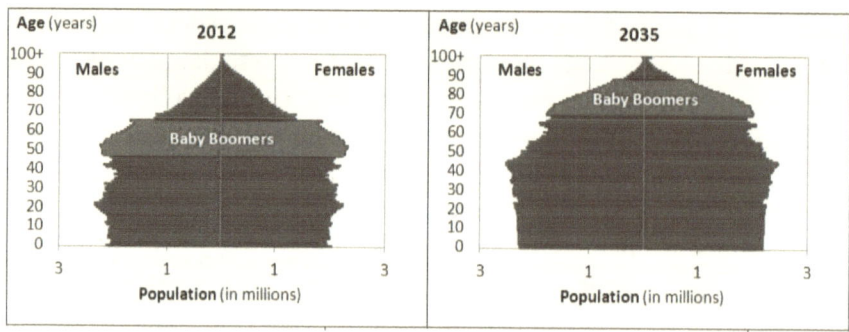

Figure 1. U. S. population by age and sex: 2012 and 2035 (U.S. Census Bureau, 2012).

As Figure 1 shows, baby boomers, defined as "persons born between 1946 and 1964", number 76.4 million in 2012 and account for about one-quarter of the population. In 2060, when the youngest of them would be 96 years old, they are projected to number around 2.4 million and represent 0.6 percent of the total population. The important point regarding the data illustrated in Figure 1 for this chapter, is that while this aging group will grow larger, the numbers of whites that will become elderly after 2035 will begin to decrease as the non-whites increase in numbers.

A More Diverse Nation

Figure 2 illustrates the changing composition of the U.S. population and the diversity within our midst that requires a culturally competent workforce and health care. For example, the non-Hispanic white population is projected to peak in 2024, at 199.6 million, up from 197.8 million in 2012. Unlike other races or ethnic groups, however, their population is projected to slowly decrease, falling by nearly 20.6 million from 2024 to 2060.

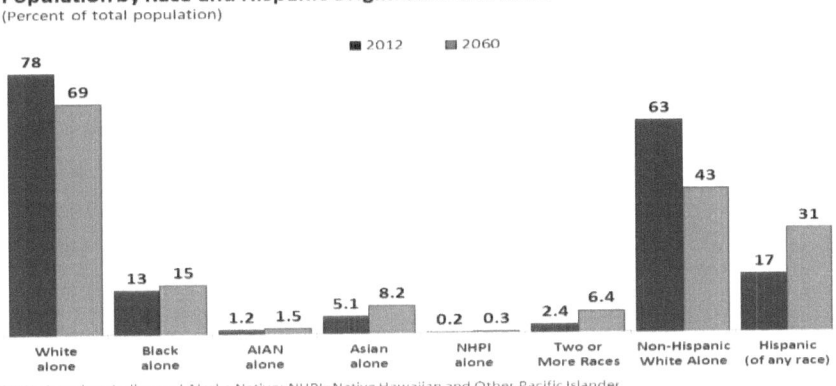

Population by Race and Hispanic Origin: 2012 and 2060
(Percent of total population)

Fig. 2. **Population by race and Hispanic origin: 2012 and 2060 (U. S. Census Bureau, 2012)**

Meanwhile, the Hispanic population would more than double, from 53.3 million in 2012 to 128.8 million in 2060. Consequently, by the end of the period, nearly one in three U.S. residents would be Hispanic, up from about one in six today.

The black population is expected to increase from 41.2 million to 61.8 million over the same period. Its share of the total population would rise slightly, from 13.1 percent in 2012 to 14.7 percent in 2060.

The Asian population is projected to more than double, from 15.9 million in 2012 to 34.4 million in 2060, with its share of the nation's total population climbing from 5.1 percent to 8.2 percent in the same period.

All in all, minorities, now 37 percent of the U.S. population, are projected to comprise 57 percent of the population in 2060. (Minorities consist of all but the single-race, non-Hispanic white population.) The total minority population would more than double, from 116.2 million to 241.3 million over the period 2012 to 2060 (US Census) 2012.

Projections show the older population would continue to be predominately non-Hispanic white, while younger ages are increasingly diverse minorities from several backgrounds. In the age group 65 and older in 2060, 56.0 percent are expected to be non-Hispanic white, 21.2 percent Hispanic and 12.5 percent non-Hispanic black. In contrast, while 52.7 percent of those younger than 18 were non-Hispanic white in 2012 that number would drop to 32.9 percent by 2060. Hispanics are projected to make up 38.0 percent of this group in 2060, up from 23.9 percent in 2012. Table I shows that Mexico is the leading country of origin for legal permanent residents to the US in 2010 with an estimated 3.3 million or roughly 25 percent of all legal residents. The next leading country is China and the Philippines followed by India and the Dominican Republic. An estimated forty two percent of legal permanent residents in 2011 were born in one of these five countries (Mexico, China, Philippines, India and the Dominican Republic).

Table I
Country of Birth of Legal Permanent Resident Population: 2011 **(Source: US Dept of Homeland Security, 2012).**

Country of birth	Legal permanent residents		Legal permanent residents eligible to naturalize	
	Number	Percent	Number	Percent
Total	13,070,000	100.0	8,530,000	100.0
Mexico	3,320,000	25.4	2,650,000	31.1
China	590,000	4.5	260,000	3.0

Philippines	590,000	4.5	330,000	3.8
India	520,000	4.0	240,000	2.8
Dominican Republic	470,000	3.6	300,000	3.5
Cuba	410,000	3.1	280,000	3.3
Vietnam	330,000	2.6	210,000	2.4
El Salvador	330,000	2.5	260,000	3.0
Canada	320,000	2.4	260,000	3.0
United Kingdom	290,000	2.2	230,000	2.7
Korea, South	280,000	2.2	170,000	2.0
Haiti	250,000	1.9	150,000	1.7
Colombia	240,000	1.8	130,000	1.5
Jamaica	240,000	1.8	160,000	1.8
Guatemala	190,000	1.4	120,000	1.5
Germany	180,000	1.4	150,000	1.7
Poland	150,000	1.2	110,000	1.3
Peru	140,000	1.1	80,000	0.9
Japan	140,000	1.1	110,000	1.3
Pakistan	140,000	1.0	60,000	0.7
Other	3,940,000	30.2	2,290,000	26.8

Other highlights are:

- The nation's total population would cross the 400 million mark in 2051, reaching 420.3 million in 2060.
- The proportion of the population younger than 18 is expected to change little over the 2012-2060 period, decreasing from 23.5 percent to 21.2 percent.
- In 2056, for the first time, the older population, ages 65 and over, is projected to outnumber the young, age under 18.
- The working-age population (18 to 64) is expected to increase by 42 million between 2012 and 2060, from 197 million to 239 million, while its share of the total population declines from 62.7 percent to 56.9 percent.

Uniformity of population changes in the era of globalization. The pattern and trend noted above is not in any way peculiar to the United States. Indeed our neighbor to the North, Canada, has seen similar dramatic shifts in its population dynamics. Fig: 3 shows the ethnic origins of the once traditional migration to North America through what can be described as "Kit and Kin" routes.

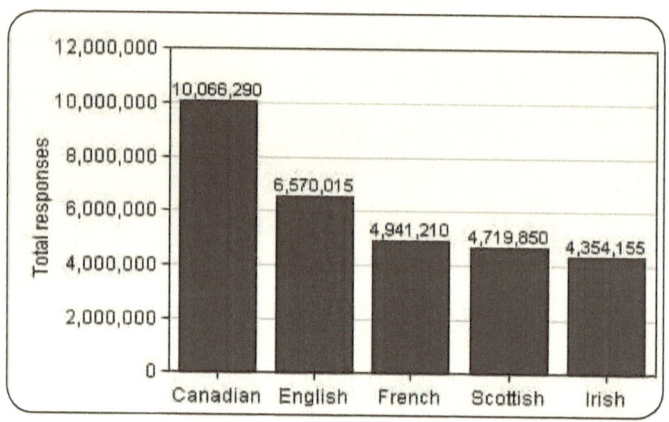

Figure 3. **Top five ethnic origins in Canada
(Source: Statistics-Canada, 2007)**

As one can see that the largest group of immigrants have been traditionally European in origin with the English being the second largest group, followed by the French, then the Scottish,and, finally, the English. The pattern of migration follows one of original immigrants migrating, followed by nuclear family members, and widening to those in the extended families of these immigrants. In some cases, close friends have followed the routes. The most important point for this discussion is that the ethnic origins of these immigrants have been European in nature. While there might have been differences in national characteristics, the prevailing context has been one of a European cultural ethos.

In contrast to Figure 3, Figure 4 illustrates the fact that Canada, like the U.S., has become a more diverse population in terms of the origins of its current population. As Figure 4 shows, the percentage of non-white groups in Canada provide interesting data with the emergence of groups of color ranging from high percentages of groups from South Asia and China as the two largest, visible, minorities. Next is the Black population with the third largest percentage. Again, the Asian groups are represented in smaller percentages by Filipinos, Southeast Asians, West Asians, Koreans, and the Japanese. Interspersed within these groups are the Latin Americans, Arabs, and, in smaller percentages, individuals from mixed, multiple, ethnic heritages. The percentages of these groups in relationship to the total population will only grow larger in the next fifty years. Herein lies the tale for cultural competency supporters; an ever changing population shift demands flexibility as well as sensitivity in the provision of services.

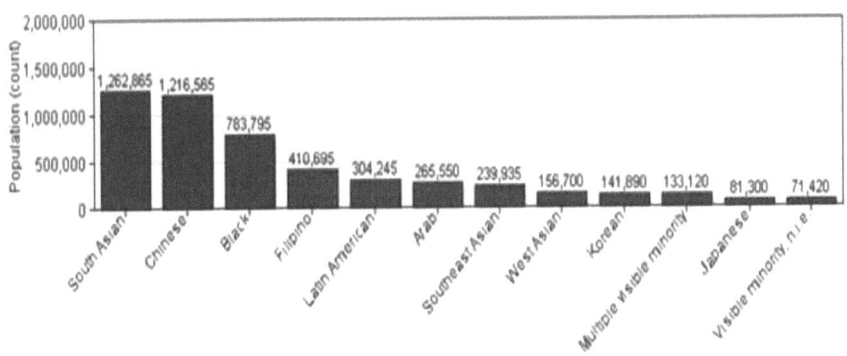

Figure 4. Visible minorities in Canada
(Source: Statistics-Canada, 2007)

A close inspection of Figure 5 shows the size and growth of the visible minority population in Canada comprises over one-fifth of the Canadian population. This percentage is going to go higher in the next fifty years as the numbers of non-whites grow exponetially while the percentage of whites begins to decrease dramatically because of lower numbers of whites being born. These data do not take into account the numbers of minorities that have not been counted because of a lack of clarity in the definitions of what it means to be a member of a minority group. If one were to take into account those numbers, the actual percentage of the visible, minority population may even be a higher number.

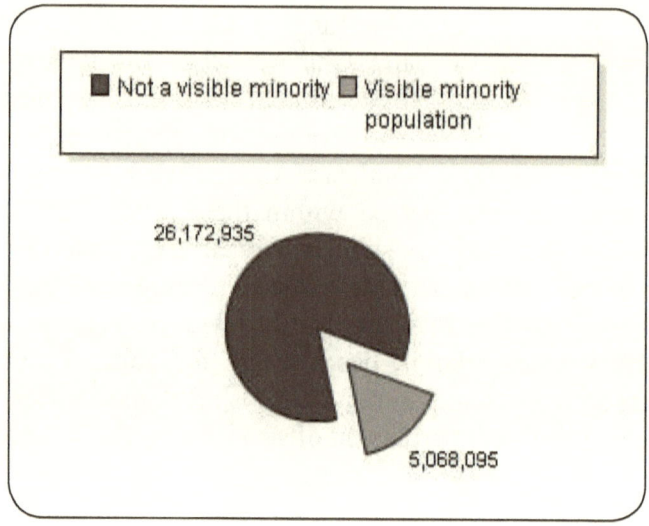

Figure 5. **Size and growth of the multi ethnic community that is now Canada (Source: Statistics-Canada, 2007).**

Research Implications

There are several important implications for this trend. These implications are presented below:

First, we must avoid notions of homogeneity in our descriptions of the new population.

Second, we must direct our research efforts towards population based investigations rather than geographical boundaries as we elucidate further cultural competencies. Thirdly, epidemiological based investigations must now focus more on indicators such as quality of care, as well as health beliefs and practices. Fourthly, we need to better understand the variability if any in the utilization of care in a culturally diverse health care delivery system as this will undoubtedly affect case management. Finally, a disaggregation of much of the available statistical data is needed for effective practice, both in terms of intervention and prevention. This has implication for the use of a wider array of Public Health Indicators.

Third, Community Based Participatory Research provides us with an opportunity to address many of the research issues thrust upon us by a diverse population requiring a culturally competent health care delivery system.

Fourth, Community Based Participatory Research (CBPR) is a collaborative approach to research that combines research methods on inquiry with community capacity building strategies to bridge the gap between knowledge produced through research and what is practiced in communities through health partners, academic partners and community partners.

Israel et. al (1998) have identified nine key principals of CBPR that support successful research partnerships:

- Recognize the community as a unit of identity;
- Build on strengths and resources within the community;
- Facilitate collaborative, equitable involvement of all partners in all phases of the research;
- Integrate knowledge and intervention for mutual benefit of all partners;
- Promote a co-learning and empowering process that attends to social inequalities;
- Involve a cyclical and iterative process;
- Address health from both positive and ecological perspectives;
- Disseminate findings and knowledge gained to all partners; and
- Involve long-term commitment by all partners.

CBPR expands the potential for transforming research findings into practice and application—commonly known as translational sciences to develop, implement and dissemination of effective interventions across diverse communities through strategies designed to reduce power imbalances, facilitate mutual benefit among community and academic partners as well as promoting reciprocal knowledge translation, thereby, incorporating community theories into research design.

Traditionally Designed Research such as:

- case studies; focus groups;
- experiments; quasi experiments
- survey research (e.g. random sampling, stratified random sampling; and
- randomized clinical trials (RCT), Double Blind Studies
- longitudinal, correlational, and factorial designed studies

Epidemiological Investigations:

- prospective investigations; retrospective investigations; cross-sectional studies;
- qualitative; and quantitative investigations

have interpreted the 'scientific method' with such rigidity that they have left no room for those whom they study to participate in the research process except as subjects. Of course the usual claim is that objectivity, that rarified term is protected. Notions of empowerment of their participants in their investigations would constitute heresy. It is this kind of view that has led to a paradigm shift as our population has become more diverse and health disparities have become more magnified.

These traditional approaches have not always served us well because of their reductionist framework and the tendency to devalue the potential contribution of more interpretive research methods as it relates to cultural competence care. In fact, there is ample evidence of disrespect. For example, the Tuskegee Experiment demonstrated inappropriateness in design and severe ethical deficiencies in the conducting of the experiment. A second example is indicated in HIV/AIDS investigations conducted in South Africa where the consent protocol was not followed. In countries where there are non-existent research protection processes such as an Institutional Review Board (IRB) or a Patient's Bill of Rights, and where Informed Consent is not adequately enforced, abuses are likely to occur. In the Caribbean, where the prevalence and incidence of non-communicable diseases are high, community-based research provides an approach that allows researchers, not just to collect data and turn our backs, but to educate and inform the population of their risk factors as related to their susceptibility. This in no way is a challenge or a danger to reliability and validity.

Role of Community Based Participatory Research

There is increased interest in research that aims to improve the health of disadvantaged (low income) populations. However, conventional research in these communities has a contentious history and offers limited opportunities to improve the health and well-being of these communities. Community Based Participatory Research directly addresses the fundamental differences in epistemology in dealing with the issue of power ignored by traditional research and aims to be compatible with the philosophy of the new public health movement.

Participatory research in disadvantaged communities has a long and successful history in the social sciences and international and rural development. There is a growing recognition of the importance and promise of this type of research within health service delivery systems, public health institutions and funding organizations. However, in spite of the increased interest expressed by communities, universities, and funders, CBPR is underutilized primarily as it is mistakenly, perceived as lacking essential features of traditional scientific method namely—scientific rigor. However, evidence from the Agency for Health Care Research and Quality presented here clearly demonstrates the broad breadth and depth of research using CBPR. Indeed it points to the growth in interdisciplinary studies that is being undertaken.

Characteristics and Consequences of Community-Based Research

Community-based research processes differ fundamentally from mainstream research in the following ways:

1. It is done in collaboration with community groups that are eager to know the research results and to use them in practical efforts to achieve constructive social change.
2. Community-based research is not only usable; it is generally used to good effect in analyzing the complexity of relationships in multi-ethnic populations.
3. Ample evidence now exists that community-based research often produces unanticipated and far reaching ancillary results, including new social relationships and trust, as well as heightened social efficacy qualities necessary in multicultural health care delivery.
4. By contrast, conventional research with its rigidity of procedures, despite some periodic spectacular successes, bears some responsibility for environmental pollution,

occasional ethical breaches (such as dangerous medical or military experiments performed on uninformed human subjects), degraded work processes, and industrial accidents.

5. By its very nature, community-based research has the potential not to produce such negative consequences; involving as it does from inception community members in planning and execution of the research process.

6. Community research projects frequently involve local groups reacting to urgent problems such as environmental pollution, local poverty and obesity. The majority of the community-based organizations often formulate a macro social analysis that informs their programmatic activities, ensuring that their projects include a proactive component or a trans-local outlook. Community-based research projects findings have practical implications often well beyond the local level.

Paradigm—Shift—Empowerment

1. Community-based research is intended to empower communities and to give everyday people influence over the direction of research and enable them to be parts of decision making processes on issues that affect them.

2. Community-based research is rooted in communities.

3. Communities often *identify* the issue or problem and participate in *defining* the research questions, *conducting* the research and, finally, *using the results* toward an action-oriented outcome. Our definition of community-based research (which we sometimes shorten to simply "community research") is: research conducted by, with, and/or for communities. Essentially, community based participatory research is encouraging all researchers whatever their method of inquiry to focus more, or give equal attention, than has previously been the practice on translational research—that is translating study findings into concrete strategies for improving practices, programs and service delivery.

Demand for Community-Based Research

There is significant demand for community-based research; however, the need is not being met due to the following issues:

1. Community-based research is seldom a component of grants applied for or awarded. For example, in Anguilla, currently, there are no Community Outreach Partnership Programs which provide data collection or analysis of trends relating to issues such as environmental pollution, beach erosion, and/or disaster risk reduction efforts.
2. CBPR encourages collaboration of "formally trained research" partners from any area of expertise, provided that the researcher provides expertise that is seen as:

    i.   useful to the investigation by the community;
    ii. fully committed to a partnership of *equals*; and
    iii. developing outcomes which are beneficial and usable for community development.

3. Equitable partnerships require sharing *power, resources*, credit, results; and *knowledge*, as well as, a reciprocal appreciation of each partner's knowledge and skills at each stage of the project (i.e., including problem definition; issue selection; research design; conducting research; interpreting the results; and determining how the results should be used for action).
4. CBPR differs from traditional *research* in many ways. For example, instead of creating knowledge for the advancement of a field or for knowledge sake, CBPR is an *iterative process*, incorporating research, reflection, and action in a cyclical process.

Examples in the Use of CBPR

Building Community-Based Participatory Research Partnerships with a Somali Refugee Community (Johnson, et al, 2009). This study examined Somali immigrant women's experiences with the

U.S. healthcare system, exploring how attitudes, perceptions, and cultural values, such as FGC, influence their use of reproductive health care.

Methods: A mixed—method community-based participatory research (CBPR) collaboration with a Somali refugee community was conducted from 2005 to 2008 incorporating surveys, semi—structured focus groups, and individual interviews. Providers caring for this community were also interviewed to gain their perspectives and experiences.

Results: The process of establishing a partnership with a Somali community is described wherein the challenges, successes, and lessons learned in the process of conducting CBPR were examined. Challenges obtaining informed consent, language barriers, and reliance on FGC self-report were surmounted through mobilization of community social networks, trust-building, and the use of a video-elicitation device. The community partnership collaborated around shared goals of voicing unique healthcare concerns of the community to inform the development of interventional programs to improve culturally-competent care.

Conclusions: Community-based participatory research using mixed-methods was critical in facilitating trust building, engaging community members as active participants in every phase of the research process, and enabling the rigorous and ethical conduct of research with refugee communities.

Community-Based Participatory Research Contributions to Intervention Research: The Intersection of Science and Practice to Improve Health Equity. (Wallerstein & Duran, 2010)

This review of community-based participatory research shows how (CBPR) has emerged in the last decades as a transformative research paradigm that bridges the gap between science and practice through community engagement and social action to increase health equity. CBPR expands the potential for the translational sciences to (a) develop, implement, and disseminate effective interventions across diverse communities through strategies to redress power imbalances; (b) facilitate mutual benefit among community and academic partners; and (c) promote reciprocal knowledge translation, incorporating community theories into the research. The authors identify the barriers and challenges within the intervention and implementation sciences, discuss how CBPR can address these challenges, provide an illustrative research example, and discuss next steps to advance the translational science of CBPR.

Examples of Community Based Participatory Research Conducted Under the Auspices of the Agency for Health Care Research and Quality (AHRQ, 2013).

Stroke Telemedicine Access Recovery Project. This career-development award provides training and mentoring in CBPR to a clinician-scientist providing pilot data for a study of barriers to successful implementation of a rural hospital's community-based Stroke Telemedicine Access Recovery, or STAR, project.

Building Health Services Research Capacity for Tribes in Montana and Wyoming. This grant provides funding for the Montana-Wyoming Tribal Leaders Council to continue to build capacity to address priority health issues identified by the tribes; build capacity and infrastructure for tribal participatory research focused on health promotion, prevention, and management of chronic diseases; and increase support for culturally appropriate health programs and for the role of traditional medicine practitioners.

Communities as Partners in Cancer Clinical Trials. Community—Campus Partnerships for Health. This grant supports a three-part conference series to create a conceptual framework for communities as partners in cancer clinical trials and explores the application of CBPR principles and approaches to key areas of cancer research.

Exploring the Role of Secondary Conditions in Nursing Home Transitions. This study uses CBPR principles to understand the role of secondary conditions in transition from the nursing home to the community and uses this understanding to modify a previously demonstrated intervention project.

A National Assisted Living CBPR Partnership to Improve Medication Management. This grant provided support to a national partnership of 10 research organizations concerned with improvement of assisted living through application of CBPR principles. Initial efforts were to improve medication management in assisted living facilities.

Community Integration After Spinal Cord Injury: Using Photo voice to Identify Barriers. This study applied participatory methodology to focus research on issues of greatest relevance to individuals with spinal cord injuries. It trained the subjects in the use of cameras to document the barriers and facilitators they encounter in the community, using semi structured individual interviews to provide additional information to subjects.

Making Chronic Kidney Disease Guidelines Work in Underserved Practices. Chronic kidney disease, a worldwide public health issue, is four times more likely to burden minority populations. This study sought to use participatory research methods to assess provider—and staff identified barriers to implementing evidence-based guidelines for chronic kidney disease in minority populations.

National Conference: Quality Health Care for Diverse Populations. This was the fourth National Conference on Quality Health Care for Culturally Diverse Populations, which highlighted the best of culturally competent health care to national health organizations and leaders, including communities.

Overcoming Health Racial Disparities. A partnership was developed between the University of North Carolina and two historically black North Carolina universities (North Carolina Central and Shaw Universities). The goal of the project was to understand and eliminate health disparities for adult cancer and other chronic illness among black adults, particularly rural black populations.

Adult Health and Disabilities in Three Housing Conditions. The project supported the National Rehabilitation Hospital's

Center for Health and Disability Research in partnering with a community-centered disability group to carry out a CBPR study on the health status and health care needs of low-income or impoverished working-age people with physical impairments living in the District of Columbia.

Conclusion

The population dynamics driving both North America and Europe present all professionals with the opportunity, not only to examine their professional practices with respect to how they provide services to those who seek care, but also present an opportunity for them to evaluate what they do. More specifically, the instruments of practice must now reflect a new reality—that is, it cannot now be business as usual. Assessment tools for measuring outcomes must become more specific as well as sensitive. In addition, tinkering with the curriculum of traditional, research strategies is not a satisfactory solution; what is required is evidence based information. Community based participatory research is an example of an approach that can provide such information.

Existing organizations, such as Medicare and Medicaid, should collect language data on all new applications which undoubtedly improve service delivery to its users. Collecting data on languages spoken by all applicants is also important in ensuring that programs comply with civil rights by not discriminating among diverse populations. In addition, having a comprehensive language database is critical to early identification and intervention, thus reducing health disparities as well as enabling comprehensive service delivery. In this regard, the Agency for Health Care Policy and Research (AHCPR) CONQUEST software, as well as its Healthcare Cost and Utilization Project Quality Care Indicators (HCUP,QIs), have several clinical performance measures that can be adopted to provide a culturally competent data system addressing as it does features such as utilization, hospital admissions, and treatment outcomes. Community Based Participatory Research has several merits for health care practitioners, community participants and researchers. *First*, it creates bridges between scientists and the communities that participate in research studies through the use of shared knowledge such as greater understanding by communities of the need for clinical trials. *Second*, when members of the community gain greater understanding of the need for a particular investigation and its research design, the community may itself contribute to the selection of the research practices, as well as the development of culturally appropriate measurement instruments. *Third*, issues such as sample selection, type of sampling would benefit from community input as it relates to oversampling in a particular population, or in the design of prevention investigations where knowledge, attitudes, and practices may very well impact outcomes. *Fourth,* recruitment is another area where communities, by being stakeholders, can enhance sample robustness.

Community Based Participatory Research provides an opportunity for researchers to more fully appreciate the need to communicate and implement their findings to a wider audience other than to their academic peers, having as its core the enhancing and adoption of best practices. It also provides an opportunity for Translation Research as well as multidisciplinary integration of basic research, patient-oriented research, and population based research with the long term goal of improving health outcomes and the reduction of health disparities. Finally, because public health problems result from complex economic political, social, biological, environmental and genetic causes, a more viable array of methods is needed for successful intervention. Thus, CBPR provides another tool to tackle these problems, particularly as elements of translational research inherent in this approach from research to practice.

References

AHRQ. (2013). *Activities using Community Based Participatory Research*-website May 28, 2013.

Anderson, L M, Fielding, P.F (2003). Cultural competent health care systems: A systemic review. *Amer J. of Prev. Medicine, 35*, 230-300.

Bell J, Standish M. Communities and health policy: A pathway for change. (2005). *Health Affairs, 24*(2), 339-342.

Buchanan DR, Miller FG, & Wallerstein N. (2007). Ethical issues in community-based participatory research: Balancing rigorous research with community participation in community intervention studies. *Programme Community Health Partnerships. 1*(2), 153-160.

Cargo M., & Mercer SL. (2008). The value and challenges of participatory research: Strengthening its practice. *Annual Review of Public Health, 29*, 325-350.

Cashman SB, Adeky S, Allen AJ, Corburn, J, Montano, J, Refelito, A, Swanson, S, Wallerstein, N, & Eng, E. (2008). The power and the promise: Working with communities to analyze data, interpret findings, and get to outcomes. *Am. J. Public Health, 98*(8), 1407-1417.

Hayes-Bautista D.E (2003). Research on cultural competency health care system. Less sensitivity, more statistics. *AM. J. Prev. Med. 24*, (3 supplement 8-9).

Irwin A. The politics of talk: Coming to terms with the "new" scientific governance. (2006). *Soc. Studies, 36*, 299-320.

Israel B., Schulz A., & Parker E. (2009). Critical issues in developing and following community based participatory research principles. In M. Minkler and N. Wallerstein (Eds), *Community based participatory research in health*. San Francisco: Jossey-Bass, 53-70.

Israel BA, Schulz AJ, Parker EA, & Becker AB. (1998). Review of community-based research: Assessing partnership approaches to improve public health. *Annual Rev. Public Health, 19*, 173-202.

Johnson C, Ali, SA, & Shipp, MP. (2009). Building CBPR partnership with a Somali refuge community. *Am J Prev Med, 37*(6), 230-236.

Jones L, Wells K. Strategies for academic and clinician engagement in community-participatory partnered research. *JAMA, 297*(4), 407-410.

Statistics, Canada. (2007). *Portrait of the Canadian population: Catalog 97-550*. Ottawa released March, 2007.

Syme, S.L. Social determinants of health: The community as an empowered partner. *Prev. Chronic Disease, 1*(1), 1-8.

US Census Bureau. (2012). *Projections: A slower growing, older, more diverse nation a half century from now*. Released Dec 12, 2012.

US Department of Homeland Security. (2012). *Estimates of the permanent resident population in 2011*, Office of Immigration Statistics, Released July, 2012.

Wallerstein, N & Duran, B. (2010) Community-Based Participatory Research Contributions to Intervention Research. The Intersection of Science and Practice to Improve Health Equity. *Amer, J. Public Health, 10*, 40-46.

Wallerstein N, Duran B, Minkler M, & Foley K. (2005). Developing and maintaining partnerships with communities. In: Israel B, Eng E, Schulz A, & Parker E, (Eds). *Methods in community based participatory research*. San Francisco, CA: Jossey-Bass, 31-51.

CHAPTER THREE

Gender and Health Care Delivery: The Intersection between Race/Ethnicity, Culture, and Structure for African American Women

Penelope J. Kinsey
The Lincoln University, PA

Denise Gaither-Hardy
The Lincoln University, PA

Theresa E. Berger
Fox Chase Cancer Center

Abstract

The literature on disparities in health care outcomes for African American women demands changes in the ways that health care professionals conceptualize their thinking regarding the manner in which these women live their everyday lives. Consequently, this chapter focuses on the need to develop a more culturally competent way of conceptualizing the lives of African American women with the presentation of a more culturally competent framework that can be used by health care professionals in their policies, research strategies, and health care practices. The chapter focuses on specific concepts that have been thought to deter progress in obtaining the most meaningful information from African American women, and describes some of the most prominent deficiencies involved in traditional approaches to research and health care. A socio-historical framework is presented and discussed for the purpose of advancing an alternative model to the current, biomedical framework. A path for a new direction in thinking and strategizing is also discussed.

Introduction

Over the past few decades, the research and health care communities have begun to pay closer attention to disparities in health care for minority groups in the United States (e.g., American Sociological Association, 2005; Kessler, Mickelson, & Williams, 1999; Smedley, Stith, & Nelson, 2003). As summarized in a 2003 report, a large number of studies have documented the existence of severe disparities in health care and health outcomes for racial and ethnic minorities (Smedley, Stith, & Nelson, 2003).

For African American women, the disparities in health outcomes have been well documented in the literature. For example, while women make up more than half of the population in the United States, African American women suffer disproportionately with higher incidences of sexually transmitted infections (STIs), the Human Immunodeficiency Virus and Acquired Immunodeficiency Syndrome (HIV/AIDS), hypertension, diabetes, and some cancers (National Cancer Institute (NCI), 2004; United States Department of Health and Human Services (U.S. DDHS), 2004; Williams, 2001).

In the case of breast cancer, while death rates for European American women have declined, they have increased for African American women. In 1975, the death rate for breast cancer was nearly 32 per 100,000, while the rate for African American women was 30 per 100,000. From 1975 to 2000, the combined efforts of researchers and health caregivers resulted in improved diagnostic procedures and treatment modalities. As a consequence, the data revealed decreased death rates for women in general. However, in 2004, a report from the Center for Disease Control and Prevention (CDC), revealed disparities in death rates for European American women and African American women. The data indicated that while the death rate for European American women from breast cancer had decreased to 25 per 100,000, there was an increase in the death rate for African American women to approximately 35 per 100,00 women. More recent studies have revealed that although African American women have a lower incidence of breast cancer (118 out of every 100,000) when compared with European American women (133 out of every 100,000), African American women are more likely to die at a higher rate (34 per 100,000) when compared with European American women (25 per 100,000) (American Cancer Society (ACS), 2008; Freeman, 2004; NCI, 2007).

Such disparities in health outcomes, as the ones presented above, have spurred researchers to look for factors that could help to explain why African Americans in general, and, African American women, specifically, manifest huge disparities in health outcomes (Chu, Tarone, & Brawley, 1999; Dignam, 2001; Jatoi, Anderson, Sowmya, & Devesa, 2005). One promising direction in research has been to investigate factors influencing the frequency with which African American women access and use health care resources (e.g., their health beliefs), their health seeking behaviors (e.g., exercise), and their experiences with the health care giving community (e.g., their perceptions of the quality of health care) (Altman & Taylor, 2001; Fuller, 2008; Institute of Medicine (IOM), 2003; Registe, 2008; Robbins, 2007; Williams, 2001).

Such an approach takes into account the central idea that the perceptions of African American women, with respect to their ideas about health, their access to health care, their health seeking behaviors, and their perceptions regarding the treatment they receive by health care professionals, may contribute to disparities in health care use, and, thereby, may contribute to disparities in health outcomes. However, this approach still does not take into account the holistic nature of the cultural context in which African American women live in their everyday lives. The traditional approach used in western medicine and research, by its very nature, does not take into account the culture of African Americans as a significant, contextual factor which may be used to develop more effective research strategies and treatment modalities (Berger, 2013).

Such an approach does not always take into account the idea that there are larger, structural factors which have influenced African American women to constrain their access to, and use of, health care resources (Combs-Jones, 2004). These factors are a shared history of racism/racial prejudice, continuing discrimination, sexism, and classicism which also may contribute to disparities in health, care use, and, consequently, disparities in health outcomes for African American women. Such an approach does not take into account the interplay between the external, structural factors confronting African American women, and their internal, cultural barometers they use to guide their everyday lives. This chapter is an attempt to illustrate, through relevant research and theoretical ideas, that incorporating this newer strategy of thinking about the role of cultural traditions, other than the western tradition, would result in more effective research strategies, more efficient health care, and greater sensitivity in health care policies (Robbins, 2007).

The first section begins with a brief review and discussion of the concepts which have been developed to traditionally define groups of people (e.g., race, ethnicity, and identity), the shortcomings of such definitions, and a discussion of the impact they have had on the development of values and definitions of health and well-being in the health care community. This review is being done to show that there are deficiencies in thinking when applied to groups of people other than those who are European American in cultural orientation. It is argued that such definitions, as applied in the current health care system, have inadvertently resulted in helping to decrease health care access and use by African Americans generally, and, specifically, by African American women.

The second section is a brief review and discussion of the traditional research and health care strategies used in western medicine to better understand how such traditions in thinking and practice, by their philosophical assumptions regarding illness, health, diagnosis, and treatment, may actually facilitate the continuance of health care disparities today for African Americans in general, and, specifically, for African American women. This review and discussion is presented to show that the deficiencies in the western point of view overlook the cultural framework out of which African Americans operate, and, consequently, overlooks vital information needed by policy makers for their health care decisions, researchers for their investigative strategies, and care givers for their health care practices.

The third section presents an alternative framework which emphasizes the importance of a shared socio-historical culture, and the influence the culture has on the ways in which African American women view health, themselves, and their communities. Where relevant, the interplay of the cultural ethos of African American women with that of such external structural factors as exposure to stress as a result of being "black," will be presented. It is hoped that by presenting such a framework, policy makers, researchers, and care givers will better understand the nuances of African American culture as they investigate patterns of health care access and use among African American women. The aim is to make the relationships between the culture of African American women and the larger social context of health care delivery specific and explicit. It is hoped that such an approach will provide professionals in the health care community with ideas they can use to improve the quality of health care for African American women, and, thereby, reduce the considerable disparities in health outcomes.

The last section presents the idea that to be culturally competent in the delivery of health care, there must be a shift in thinking and strategizing from the current paradigm that is based on an illness model. It is argued that this paradigm must include the key factors emerging from the socio-historical background of African American women as central elements with respect to the reduction of disparities in their health care outcomes. A path for a new direction is presented

Concepts Used to Define Groups of People: Their Relationships to Culturally Competent Health Care

The terms and concepts used in the introduction to report differences in health care outcomes for African American women and European American women are rooted in a western, philosophical system of historically classifying groups of people based on the concept of "race." In recent years, the concept of "ethnicity" has been added to indicate differences based on certain definable characteristics. A second concept, "culture," has also been used to define groups of people. The issues of race and ethnicity are discussed in relationship to the definitions of culture. It is argued in this section that it is important to define and delineate the usefulness of each concept as a defining factor in research on health care outcomes for African Americans generally, and, specifically for African American women. The fact that the research strategies developed so far have relied on concepts that may not reflect the realities of the people who are being investigated, strongly suggests the need for alternative ways of thinking. This discussion sets the stage for the rationale and concepts used in the alternative framework presented later in this chapter.

The Concept of Race

The classification of race, based on visual observations of people, particularly their skin color, has a long history in Western Europe, but is discounted today from a scientific perspective (Berger, 2013). As a concept, Banton (1987) notes the term "race" emerged in Europe during the sixteenth century. The Bible was accepted as the authority for judging human interactions, and it was used to designate lineage ordained by God. With the rise of European power in the world, the term came to connote differences in diverse groups of people based on delineating the "other" such as Muslims. The major philosophers in Europe began to voice ideas regarding racial superiority based on the so-called "white" people of northern and central Europe. The ideas of superiority were couched in terms that embodied the Enlightenment like "reason" and "civilized." In contrast, the other so-called "non-white" groups of people were viewed as "savage" and "superstitious." The idea of associating the skin color of a group of people with that of mental capacity was reflected in the writings of David Hume and Immanuel Kant, two noted philosophers of the time (Fernando, 2010).

Berger (2013) explains that in the nineteenth century, as Darwinian concepts became accepted in European thinking, race was entered to designate and rank groups of people. She argues that "race," while a sociological concept as opposed to a biological concept, continued to play a significant role in structuring the research strategies of scientists. This was especially the case in the search for causes of diseases in medicine. Today, the ideas about "race" as a biologically based, or socially based, concept have led to confusion. For example, Fernando (2010) indicates the following admonition:

> . . . race as lineage may be a satisfactory explanation of physical differentiation of populations that are relatively isolated from each other, but cannot interpret differentiation in an increasingly globalized 'mixed' world, except by assuming that ecological forces determine behavior of human beings in the way they determine social life of domesticated animals, whereby for, example, different breeds of dogs persist (p.8).

The implications for such thinking are to (a) believe in the assumptions about inferior/superior "races," (b) make value judgments about people solely based on the fact that they are "different," (c) assume that domination over another group of people is reasonable, and (d) believe in the power and domination of one group of people over other groups. Berger, (2013) summarizes the scientific findings in the following ways:

- Differences within races are greater than the differences between races on important physical characteristics apart from those used to define race.

- There is no evidence for designating any race as superior or inferior in terms of ability in any particular area or in adaptation to the environment.
- There are no pure races that have unique genetic characteristics.
- Physical characteristics, such as thick lips, are found in all races.

The consequences of such thinking about race in developing appropriate research strategies for investigating diverse groups of people is that it will take time for those health care professionals in the health care community to overcome such a distorted way of thinking about diverse groups of people. Against a solid backdrop of a distorted history regarding the achievements of ancient civilizations other than those in western cultures, health care professionals must remain vigilant lest they slip back into the old way of thinking about diverse groups of people. For example, Fernando (2010) reports that with the breakdown of direct racial domination and physical oppression in the United States during the 1960s, racism became institutionalized through technocratic means so that the economic position of African Americans actually dropped between 1970 and 1980 in comparison to their European American counterparts. The association of African Americans with falling educational standards, decline in moral values, and street crime has crept into the American consciousness. Health care policy makers and health care professionals are products of that consciousness, and, are therefore, susceptible to the negative impact of such cultural "facts." Since the nineties, there has been some effort to shift thinking about "race" as a potentially, important differentiating factor when investigating African Americans generally, and African American women, specifically. This shift may result in eroding the current, color-based racism, and perhaps the elimination of race thinking itself.

The Concept of Culture: Issues of Race and Ethnicity

The concept of "culture" plays a significant role in the alternative framework presented in this chapter. A perusal of the many ways in which the term has been used in health care research indicates a need to being some clarity with respect to how it is used to describe the socio-historical background of African American women. For example, while culture originally meant "to cultivate," it recently has come to signify a mixture of behavior and cognitions arising from shared patterns of belief, feeling, and adaptation which people carry mentally (e.g., Leighton & Hughes, 1961). The concept has been used to convey references ranging from families, communities, or even nations. Therefore, in a multicultural society such as the United States, the term implies differences between groups of people with different backgrounds, traditions, and worldviews.

Fernando (2010) goes even further when he states that culture "means the ethos or the intangible underlying determinants of people's behavior in a particular context (p. 9)." It is a way of life common to a group which may or may not be defined as a "community." For people living within that culture, the concept represents conceptual structures that determine the total reality in their lives and of their families, and their larger communities. Sometimes the term has come to encompass all features of an individual's environment that are held in common by that individual with others forming a distinct group. For example, family systems and ethical values would be common to a group.

Since the middle of the 1980s, there have been major changes in the manner in which the term "culture" has been used in the health care literature. Increasingly, investigators have become aware of the need to recognize that individuals or groups are not passive recipients of "culture." Culture is made by people, both as individuals and as groups, with systems of values and identities that continually being constructed (Fernando, 2010).

For health care professionals, it is important to ensure that there is no confusion when referring to "race" or "culture" in the description of groups of people. In the public arena, people seen as racially different may be assumed to have different cultures, and value judgments attached to "race" are transferred to "culture." Another problem is that when people are identified in ethnic terms-ethnicity containing both cultural and racial connotations that are not clearly differentiated-there may be a tendency to impose culture on people because of the way they look "racially" instead of allowing them to position themselves within their specific culture (Fernando, 2010).

Hall (1992) indicates ethnicity overlaps in meaning with both culture and race. As a construct, ethnicity has been defined as involving physical appearance (race) or social similarity (culture) alone or in combination. The subjective feelings of people are important in the sense that they represent a sense of belonging to a group where cultural or racial similarity plays a significant role. Yet, belonging to a group may not be based on an individual's subjective sense of belonging, but may be based on the way other people view that individual. Thus, a society that has a racist underpinning may promote an ethnicity based primarily on race as perceived by the society rather than by individual members of a cultural group. Berger (2010) adds that for too long there has been a confusion of logic regarding race and ethnicity in health policy, research, and practice. She notes the illogical, historical legacy, and the current incorporation of that legacy into a tradition which relies so heavily on terms like "race" and/or "ethnicity" to convey identifying characteristics of individuals in the relative absence of genetic corroboration.

Fernando (2010) provides an example that is instructive for the health care researcher. In collecting data for ethnic identification, the choice of one ethnic category for identifying each person as a member of an ethnic group is often pushed onto people as representing that person's subjective self-perception which is assumed to be indicative of their personal identity. The forced choice of one's ethnicity may have a very practical purpose of obtaining clear-cut, numerical quantities, but may lead to problems in terms of cooperation from subjects, and, consequently, errors in the data. Such forced choices in methodology have resulted in "objective" data with little meaningful information for the very group of people who are being investigated. This is a cautionary tale for health care researchers and is one of the major reasons why some investigators have begun to develop research strategies that take into account the subjective perceptions of individuals within their own cultural ethos and not from the investigators' research protocols. The framework presented in this chapter is an attempt to bridge the gap between the requirements of a biomedical model and the imperatives of a socio-historical framework in the study of health care use among African American women. It is argued that the latter framework is a better departure for health care professionals as they target African Americans generally and, specifically, African American women.

Traditional Approaches to Health Care

The approaches to health care in the United States today are based on a biomedical model that originated in Europe and is viewed as *western* in cultural orientation. Capra (1982) states that this view of medicine and health care tends to dominate the world. Capra notes that this singular, western point of view has been termed the scientific tradition. This tradition is rooted in what is called a scientific paradigm-i.e., a system of beliefs and assumptions that determines fact-gathering within a science (Kuhn, 1962). The rules set down in the paradigm determine the rules that are more often implicit, rather than being clearly stated, and are more like shared beliefs. Ingleby (1980) points out that the paradigm determines what researchers "can use as useful and respectable data, what form theories within specific disciplines should take, what sort of language scientists should use, ... and so on (p.25)"

Table I shows the key elements of the scientific paradigm which developed out of a European philosophical understanding of the world. **Positivism** is viewed as the belief that "reality" is rooted only in regard to what can be observed, and knowledge is limited to demonstrable events and their empirically verifiable connections. Martin-Baro (1994) notes this means ignoring everything other than a verifiable "reality". **Causality** refers to cause and effect, or the implication that nothing is truly random and nothing is beyond understanding (e.g., the divine). **Objectivism** is viewed as describing events, people, organs, etc as objects without moral judgments. **Rationality** refers to the idea that the final judge of "truth" is reason, and that all assertions must be verified by logical reasoning. Fernando (2010) indicates that the (a) current methods of investigating phenomena are based on a legacy of the mechanistic approach of physics advanced by Newton; (b) the reduction of complex systems into their parts; and (c) the use of logical reasoning as opposed to other type of cognitive processing like intuition. Since its inception, the major parts of this paradigm continue to be used as the basis for the investigation of any phenomena in the physical universe.

Table I. *Scientific Paradigm* (Source: Fernando (2010))

Beliefs

Positivism
Reality is rooted in what can be observed

Causality
Nothing occurs randomly
Natural causes for all events and effects

Objectivism
Feelings, thoughts etc. regarded as objects

Rationality
Reason superior to emotion
All assertions verifiable by logical proof

Approaches

Mechanistic
Newtonian physics as opposed to modern physics

Reductionist
Sum of the parts equals to whole

Logical reasoning
Intellectual exercise

During the past three centuries in western culture, the scientific paradigm has been the basis for discovering most of what is known about the physical universe. The paradigm has been adjusted from time to time, allowing for new discoveries in physics and biology. For medicine, the work of Darwin and Galton remain the two most important progenitors of the view that one should look to biology, natural selection, variation, and adaptation in the investigation of humans and "races." Set against a philosophical basis of evolutionary advantage and "survival of the fittest," hereditary factors have been viewed as the basis for investigating such phenomena as differences in susceptibility to disease. In the twentieth century, the discovery and use of drugs to "cure" people is based on the scientific paradigm (Berger, 2013; Fernando, 2010).

Today, the traditions of disease causation and health care are taught by academic institutions derived from the western tradition; non-western traditions, like African philosophies, are consigned to specific areas such as cultural studies, and are seldom recognized as "true" medicine and health care. Historically, other traditions have been dismissed as philosophies and practices which are viewed as "cult-like" in their manifestations (Berger, 2013; Fernando, 2010). This section is a brief discussion of some of the more prominent traditions of western medicine and health care, and a discussion of why other traditions of investigation and practice should be considered as viable resources. It is hoped that such a discussion will provide a basis for acknowledging that, in its current state, the western, biomedical model is not particularly helpful to address the significant disparities in health care outcomes for the African American population in general, and, specifically, for African American women

Description of the Western View and its Implications for Health Care

Berger (2013) has advanced the idea that the concepts of "health" and "illness" have been built on foundations that incorporate traditional, western ideas about the nature of human beings. Today, western medicine and health care claim to be "scientific" because of their reliance on objectifying as much as possible their observations about human beings, based on a predetermined, biomedical model, and presenting them in the form of quantification. Fernando (2010) also indicates that experts in medicine and health care maintain their status as health care "specialists" by using scientific methods of study and research, apparent, "objective" techniques of observation and assessment of people designated as patients, and an "open," mind about their information base. Underlying this philosophy is a theme that "illnesses" should be classified in terms of their types or diagnoses.

Capra (1982) notes that the approach of the western, biomedical model of illness is to understand how the body works by focusing on its subdivisions-i.e., different organs and parts of organs, and identifying functions of each part in precise detail. This approach is essentially a reductionist one. Illnesses are located in one or more parts, never in terms of the whole as a whole. Health care interventions (treatments) are developed and targeted at correcting one or more faults in one or another part (e.g., right ventricle of the heart).

The targeting of treatments is based on diagnosis, which represent the analysis conducted by a host of "experts" and "practitioners" within the context of the biomedical framework. The precursors to diagnoses are assessments of what are perceived as symptoms and signs, which are really evaluations Kleinman (1987). Fernando (2010) adds that the practical importance of diagnosis arises from the needs of the diagnostician to be sufficiently informed so as to prescribe the "best" treatment. As Fernando indicates, in a biomedical model of thinking and practice, treatment is geared toward diagnosis.

In attempting to be "objective" and "reliable," health care practices are separated from diagnoses, although in practice the two processes blend together and influence each other. Treatment is separated from "management" or "care." The latter two terms are used within a biomedical model as patients being advised, the context in which treatment is given, and the way staff and patients interact with each other (Kleinman, 1995).

Janzen (1978) points out that the two processes of diagnosis and treatment have emerged from a medical belief system that may not be appropriate for different cultural groups. Every culture seems to include a concept of illness and ways of dealing with illness, and may be viewed as distinct medical systems. However, in some cultures, the medical systems cannot be clearly separated from religious or social systems. At the micro level, there are specific health beliefs and practices, models of illness, and the roles and status of health care providers. At the macro level, there are socio-economic conditions, political systems, power relationships between and within institutions, and allocation of resources. The impact of cultural differences may apply at both levels in somewhat different ways. For example, the value attached to one type of belief or practice in the United States, a multicultural and racist society, is often determined within the health care system by its supposed racial connection rather than its cultural importance. Therefore, the family life of African American women is often seen as deficient in terms of weight concerns and patterns of health care use (Robbins, 2007).

Fernando (2010) explains that cultural differences in medical belief systems (i.e., ideas about illness) may be viewed in different ways. However, if one uses concepts based on western culture, the significance of other ways of culturally defining illness may be missed Kleinman (1978). From a western standpoint, other culturally defined, medical systems are seen as "magical" and "supernatural", while the biomedical model is viewed as "objective" and "natural". This particular point of view has direct implications for health care directed toward African Americans. This point is illustrated in the next section which presents an alternative framework that may be used as a basis for reducing disparities in health care outcomes for African American women.

A Socio-Historical Context for Health: African American Women, Their Culture, and the Health Care System

Robbins (2007) notes culture and the larger social context may often mean different things to different people. Sewell (1992) defines culture as the practices and enactment of the "rules of social life." Culture is what gives meaning to the experiences that people have, and, humans are the only species that attribute such meaning to their experiences. The larger social context is defined by Sewell as sets of "schemas and resources which empower and constrain social action and that tend to be reproduced by that social action (p. 19)." Martin (2003) maintains that the two factors overlap and interact. Robbins notes that the two sets of factors are reciprocal and reinforce each other. For example, she states that gendered practices provide "an example of how culture reproduces context." This practice is best exemplified in the case of the expectation that professional females will do the subservient tasks in organizations, such as making coffee. By doing so, such a practice reinforces the contextual institution of men having dominant positions that confer power to them. Barrett and Robbins (2007), note that when a female person occupies a lower position in a system of inequality, this tends to increase the probability that the person will increasingly be exposed to dual stress in the form of sexism and classism. For African American women, this duality is increased to a triad when one takes into account the stress of exposure to racism/discrimination. As related to their health beliefs, their behaviors, and their perceptions of the health care system, this triad of stress is important to include in any research strategy or health care protocol designed to reduce health disparities for African American women.

Rationale for Framework

Most of the research examples presented in the introduction are based on biomedical models of health that compare African American women to European American women on a number of "objective" dimensions (e.g., Robbins, Jackson, Dimperio, et al., 2006; Salganicoff, Beckerman, Wyn, & Ojeda, 2002; Shive, Ma, Tan, et al., 2006). These examples represent a large body of literature conducted to confirm that the dimensions really provide meaningful information about African Americans. Irrespective of the important information that one may obtain from the literature regarding the health use behaviors of African American women, there still may be a tendency to label outcomes for black women as pathological and/ or deficient (Whitfield & Baker-Thomas, 1999). Such a direction obscures some important factors that health care professionals may miss in their collective quest to improve health care for African American women. As Combs-Jones (2004), explains, the research outcomes, no matter how laudable, may serve to bolster the power inadvertently to those individuals in the health care community who possess that power and make the decisions about the source and the content of legitimate knowledge.

Role of Values. A major issue when considering the need to include the socio-historical culture of African American women is one of values which is expressed differently in different cultures. Awareness of values necessarily implies there is recognition that the role of values must play a role alongside evidence in all areas of health policy and practice. In addition, there must be a respect for diversity of values which encompasses specific policies and principles concerned with decreasing the power of one dominant group, and with increasing the equality and diversity of groups in need of health care (Berger, 2013). The cultural values of African Americans generally, and of African American women, specifically, form a continuum that ranges from basic philosophies about life itself, the nature of "truth," the essence of the human condition, and the everyday decisions they make. Berger notes the values in health research and health care giving arose entirely out of a European, western, cultural context. For example, in most traditional, research strategies and care giving procedures, historically there has been little input from African Americans with respect to their philosophies about life and health. Fernando (2010) states that the concept for human rights, the central element of European thinking, was largely determined during the Enlightenment with its emphasis on the individual rather than the community. Racism was not even a part of the thinking since it was reinforced during the Enlightenment.

Berger (2013) adds that certain values come down from traditions to form the basis for the way health is perceived, research is developed, and health care services are organized. She notes that these values determine what is held to be the standard or the "right" way of thinking (e.g., the importance of individuality, self-efficacy, and "race" as a determinant of differences in assessing health outcomes). Western ethics, as embedded in the biomedical ideal, are unlikely to address much of what is important to African Americans (e.g., family connection, need for community, and the religious/spiritual impulse). Specifically, Berger argues that there appears to be little evidence for the *recognition* of the role of values in the African American community alongside the evidence in all areas of health care policy and practice. There is little evidence of an *awareness* of the values involved in the African American community, the roles they play and their impact on health care delivery. She also adds that there is little evidence observed within the health care community of a *respect* for the values within the African American community such that it is reflected in a service-user focus as a unifying focus for health care policies, research, and health care delivery. The justification for the inclusion of a socio-historical context, which should be used when addressing the health care concerns of African American women, implies that the values of each individual service user and their communities must be the starting point and a key determinant for all actions by health care professionals.

Concept of Health. The concept of "health," has been used for research and provision of health care services for decades (Becker, 1974). However, there may be differences in how health is defined in different cultural settings. Differences in perceptions of health may relate to what people value and this may vary in terms of the importance given to material prosperity, spiritual development, and family connection (Fernando, 2010). For example, African American women, when compared with European American women, may have very different ideas about what is important for health from living in a society where they share a socio-cultural history of exposure to stress from racism/discrimination. Moreover, these women may look to external factors such as the intergenerational relationships they have in their families and in their community institutions as sources of well-being rather than to internal factors such as their personal emotions. When comparing African American women to European American women, the concept of "health" should not be viewed as an "objective" index measuring primarily "illness" or "absence of disease." It may be that the concept of "health" should be "open to the whole range of human experience, social, mental, and spiritual, as well as material" (Chambers, 1997). It is a central tenet of the framework being presented here that the socio-historical culture of African American women is a factor which should be included in all conceptions of health and illness. It is argued that such an approach will increase meaningful, cultural competence in health care delivery.

Table II: *Influence of Holism on Illness Experiences*
(Source: Fernando, 2010))

	Cultural tradition	
	Holistic	**Non-holistic**
External vs. internal experiences/Subjective vs. objective experiences	Intertwined and interposed within each other	Distinct and separate from one another
Causes of ill health	Experienced as both internal and external *at the same time*	Experienced as either external or internal, one impacting on the other
Experience of health	Sense of harmonious balance between different aspects of self and environment	Sense of subjective well-being distinct from external influences

Table II shows the differences between a holistic and traditional view of health. With respect to culturally competent health care delivery for African American women, the table illustrates that the values of their community instill a philosophy which may enable them to experience external and internal experiences as *one and the same*; their experiences may be both "objective" and "subjective" at the same time. In this way, they may look at the world in terms of its interconnectedness rather than as its separate parts. Nobles (1991) notes that this lack of separateness is not like the illusion of mathematical normality observed in western culture. For Nobles, normality, as reflected in African thought, is equivalent to one's nature and not one's separate parts of a personal identity.

Table II also shows that the experience of health and ill health, as reflected in the African American tradition (a holistic culture), may not include an *inside-outside* division, or if it does, the inside and outside are so interwoven that they cannot be usefully separated. Fernando (2010) argues that a traditionally western, non-holistic approach promotes the attribution of ill health to either an external cause or an internal one, but not both at the same time. He also argues that the holistic tradition of African Americans, and similar cultures, promote a sense of health as a balance between various forces in the person and the social context as opposed to viewing health in an individualized sense. While the divisions regarding the holistic tradition of African Americans may not be as relevant for every African American woman as she accesses and uses the health care system, it is important to note that African American women emerge from a culture that has holistic traditions, and this may extend to the concept of "health."

Socio-Historical Culture of African American Women

The inclusion of the socio-historical culture of African American women, as an underlying part of a framework to be used in research and care giving efforts, is an acknowledgment that the cultural capital of the African American experience is necessary. Mills (1959) argues that when considering why and how people from differing cultures may operate differently, one must consider the historical, political, and social structure out of which people emerge to perceive and act accordingly. As this relates to African American women, one must, as a researcher and care giver, be continually aware that their socio-cultural history, which includes historical and current experiences with slavery, institutional racism, and sexism, may influence why and how African American women filter their perceptions of American, generally, and, specifically, of the health care system.

Awareness and knowledge must be explicit in the minds of caregivers as they attempt to provide the best care giving service possible. Awareness and knowledge must also be explicit in the minds of researchers as they attempt to develop valid research frameworks that will connect health disparities to the individual and structural circumstances of African American women. In this section, attention is paid to three important factors within the African American culture that may serve as vital sources of information for researchers and care givers as they develop strategies to reduce health care disparities for African American women. These interrelated factors are (a) the social constructions of health and health care use as related to the stress of being "black;"

(b) the impact of intergenerational transmission of values and behaviors; and (c) the role of religiousness/spirituality. Figure 1 shows the factors that represent these interrelated factors.

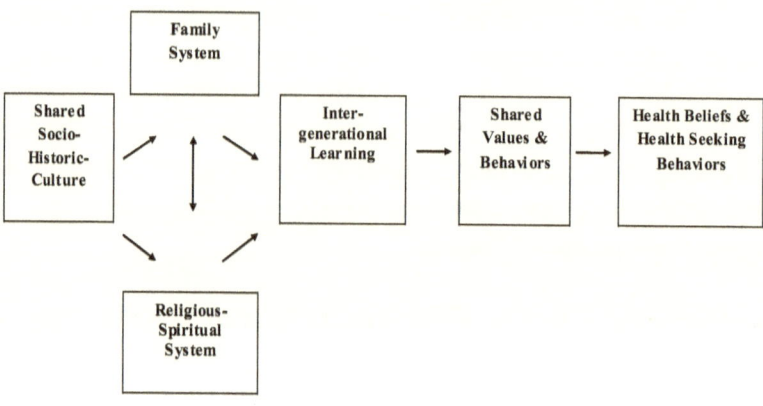

Figure 1. Socio-historical framework for health beliefs and health-seeking behaviors.

Cultural Constructions of Health and Health Care Use: Relationships to the Stress of Being "Black." What are the cultural constructions of health and health care use within the African American community? As social constructs, beliefs about health and illness develop within a specific, cultural environment (Anderson, 1988). If one assumes that African American women develop views about health specific to their socio-historical experience as black and female in America, then these views must reflect the typical realities of their lives. For example, if one asks an African American woman to define health, her accounts might be filled with the stress and pressures of being "black." From the standpoint of a cultural context, this stress may predispose her to illnesses at earlier ages and at higher rates than her European American counterpart. Even if she was middle class, the fact that most middle-class African American women are in jobs that put them near the lower end of the middle class, might impact her decisions to use the health care system with less frequency than her European American counterpart.

For this "woman," the social context of being "black" (i.e., a woman with unequal, financial resources, subjected to the stress of exposure to continued racism/discrimination) also should be included when considering the definition of health to her. It is important for health care professionals to understand that the health status and health care usage patterns of African American women are made more complex when considering overlapping, structural factors such as the socioeconomic status of African American women. One would want to make sure the use of such structural, differentiating variables as socioeconomic status, does not lead to superficial knowledge that provides "significant results" but little true meaning about the factors that relate to the health of African American women. Thus, in this hypothetical case, the example is instructive because the intersection of culture and larger social structures may not be reflected in the comparative research on differential rates of health care use presented in the introduction.

The social constructions of health seeking among African American women may also interact with perceived barriers to ready access to health care. For example, residential segregation may play a significant role in the extent to which African women may seek health care from the health care system. For example, Combs-Jones (2004) notes that in her study of middle-aged, African American women, some of the participants in the south indicated that they had difficulty seeking help. These women lived in segregated neighborhoods, resulting in them remaining outside the influence of the larger, European American culture. Their descriptions of educational and social interactions expressed a separateness that prevented them from seeking help. Thus, this example demonstrates that African American women often feel that when they attempt to access the health care system, they feel as if they are accessing a "foreign" culture. The professional, care-giving culture which relies so heavily on "objective," health assessments and protocols does not pick up, for example, justified anger arising from racism and bias in the care-giving system. What is picked up is "hostility," or characteristics of the "angry, black woman."

If one listens to African American women as they go about their lives, a persistent theme occurs, and that is the stress associated with being "black," and its link to their overall health. As Combs-Jones (2004) notes, the stress of being "black" in America should be included in research protocols by having African American women disclose how such stress is related to their health outcomes. For example, in her interview of middle-class, African American women, Combs-Jones indicates that explicit references to stress and health occurred frequently during her interviews. These references involved statements about conditions which were stress producing to the women. Combs-Jones notes that generally, the stressful incidents at work were not explicitly connected to health. There were more implicit connections made with respect to operating as "black" women in "white" environments. Combs-Jones provides an interesting example of one woman that vividly illustrates the dilemma African American women feel when interacting outside their cultural context. It is presented below:

> We live in the world of being black. When you walk out the door, you take on the world of whiteness. You have to learn the survival skills of the white world. Education is important. It is like going in the battlefield-you need to strategize. Some days you walk in (to work) beat up. We live in two worlds. From the time you grow up, you learn that. The person you are at home is not the person that is at the air force base. (For example), my hair; I couldn't wait to get out of the military. (Now) I can do it as I please. We are the only group that lives in two worlds (p. 76).

The vignette described above indicates a type of "shifting" that Jones and Shorter-Gordon (2003) call a kind of adaptive behavior in which African American women are "relentlessly pushed to serve and satisfy others and made to hide their true selves to placate (others)." (p.7). Combs-Jones notes that leading double lives implicitly exposes African American women to consistent stress. Consequently, this stress, as reported in the first section, appears to have a negative and cumulative impact on health. The experience reported above has been, and continues to be, a prominent feature of a shared socio-historical culture that occurs to most, if not all, African American women. The results of some research findings indicate that the stress of being "black" in America has been associated with producing higher rates of illness (e.g., Feagin & McKinney, 2003; Williams & Williams-Morris, 2000).

Such findings, as the ones presented above, may be mediated when one takes into account the extent to which exposure to racial discrimination varies with such structural factors as geography, class, and type of neighborhood, and, whether the frequency, duration, and intensity of exposure may result in different health outcomes for different African American women. Combs-Jones (2004), in her landmark study of middle-aged, African American women, reports some interesting results with respect to some intra-group differences in access to health care and treatment. These differences centered on class (i.e., differences based on education, occupation, and income). Against a historical backdrop of a shared history that points to disparate treatment of African Americans at both the practitioner and user levels of the health care system, there seem to be some differences with respect to health care treatment and use by her participants.

For the middle-class women in her study, Combs-Jones found that they mentioned education as the single most important factor in determining adequate medical care, as well as a significant factor in gaining access to medical information. Combs-Jones notes that education is highly prized in the African American community, and it is considered the best opportunity for African Americans to obtain higher status jobs and increased income. Of the 96 women in her study, 96% worked. Combs-Jones concluded that education acted as a proxy for both occupation and income. This may have accounted for some key points made in their reports with respect to health care delivery. These points were (a) their health care plans were adequate in meeting their medical needs; (b) their experiences with racial discrimination were based on the accounts of other African American women who had received disparate treatment, and not on their own personal experiences; and (c) the privileges of being middle-class served to minimize race and gender discrimination in their experiences with the health care system.

One participant in Combs-Jones's study that vividly illustrates the three points presented above is indicated in the comments made by one participant in response to a question regarding confidence in doctors. This woman reported the comments presented below.

> (Usually) it's about something that they have heard
> from somebody or a friend or somebody. I've never run
> across a black woman that has any personal experiences
> (of discrimination) with the doctor. Women that are my

age, well I sit down and talk and a couple of them are
from really low-income areas. I don't think that they had
medical insurance like most women my age would have.
There are a couple of them that do have good insurance.
One (woman) in particular hasn't had personal medical
experiences with the doctor, but she doesn't go to
doctors unless she really feels like it (p.95)

The most important feature of the comments presented above is
that the woman's account reveals that some middle-class, African
American women still do not have confidence in "the doctor,"
even though they have the money to pay for medical care. Such a
perception appears to be rooted in a shared history of disparate
treatment in health care delivery for African Americans (e.g., Byrd
& Clayton, 2000).

Despite the variations due to class, the essential point to be
made is that the historical barriers to health care, and continuing
discrimination toward African Americans, may serve as barriers
to health care access and use. It is important for health care
professionals to understand the internal worlds of African American
women, and not just their responses to "objective" assessments
conducted by the health care community. Some investigators have
begun to tease out such "subjective" factors, as the stress of being
"black," and others like "mistrust" and "fear of the health care
system." The research results have proved promising in enabling
researchers to provide the kinds of culturally amplified information
required to reduce disparities in health care outcomes for African
American women (e.g., Brett & Hays, 2004; IOM, 2003; Mensah,
2005). Figure 1 also shows that health beliefs and health seeking
behaviors are results of a shared, socio-historical background. Again,
this is a vital part of a new framework that must be integrated into
the protocols of future research efforts and health care practices.

Role of Intergenerational Learning. It is argued here that the
cultural constructions of being "black" in America made by African
American women, may serve as sources of stress, and, therefore,
may be considered vitally important sources of information for
health care researchers and care givers in their quest to reduce health
disparities. For African American women, one must necessarily

include the social structures within their communities that may serve to influence their health seeking behaviors. These kinds of information are missing from traditional types of research strategies. As Combs-Jones (2004) notes, the simple reporting of numbers does not necessarily consider such factors as the support networks in black families and their influence on health seeking behavior. After all, the transfer of knowledge and beliefs begins in families.

For African American women, the family and extended family are vital keys in understanding the nuances of their health seeking behaviors. In African American families, there is some evidence of intergenerational learning within the context of intergenerational relationships that has provided for greater opportunity to transfer information, values, and beliefs than among European American families (Glass, Bengston, & Dunham, 1986; Laditka, 2000). Such evidence suggests that African American families may exhibit a cohesive characteristic, which in turn, may influence the development of a system for the transfer of knowledge and beliefs about health and health seeking behaviors. This filtering system is transferred through a collective memory of racism and discrimination.

The stereotypical image of the strong, black matriarch as the dominant person in the black household began in slavery, and has been maintained even into the twenty-first century. In part, this stereotype came about because black women worked alongside their black men, and this idea did not conform to Eurocentric views of women as wives, mothers, and homemakers. Combs-Jones (2004) notes this image of African American family life continues into the twenty-first century to include these mythical images of black womanhood that overburden black women. Questions about health and experiences with the health care system do not generally support research efforts to disclose patterns in lifestyles and the social environments of African American women. As presented in previous sections, the recent efforts to investigate such life style variables as the extent to which African American women within family systems exercise are steps in the right direction. However, investigators must include the role of intergenerational learning to determine how the dynamics of black family life impact on the collective memories of African American women, and, subsequently, on their perceptions of health and health seeking behaviors. This factor is also shown in Figure 1.

St Jean and Feagin (1998) advance the idea that the "collective memory" of African American women reflects their historically shared experiences with overt discrimination in the past, and in the less overt patterns of discrimination today. Such a collectively shared memory is thought to culturally bond African American women (Feagin & McKinney, 2003). In some areas of life, one can take the position that this bonding may often override differences in socioeconomic status, age, and geography. These shared experiences may develop into a black, female consciousness that is used to define health beliefs and health seeking behaviors which should be considered an integral part of a shared historical heritage and cultural environment (Combs-Jones, 2004). As Ani (1994) notes, this "group identification" has developed through shared values, attitudes, and beliefs. However, it is important for researchers and care givers to tease out the extent to which such a shared identification is explicitly or implicitly associated with health beliefs and health seeking behavior among African American women.

Combs-Jones (2004), in her study of aging among African women, provides an important insight regarding the nuances of intergenerational learning in the formation of body images, weight concerns, obesity, and dietary practices. The research examples presented in the introduction indicate that obesity is a problem of epidemic proportions among African American women, and has resulted in poor, health outcomes. The interviewed women in the study indicated that they were concerned about being overweight and, in some cases, were obese. They seemed to understand that there are many African American women who are overweight. They appeared to tie their concerns to their dietary practices. However, Combs-Jones notes that despite the warnings and concerns, the study participants pointed to one strong cultural reason for acceptance of high body mass indices among African Americans. There was the perception that a certain level of weight was considered attractive. For these interviewees, "to be thin (was) to be poor. (p. 449)." In addition, one interviewee's responses illustrate the role of intergenerational learning on their concerns about weight. The vignette is presented as follows:

> Culture. The way you are brought up. To us, food would make you happy. When I am around my mother

and siblings we will say, 'wasn't Laura's baking the best . . . ?' I don't think white women talk about the food at Thanksgiving. We will sit around and talk about food all the time. (For example), when you said you were coming I said I would make something. White women don't care about it (p. 73).

The most important thing about what is revealed above is that, within African American culture, eating and sharing food, is viewed as a ritual and not a problem. If there are going to be significant changes in the approaches researchers and care givers use to lessen the impact of poor health outcomes resulting from obesity, they must direct their efforts to include the ways in which cultural values are interwoven into the intergenerational learning processes of African American women. In particular, Louden (2013) suggests that, within the lives of African Americans, broadening the scope of research to include significant parts of the family and community systems will go a long way in developing the kinds of strategies needed to significantly decrease the disparities in health outcomes.

Role of Religiousness/Spirituality. The cultural construction of spirituality (i.e., the private, human impulse to know and be connected with the divine), and the manner in which religiousness is expressed (i.e., the institutionalized ways of becoming connected with the divine) are important imperatives operating in the lives of African American women (Kinsey, 2005). The stressful events of poor health, issues of access to health care, issues relating to use of the health care system, the use of religion are closely interrelated. Historically, religious traditions have served African Americans as resources which have been used in moments of intense stress. These traditions have provided ready-made prescriptions for how African Americans have responded to such negative life events as experience with intense physical pain and personal loss (Koening, 2000; Loefler, 2003). Figure 1 also shows this component of the socio-historical framework for African American health beliefs and health seeking behaviors.

Pargament (1995), a theorist and investigator in the psychology of religion, offers the view that "while different religions (offer) different solutions, every religious tradition (has offered) a way to come to terms with tragedy, suffering, and the most significant issues in life (p. 3)." This position is reflected in the case of African Americans. The cultural patterns of African Americans suggest that religion and/or spirituality are significant, community forces which provide them with acceptable rationales, plans, and coping behaviors in response to stress (Cooper, Brown, ThiVu, Ford & Powe, 2001). These patterns appear to be derived from a West African worldview in which religiousness and spirituality are considered as critical elements of personal identity, and are viewed as essential in the normal development of attitudes, values, and beliefs (Mbiti, 1991; Onunwa, 1994).

Kinsey (2005) notes the unique history of Africans in the American Diaspora also provides additional support for the assumption that religiousness and spirituality are significant forces operating within the lives of many African Americans in general, and, specifically, in the everyday lives of many African American women. African Americans have a history which includes the lack of personal and collective freedom, physical hardship, and mental and physical suffering brought on by slavery and its aftermath in the forms of historical discrimination, both economic and social in nature. The vestiges of such discrimination have continued even into the twenty-first century. This unique history has also included a lack of relative access to the resources provided within the general American culture for assistance in coping with stress, and, subsequently, a lack of access to health care when it has been needed. Pargament (1995) notes that the combination of a culturally derived tradition of readiness to respond to health crises in religious and/or spiritual ways make it reasonable to assume that religious and/or spiritual components may be integral parts of a general orienting system operating in many African Americans generally, and, in many African American women, specifically.

Since the early eighties, a growing group of theorists and researchers in the "psychology of religion" and the "psychology of spirituality" and their impact on coping with stress, have asserted that religiousness and spirituality are "person action constructs" that can be used to identify those aspects of the African American personality structure and function (Akbar, 1995; Baldwin, 1991; Phillips, 1990). Pargament explains that while the means used to search for significance in life are important, it is their use as strategies to achieve valued goals which are their most important value.

Results from the religiousness and coping literature have identified several important goals, but it is the search for community (i.e., the search for intimacy, a feeling of connectedness to other people) that is the most salient for this discussion. The goal of search for community is emphasized because of its singular importance in the lives of the African American community, generally, and in the everyday lives of African American women, specifically. It is argued that African American women use religious coping to master situations which are stressful, and religion to them is, at heart, a social, as well as a psychological, emotional, or physical matter. Religion provides a representation of society, and of the members' relationships to it. Most importantly, religious beliefs and rituals unite African American women into a common view of life. If religion has given birth to all that is essential in African American society, it is because the central element of that society is the soul of religion (Kinsey, 2005).

Theorists emerging from the traditional paradigm of thinking about spirituality and religion draw distinctions between the two concepts. However, these distinctions may not reflect the realities of people in the real world. For example, the results of a study conducted by Zinnbauer, Pargament, Cowell, et al (1996) support this assertion. In that study, in response to a question, most respondents from different groups (i.e., hospice nurses, nursing home residents, conservative Christians, establishment Christians) served by professionals from the health care professions, reported they were spiritual and religious. In contrast, most of the health care professionals serving them reported they perceived themselves to be spiritual, but not religious. For most of the respondents, there did not appear to be differences between their individualized, personal experiences of spirituality and their institutionalized expressions of religion. The investigators concluded the responses of the health care professionals seemed to suggest an anti-institutional, religious bias that distanced them from the people they served.

The results presented above indicate that the distinctions between religiousness and spirituality may be overdrawn in academic and professional circles. As Pargament (1995) explains, for many people, the individualization of religious experience, in terms of spirituality, is likely to occur within a social context that also encourages the expression of personal experiences with the divine within the context of an institutional system of beliefs and practices. Religiousness, then, is experienced and expressed not only privately, but publicly as well. With the exception of the Native Americans, no other ethnic group in American has built a culture on the firm belief that the divine is real, and the human's relationship with the divine is not only spiritual in nature but is religious as well.

Pargament's (1995) approach is especially applicable to developing ways in which health care professions can understand when, how, and why many African American women may engage in religious and/or spiritual strategies in their health seeking behaviors. In his review of the literature, he indicates that results from many investigations in this area report relationships between religious-spiritual coping among African American women and positive, health outcomes. For example, one common finding is that religious-spiritual coping is more common among women, older people, Southerners, and those who are religiously committed and involved. A study conducted by Ellison and Taylor (1996) found that, for a large sample of African American women, individuals with a self-reported high level of subjective religiousness were more likely to use prayer as a coping mechanism in stress-producing, health situations.

Other investigators have focused on the relationships between personal religious expressions (i.e., religious beliefs, faith, and salience of prayer) and the outcomes of stress-producing, health-related situations. For example, in one study, O'Brien (1982) investigated the importance of faith in the lives of 126 dialysis patients who were mostly African American. Of all the subgroups in the study, African American women were the most likely to report that the importance of faith was tied more to interactional behavior with medical staff and others, better quality of interactions, less alienation, and more compliance.

For African American women, the use of religious-spiritual strategies to cope with the stress of poor health, and the stress of accessing and using the health care system, illustrates that their individual, orienting systems of coping with the status of their health are derived from a background of limited resources and shared, prior experiences. Therefore, it is reasonable to assume that when religiousness/spirituality is embedded in the individual's framework for living, the more quickly it will be used to cope with the stress of poor health, and problems in accessing a health care system that may appear at times, careless and negligent (Kinsey, 2005).

While the religious/spiritual strategies may be available for access and use, there is one resource that African American women have used historically as an integral element of their health seeking behaviors. This resource is the black church. Historically, African Americans in the American Diaspora have had limited options for action and fewer alternatives for assistance in negotiating the health care system (Combs-Jones, 2004; Taylor, 2001). The black church has emerged as one of the few resources available to assist in coping with stressful, health crises (Coleman, 1997). Beginning with slavery up to the current time, the influence of the black church remains the most central resource for African Americans; it remains as a symbol of strength and hope, an institution in which mechanisms for social change emerge, and a resource in religious faith and practice is an integral part of the African American community. Combs-Jones (2004) indicates that the:

> (Black church) continue(s) to symbolize home, close family relationships, and solidarity not often experienced in other organizations. In addition to providing a sense of solidarity, continuity, and leadership among American blacks, the black church (community) also (has) a history of responding to issues of health affecting the black community. Moreover, the church has always espoused a connection between faith and good health (p.105).

However, when one reads the literature that focuses on religiousness/spirituality, there is little attention paid to this most important resource operating in the lives of African American women. The black church, as a resource, is overlooked because the current paradigm used to assess health care outcomes is based on an illness model that dominates today, one that is secular (non-spiritual), genetic-biomedical, and reliant almost entirely on the natural rather than the supernatural. In the quest for objective fact, groups of "experts" have emerged to control the policy decisions, research agendas, and health care protocols. When the black church is included, it is usually as an afterthought,-another way to obtain subjects for investigations, or an obstacle that needs to be overcome to achieve a particular goal (Kinsey, 2005). The consequence is that health care professionals continue to pursue their goals from their traditional positions of power, and, therefore, miss golden opportunities to inform their health care agendas in ways that would provide the kind of nuanced information needed so badly to facilitate the easing of disparities in health care outcomes for African American women.

Conclusion: A Path for a New Direction

Because African American women are more acutely aware of their human resources to cope with the boundary conditions of life, they appear to be more committed to using their families and communities as sources of help during times of stress, while in poor health, and in their search for a connection to the divine that transcends their immediate worlds. There is, of course, more to understanding the socio-historical factors operating within the lives of African American women than what has been captured in the framework described in this chapter. However, conceptualizing health beliefs and health seeking behaviors within the context of a shared, socio-historical perspective provides some conceptual tools and guidelines for locating the essential character of a collective, "black female consciousness." In so doing, significant advances may be realized onto a broader, organizational framework.

Following the lead of Griffith (1986), the health care professionals who try to understand cultural groups distinct from their own without allowing for the importance of cultural values and behaviors as significant variables to investigate and use, face the same problem as earlier scientists who tried to find a cure for yellow fever. They were unable to cure yellow fever until they realized that the disease was not due to the night air, but to the mosquitoes that were in the background of their daily lives. It is argued here that this inattention to the "background" in which African American women live must be corrected.

A major contention of this chapter is that the health beliefs and health seeking behaviors of African American women must be assessed within a broader personal, situational, and social context.

Health beliefs and health seeking behaviors cannot be evaluated apart from the larger culture of African Americans. The merits of a specific intervention procedure cannot be assessed apart from the larger cultural context of African Americans. While there are no simple formulas, the policy maker, the health care researcher, and the health care giver must gather information about many aspects of the individual woman who happens to be African American. This requires a change in the biomedical model currently used to determine the kinds of information and policies needed to facilitate a decrease in the disparities in health care outcomes that occur today.

The most central issue for the advancement of an alternative framework is how to shift thinking on the part of health care professionals and policy makers. The major issue for health care professionals and African American women who access and use health care is whether—and how—such a framework can get translated into practical change. This change really means changing medicine and the allied health areas (psychology, sociology, and nursing), the disciplines that form the basis for professional practice in health care. Fernando (2010) indicates that in the United States today, there is little in the way of top-down direction to professionals on how to implement-or even whether they should implement-such new ways of thinking as the values approach embedded in the framework presented in this chapter. He adds that for change to occur, one must look to influencing professional training and getting legal backing through legislation.

In the United States today, the recent political controversies surrounding passage and implantation of the Affordable Care Act (Robinson & Finegold, 2012) strongly indicate there is very little in the way of a coordinated, top-down direction to professionals on the need to change health care delivery to meet the needs of a culturally, diverse population (Louden, 2013). This is not encouraging news for African American women, the central focus of this chapter. The lack of legal reasons for health care professionals to change is a drawback, especially since many professionals today feel over-cautious about veering from the traditional ways of thinking and doing things because of the "blame culture" they work in. However, there appears to be some change with respect to incorporating a values-based approach that embraces the idea of diversity. These changes are being instituted in various universities and health care, training institutions across the United States (Anderson, Scrimshaw, Fullilove, et al, 2003). If such training is sufficiently strong, and resources allow, there is hope that the framework presented and discussed in this chapter, in spite of the limitations discussed above, may make a significant difference in providing culturally competent health care for African American women, and, thereby, reducing disparities in their health care outcomes

References

Akbar, N. (1995). *The community of self* (Rev. Ed.). Tallahassee: FL: Mind Productions & Associates.

Altman, BM & Taylor, AK. (2001). Women in the health care system: Health status, insurance, and access to care. *MEPS Research Findings, 17*. Rockville: MD, Publication No. 02-0004.

American Cancer Society. (2008). *Breast cancer facts and figures: 2007-2008*. Atlanta, GA: American Cancer Society, Inc.

American Sociological Association. (2005). *Race, ethnicity, and the health of Americans*. Sidney S Spivack Program in Applied Social Research and Social Policy, July. Retrieved January 10, 2012, http://www.asanet.org/galleries/default-file/race_ethnicity_health.pdf.

Anderson, ML. (1988). *Thinking about women: Sociological perspectives on sex and gender* (2nd ed). New York: Macmillan.

Anderson, M, Scrimshaw, SC, Fullilove, MT, Fielding, JE, Normand, J. (2003). Culturally competent healthcare systems: A systematic review. *Am J Prev Med, 24*(3S) 68-79.

Ani, M. (1994). Yarugu: *An African centered critique of European cultural thought and behavior.* Trenton, NJ: African World.

Baldwin, JA. (1991). African (black) psychology: Issues and synthesis. In RL Jones (ed), *Black psychology*. Berkeley, CA: Cobb and Henry, pp. 125-135.

Banton, M. (1987). Racial theories. Cambridge, England: Cambridge University Press.

Barrett, A & Robbins, C. (2007). The multiple sources of women's aging anxiety and their relationship with psychological distress. *Journal of Aging and Health, 3*, 119-135.

Becker, M. (1974). The Health Belief Model and personal health behavior. *Health Education Monograph, 2*, 324-473.

Berger, TE (2013). L.O.G.I.C.: A model for diversity in health care delivery in the twenty-first century. Philadelphia, PA:, Unpublished manuscript.

Brett, KM & Hayes, SG. (2004). *Women's health and mortality chartbook*. Washington, DC: DHHS Office on Women's Health.

Byrd, WM & Clayton, LA (2000). *An American health dilemma, Vol. 1: A medical history of African Americans and the problems of race-beginnings to 1900*. New York: Routledge.

Capra, E. (1982). *The turning point: Science, society, and the rising culture*. London: Wildwood House.

Centers for Disease Control and Prevention. (2004). *Vital statistics data, and underlying causes of death: 1997-2001*. Washington, DC: National Center for Health Statistics, (Author).

Chambers, R. (1997). *Whose reality counts? Putting the first last*. London: ITDG Publishing.

Chu, K, Tarone, R, & Brawley, O. (1999). Breast cancer trends of black women compared with white women. *Archives of Family Med, 8*, 521-528.

Coleman, W. (1997). West African roots of African American spirituality. *Psychological Review, 9*(4), 533-539.

Combs-Jones, Y. (2004). African American women at midlife: The social construction of health and aging. *Electronic Theses, Treatises, and Dissertations*. Retrieved from http://diginole.lib.fsu/etd.

Cooper, LA, Brown, C, ThiVu, H, Ford, DE, & Powe, NR. (2001). How important is intrinsic spirituality in depression care? A comparison of white and African American primary care patients. *Journal of Gen Internal Med, 16*(9), 634-638.

Davis, A. (1983). *Women, race, and class*. New York: Vintage.

Dignam, J. (2001). Adjuvant therapy for breast cancer in African American and Caucasian women. *Journal of the Nat Cancer Inst Monographs, 30*, 36-43.

Dill, BT. (1988). Making your job for yourself: Domestic service and the construction of personal dignity. In A Beckman & S. Morgen, (Eds), *Women and the politics of empowerment*. Philadelphia: Temple University Press.

Ellison, CW & Taylor, RJ. (1996). Turning to prayer: Social and situational antecedents of religious coping among African Americans. *Review of Religious Research, 38*, 111-131.

Feagin, JR & McKinnsey, KD. (2003). *The many costs of racism.* Lanham: Rowan and Littlefield.

Fernando, S. (2010). *Mental health, race and culture* (Third Ed). New York: Palgrave Macmillan.

Freeman, HP. (2004). Poverty, culture, and social injustice: Determinants of cancer disparities. *Cancer Journal for Clinicians, 54,* 72-77.

Fuller, ME. (2008). A comparison study between African American and Caucasian women in their health beliefs and locus of control concerning breast cancer in North Florida. *Electronic Theses and Dissertations* Paper 4378. Retrieved from http://diginole.lib.fsu.edu/etd.

Glass, J, Bengston, VL, & Dunham, CC. (1986). Attitude similarity in three-generation families: Socialization, status inheritance, or reciprocal influence? *American Soc Review, 51*(5), 685-698.

Glenn, EN. (2002). *Unequal freedom: How race and gender shaped American citizenship and labor.* Cambridge, MA: Harvard University Press.

Griffith, JL (1986). Employing the God-family relationship therapy with religious families. *Family Process, 25,* 609-618.

Hall, S. (1992). "New Ethnicities." In J Donald & A Ratansi (Eds), *"Race, culture and difference.* London: Sage, pp. 252-259.

Ingleby, D. (1980). *Critical psychiatry: The politics of mental health.* New York: Pantheon Books.

Institute of Medicine. (2003). *Unequal treatment: Confronting racial and ethnic disparities in health care.* Washington, DC: The National Academies Press.

Janzen, JM. (1978). The comparative study of medical systems as changing social systems. *Social Science and Medicine, 12,* 121-129.

Jatoi, I, Anderson, W, Sowmya, R, & Devesa. (2005). Breast cancer trends among black and white women in the United States. *Journal of Clinical Oncology, 23*(31), 7836-7841.

Jones, C & Shorter-Gordon, K. (2003). Shifting: *The double lives of black women in America.* New York: HarperCollins.

Kessler, RC, Michelson, KD, & Williams, DR. (1999). The prevalence, distribution, and mental health correlates of perceived discrimination in the United States. *Journal of Health and Social Behavior, 40*(3), 208-230.

Kinsey, PJ. (2005). The religious-spiritual orienting system and coping: Implications for the assessment of African Americans. In A Carter-Obayuwana, S Gopaul-McNicol, & D Louden (Eds), *Personality assessment and culture*. Lincoln University, PA: Office of Research, Development, Planning and Coordination.

Kleinman, A. (1978). Concepts and a model for the comparison of medical systems as cultural systems. *Social Science and Medicine, 12*, 85-93.

Kleinman, A. (1987). Culture and clinical reality: Commentary on culture-bound syndromes and international disease classifications. *Culture, Medicine, and Psychiatry, 11*(1), 49-52.

Kleinman, A. (1995). *Writing at the margin: Discourse between anthropology and medicine*. Berkeley, CA: University of California Press.

Koenig, HG. (2000). Religion, spirituality, and medicine: Application to clinical practice. *JAMA, 284*(13), 1708.

Kuhn, TS. (1962). *The structure of scientific revolutions* (Third Ed). Chicago, IL: University of Chicago Press.

Laditha, JN. (2000). Adult children helping older parents: Variations in likelihood and hours by gender, race, and family role. *Research on Aging, 23*(4), 429-456.

Leighton, AH & Hughes, JM. (1961). Cultures as causative of mental disorder. Millbank *Memorial Fund Quarterly, 39*(3), 446-470.

Lewis, G. (1986). Concepts of health and illness. In C Curter & M Stacey (Eds), *Concepts of health, illness, and disease: A comparative perspective*. London: Berg, pp. 119-135.

Loefler, I. (2003). Health, science, and religion in contemporary American culture. *Mayo Clinic Proceedings, 78*(7), 893-895.

Louden, D. (2013). Epidemiological issues: Critical factors in culturally competent health care. In PJ Kinsey & D Louden (Eds), Health, ethnicity, and well-being: An African American perspective. Bloomington, IN: Xlibris (In Press).

Martin, P. (2003). "Said and done" versus 'saying and doing:" Gendering practices, practicing gender at work. *Gender & Society, 17* (June), 342-366.

Martin-Baro, I. (1994). Towards a liberation psychology. In A Aron & S Corne (Eds), *Writings for a liberation psychology*. Cambridge, MA: Harvard University Press.

Mbiti, JS. (1991). *Introduction to African religion* (2nd Ed). London: Heinemann.

Mensah, GA. (2005). Eliminating disparities in cardiovascular health: Six strategic imperatives and a framework for action. *Circulation, 111*(10), 1332-1336.

Mills, CW. (1959). *The sociological imagination*. New York: Oxford University Press.

National Cancer Institute. (2004). *Surveillance epidemiology and end results: SEER Program*. Bethesda, MD, Division of Cancer Control and Population Sciences (Author).

National Cancer Institute. (2007). *Breast cancer facts and figures: 2007*. Bethesda, MD: Division of Cancer Control and Population Sciences (Author).

Nobles, W. (1991). African philosophy: Foundations for black psychology. In RL Jones (Ed), *Black psychology*, 3rd Ed. Berkeley, CA; Cobb & Henry, pp. 47-63.

O'Brien, M. (1982). Religious faith and adjustment to long-term hemodialysis. *Journal of Religion & Health, 21,* 68-80.

Onunwa, U. (1994). The individual and community in African traditional religion and society. *Mankind Quarterly, 34*(3), 249-260.

Pargament, K. (1995). *The psychology of religion and coping*. New York: Guilford Press.

Phillips, FB. (1990). NTU psychotherapy: An Afrocentric perspective. *J of Black Psychology, 17,* 55-74.

Registe, MF. (2008). The relationship between health beliefs and the performance of breast self-examination among African American women. *Electronic Theses, Treatises, and Dissertations.* Paper 1904. Retrieved from http://diginole.lib.fsu/edu/etd.

Robbins, CL. (2007). Cultural and structural explanations of racial and ethnic differences in women's health care. Electronic Theses, Treatises, and Dissertations. Paper 1830. Retrieved from http://diginole.lib.fsu.edu/etd.

Robbins, C, Jackson, P, Dimperio, D, Hackney, M, Harker, B, Johnson-Cornett, B, & Thompson, D. (2006). *Women's health data report: 2006*. Tallahassee, FL: Florida Department of Health.

Robinson, W & Finegold, K. (2012). The affordable care act and African Americans. *ASPE Research Brief.* Dept of Health & Human Services. Retrieved from http://aspe.hhs.gov

Salganicoff, AJ, Beckerman, Z, Wyn, R, & Ojeda, VD. (2002). *Women's health in the United States: Health coverage and access to health care.* Menlo Park, CA; Center for Health Policy Research.

Sewell, WH, Jr. (1992). A theory of structure: Duality, agency, and transformation. *Amer. J. of Sociology, 98*(1), 1-29.

Shive, SE, Ma, GX, Tan, Y, Toubbeh, JI, Parameswaran, L, & Halowich, J. (2006). Racial differences in preventive and complementary health behaviors and attitudes. *J of Health Disparities Research and Practice, 1*(1), 75-92.

Smedley, AY, Stith, AR, & Nelson (Eds). (2003). Unequal treatment: Confronting racial and ethnic disparities in health care. Washington, DC: National Academies Press.

St. Jean, Y & Feagin, JR. (1998). *Double burden: Black women and everyday racism.* New York: ME Sharpe.

Taylor, SE. (2001). The health status of black women. In RL Braithwaite & SE Taylor (Eds), Health issues in the black community. San Francisco: Josey-Bass, pp. 44-61.

U.S. Department of Health & Human Services. (2004). *Women's health USA: 2004.* Rockville, MD: Health Resources and Services Administration (Author).

Whitfield, K & Baker-Thomas, T. (1999). Individual differences in aging minorities. *International J of Aging and Human Development, 48*(1), 243-268.

Williams, MP. (2001). Promoting early breast cancer screening: Strategies with rural African American women. *American J of Health Studies.* Retrieved Oct 10, 2012 from http://www.findarticles.com/p/articles/mi_m0CTG/is/2/17/ai_85.

Williams DR & Williams-Morris, R. (2000). Racism and mental health: The African American experience. *Ethnicity and Health, 5*(3/4), 243.268.

Zinnbauer, B, Pargament, K, Cowell, B, Rye, M, & Scott, A. (1996-August). Religion and spirituality: Unfuzzying the fuzzy. Paper presented at the meeting of the American Psychological Association, Toronto, Canada.

CHAPTER FOUR

Age and Health Care Delivery: Critical Issues Affecting the African American Senior

Virginia J. Smith
The Lincoln University, PA

Frank P. Worts
The Lincoln University, PA

Jennifer D. Smith
Temple University

Abstract

This chapter focuses on key factors impacting the African American senior in today's world. Specifically, attention is paid to the contextual and cultural factors that affect the health status of the elderly, especially those factors associated with causes of deaths among older African Americans and the role that quality of care, insurance, disabilities, and specific health conditions. Special attention is paid to health disparities and the factors that influence the health status of older adults, especially the fact that there is an insufficient amount of research directed toward racial and ethnic differences among the elderly. The consequence of health disparities observed for elderly African Americans with respect to a variety of issues is discussed, with special attention paid to the barriers to a quality health status. The factors of oral health and immunizations are presented with the purpose of demonstrating that such factors have long been overlooked when accounting for health disparities among the African American elderly. Finally, recommendations for reducing health disparities among the elderly are made with respect to recommendations for public policy, communities, and health care providers.

Introduction

Advances in health care and health prevention efforts have been major factors in the dramatic increases in life expectancy in the United States over the past century. Additionally, there have been major shifts in the leading causes of death for all age groups, including older adults, from infectious diseases and acute illnesses to chronic diseases and degenerative illnesses. It is estimated that 80% of Americans over the age of 65 are living with at least one chronic condition. This growth in the number and proportion of older adults is unprecedented in the history of the United States. In addition to the longer life spans, the aging of the baby boomers will combine to double the population of Americans aged 65 and older during the next 25 years. Projections by the U. S. Census Bureau (2008) are that the nation will be more racially and ethnically diverse, as well as much older, by midcentury.

Figure 1 shows the projected trends for population growth among older adults through 2050. The African American older population was 3.2 million in 2008 and is projected to grow to over 9.9 million by 2050. In 2008, African American persons made up 8.3 percent of the older population. Census Bureau estimates suggest that by 2050, 11% of the older American population will be African American. This population is projected to increase to 88.5 million in 2050, more than doubling the number in 2008 (38.7 million). Within this aging group, the oldest of the old (those over the age of 85 years) is the fastest growing segment. Projections by the U. S. Census Bureau (2008) estimate that the 85 and older population will more than triple from 5.4 million to 19 million between 2008 and 2050. Additionally, whereas living to be 100 was in the past an unexpected occasion, it is becoming a much more frequent event among older Americans.

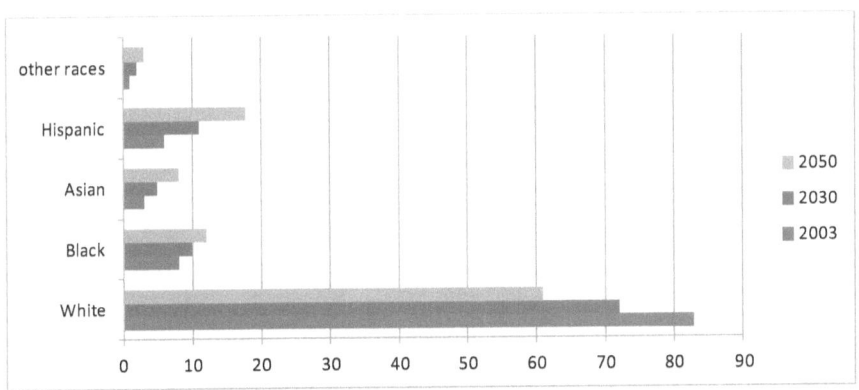

Figure 1. **Population projections by percentage of older persons by race**

In summary, by 2030, there will be 71 million American older adults accounting for roughly 20% of the U.S. population. Additionally, there is a trend of shifting among the racial/ethnic groups in the United States. In 2003, 83% of older adults in America were white non-Hispanic. By 2030, it is estimated that this percentage will reduce to 72%. It is projected that by 2050, the total number of non-Hispanic whites, aged 65 and over will double, while the number of African-Americans, aged 65 and over will triple (U. S. Census Bureau, 2008). With this older and more diverse population, health disparities become more important to practitioners and policy makers in the health care arena. Health status is associated with being a member of a racial/ethnic group in several ways. Quality of health status can be linked to genetic differences, socio-economic issues, access to care issues, responsiveness on the part of the health care delivery system, and personal habits and behaviors consistent with the group identity.

Health Status of the Elderly

The improvements in life expectancy among all Americans over the past century are generally attributed to advances in medical care and preventive efforts in the areas of public and personal health. Accompanying these increases in life expectancy is the shift from the leading causes of death. At the turn of the 20th Century, the major causes of death were infectious diseases and acute illnesses. As people live longer and received better medical care, their health issues are controlled and maintenance plans are in place to manage the chronic conditions that they experience. They live longer with these chronic conditions that have also become the leading causes of death among those Americans aged 65 years and older. According to the Centers for Disease Control and Prevention (2007), the three leading causes of death for this population are heart disease, cancer, and stroke, together accounting for 61% of all deaths among older Americans. All three of these conditions are now maintained for longer periods of time than they were in several decades ago.

In addition to causing more than one half of the deaths among older Americans, these three illnesses contribute to the rate of disability, pain, and reductions in functional status among this population, affecting their quality of life and their levels of independence. According to a 2004 survey conducted by the Centers for Disease Control and Prevention, older adults suffer the highest rates of poor physical health and activity limitation (Centers for Disease Control and Prevention, 2007).

Figure 2 shows the distribution of chronic conditions among older adults by race and ethnicity for 2002-2003 based on the 2006 National Health Survey conducted by the Centers for Disease Control and Prevention.

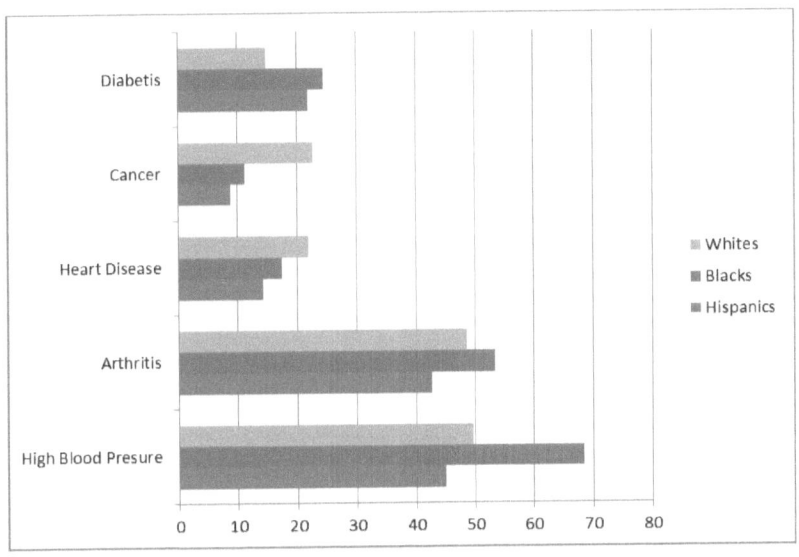

Figure 2. **Prevalence in percentages of chronic conditions among persons age 65+ by race**

Based on data releases from the National Center for Health Statistics and the Bureau of Labor Statistics, from 2006 through 2009, (Centers for Disease Control and Prevention, 2007) the Administration on Aging profiled the health status of older Americans in 2010 as follows:

- Most older persons have at least one chronic condition and many have multiple conditions. The most frequently occurring conditions among older persons were: hypertension (38%), diagnosed arthritis (50%), all types of heart disease (32%), any cancer (22%), diabetes (18%), and sinusitis (14%).

- 41.6% of non-institutionalized older persons assessed their heath as excellent or very good (compared to 64.5% for all persons aged 18-64 years).
- About 12.9 million persons aged 65 and older were discharged from short stay hospitals. This is a rate of 3,395 for every 10,000 persons aged 65+ which is about three times the comparable rate for persons of all ages (which was 1,149 per 10,000). The average length of stay for persons aged 65+ was 5.6 days; the comparable rate for persons of all ages was 4.8 days.
- Older persons averaged more office visits with doctors: 7.1 office visits for those aged 65 and over while persons aged 45-65 averaged only 3.7 office visits during that year. Almost 97% of older persons reported that they did have a usual place to go for medical care and only 2.6% said that they failed to obtain needed medical care during the previous 12 months due to financial barriers.
- Older consumers averaged out-of-pocket health care expenditures of $4,846, an increase of 61% over 10 years ago. In contrast, the total population spent considerably less, averaging $3,126 in out-of-pocket costs. Older Americans spent 12.9% of their total expenditures on health, more than twice the proportion spent by all consumers (6.4%). Health costs incurred on average by older consumers in 2009 consisted of $3,027 (63%) for insurance, $821 (17%) for medical services, $828 (17%) for drugs, and $170 (3.5%) for medical supplies.
- Among older adults, chronic diseases can lead to limitations in daily activities and thus often reduce health-related quality of life for seniors. The percentage of older U.S. adults who report very good or excellent health decreases with age.

The Behavioral Risk Factor Surveillance System (BRFSS) is a survey conducted by the Centers for Disease Control in the 50 United States and its territories. It is the world's largest telephone health survey system and it tracks health risk factors on an annual basis. The BRFSS has been in existence since 1984. Below is a list of findings from this survey based on 2007 data about risk factors that relate to the older adult population (Centers for Disease Control and Prevention, 2007).

- 36.6% of older adults reported having a disability (defined as being limited in any way in any activities because of physical, mental, or emotional problems or having a health problem that requires the use special equipment, such as a cane, a wheelchair, a special bed, or a special telephone).
- Older persons with disabilities are less likely to be physically active and more likely to be obese.
- In 2004, among adults aged 65 or older, the average number of physically unhealthy days per month (based on self reported data) was 5.3.
- 72% of older Americans reported having an influenza shot within the past year.
- 67.3% of older Americans reported having had pneumonia vaccination.
- Although most older adults who were once regular smokers have quit, about 9% of adults aged 65 or older were still smoking cigarettes in 2004.
- 93.7% of older adults reported having their cholesterol checked in the past five years.
- Mammograms for women aged 65 or older are covered by Medicare, but many women are still not taking advantage of this opportunity. The risk of getting breast cancer increases as a woman gets older. Nearly 8 of 10 cases of breast cancer are found in women over age 50.
- Compared with other age groups, a greater proportion of adults aged 65 or older eat five or more fruits and vegetables daily.
- 28.1% of older Americans report eating 2-5 servings of fruit and vegetables per day.
- 32.5% report not having any leisure time physical activity in the past month.
- Hospitalization for hip fracture occurred at the rate of 450 per 100,000 men and 1026 per 100,000 women.

In addition to these demographic and risk factor data, there are several other characteristics of an aging population that impact health. For example, when asked about living preferences, the older population is more likely to express a preference to remain in their own homes, or at least in their own neighborhoods. This preference is expressed even when health status is poor. Those who are disabled and remain in their own homes, are at less risk when there is an informal system of care available to assist them on a daily basis. Only a small portion of these persons utilize the formal system for in-home care. Additionally, older Americans have varying degrees of limitations on their activities of daily living. How they assess their health status depends on the level of their functional status as defined by the number of areas in which they experience limitations or difficulty performing on a daily basis. Therefore, to meet the health needs of the older Americans, a continuum of services should be available to address their varying needs. There is no boiler plate solution to the variety of health issues that they face.

Health Disparities and African American Older Persons

In spite of the increase in life expectancy among minority older persons, there are major disparities in health status between African-Americans and their white counterparts. As with the general population (all ages), the disparities in health among older African-Americans are traced to a range of complex factors, including, access to care, diagnosis, progression, response to treatment, caregiving, and overall quality of life. All of these factors can be affected by socio-economic issues. Consequently variables such as income status and educational level have been studied in various attempts to explain the disparities. In some cases improvements in socio-economic status or educational level contribute to reduced disparities. However, even controlling for factors such as poverty, educational level, geographic location, the disparities among African-American elders remain.

The Centers for Disease Control and Prevention has observed a variety factors that influence health status of older adults. These factors are consistent with those that are observed in the general population. However, they speculate that older adults may experience the effects of health disparities more dramatically than any other population group because they are more likely to have chronic illness and require frequent contact with the health care system. Additionally, advancing age puts one more at risk for poverty, affecting access to health care services. "The care of older adults who are chronically ill, poor and members of an ethnic community is an increasingly urgent health priority" (Centers for Disease Control and Prevention, 2007).

A major issue facing health care providers and policy makers is the insufficient amount research on racial and ethnic differences directed specifically towards the elderly, despite population, despite the projections that show that the population aged 65 and over is becoming increasingly diverse. In response to this concern, the National Institutes of Aging commissioned a two-day conference. Findings from this event indicate that health differences involve a "complexity of factors." From an examination of the differences among five racial/ethnic groups—Hispanics, whites, blacks, Asians, and American Indians and Alaska Natives—emerged clear indication of this complexity. However, the disparities were summarized as follows: "Blacks generally have worse health than other groups. American Indians and Alaska Natives, especially those on reservations, are also less healthy than other groups except blacks" (Bulatao & Anderson, 2004).

Low socioeconomic status is a risk factor for poor health. This is confounded by the fact that sometimes illnesses or disabilities (which are more common among the older population) impose additional costs, impacting economic status. However, in examining the factors affecting health status of older persons, socioeconomic status is not always the most important factor. (Bulatao & Anderson, 2004).

Risk factors associated with behaviors such as smoking, poor diet, lack of exercise, and drug and alcohol abuse have been examined in relation health status of older persons. Although these behaviors clearly impact health statue, their roles in racial health disparities among older adults have not been consistently documented. (Bulatao & Anderson, 2004).

Another factor discussed by this group is prejudice and discrimination that may impact health disparities. The direct impact of these variables on health status of African-American older persons is not understood or documented. There have been some studies that suggest discrimination and prejudice among health care providers may lead to stress and elevated blood pressure among older African-Americans. Related to this issue is the amount of stress caused by socio-economic factors and its impact on health status. Additionally, the effect of stereotypes held by providers has been considered but not clearly documented. Additionally, patient compliance has be studied as a factor in quality health care, but again, its contribution to the knowledge about health disparities has not been documented. (Bulatao & Anderson, 2004)

Another factor that emerged from the discussion was the suggestion that differences in access to quality health care related to racial and cultural barriers may impact the quality of health status among minority older persons. However, the extent of the impact of access this accounts for disparities is not clear. (Bulatao, and Anderson, 2004).

These conferees concluded that "the influence of each of these factors can cumulate over the life course, so that the health status of older cohorts reflects their entire life experiences." There was the suggestion that events resulting from these health disparities over the life span have a cumulative effect on life expectancy and health status during the older years. (Bulatao & Anderson, 2004).

Consequences of Health Disparities

It is said that if one lives long enough, he/she will face poor health. Although some older persons live out healthy lives, the majority of them face some illness. Also, being a member of a minority racial or ethnic group places the older adult at greater risk for poor health. Comparing the health status data on African American older adults to their white counterparts shows the following disparities:

- On the BRFSS, African Americans reported an average of 6.8 physically unhealthy days per month, compared to 5.5 days per month reported by their white counterparts; African Americans have the lowest rates of influenza and pneumonia vaccinations; 25% percent of older African Americans compared to 31% of whites report eating five or more fruits and vegetables per day; the prevalence of Frequent Mental Distress (FMD) varies by racial and ethnic groups among Americans aged 65 or older. The prevalence of FMD was lower among whites (5.9%) as compared African Americans (9.8%).
- Data on causes of death show higher mortality rates among older African Americans than whites; the death rate for

African Americans (both male and female) ages 65-79 is at least 30% higher than the death rate for whites in the same age group; life expectancy for blacks is nearly 7 years shorter than for whites; older blacks have higher death rates than older whites from the two leading causes, heart diseases and cancer; older blacks are also more likely than whites to die from diabetes, nephritis, and septicemia (Bulatao & Anderson, 2004).

- It is estimated that deaths from hypertension contribute the most to black-white differences (Bulatao & Anderson, 2004).
- Self-rated health status on the National Health Interview Survey was generally the worst for African Americans among all racial and ethnic groups; older African Americans reported a diagnosis of hypertension much more often than whites; African American older persons reported a previous stroke more often than whites; African American older persons more frequently reported diagnoses of diabetes (See Table I).
- In other studies, African Americans aged 50 and older reported higher levels than whites of hypertension, diabetes, stroke, kidney disease, bladder problems, lung problems, asthma, back problems, foot and leg problems, and vision and hearing problems (Crimmins, 2004).

Table I. *Self-Rated Health and Activity Limitations by Race and Age*

Racial or Ethnic Group	Male			Female		
	65-74	75-84	85+	65-74	75-84	85+
Self-Rated Health: Percent Fair or Poor						
White	24.5	30.8	32.0	23.0	29.1	34.0
Black	41.3	47.3	51.4	41.0	45.8	46.2
Percent with Activity Limitations						
White	35.0	39.5	49.6	32.8	41.0	60.8
Black	41.6	48.1	59.5	43.2	51.1	65.7

Barriers to Quality Health Status

In an introduction to the proceedings from the First National Conference on Behavioral and Sociocultural Perspectives on Ethnicity and Health, convened in 1992, Anderson (1995) suggests that the causes of health disparities fall into five broad categories of factors (Anderson, 1995):

- social influences such as culture and institutions
- behavioral risk factors, including diet, exercise, substance abuse, and smoking that lead to chronic disease
- risky behaviors that cause infectious disease and injury
- adaptive health behaviors and protective cultural practices
- health care behavior including compliance with medical instructions

These factors addressed by Anderson are important to health status and in some ways contribute to differences in health outcomes. However, they imply that the burden of reducing the discrepancies lies with the individual and his sub-group. Others, as well as these authors, suggest that there is a broader list of factors that include genetics, racism and discrimination, inflexibility in the health care delivery system, cultural barriers, and poor access to care. In this section, we discuss the broader perspective that combines the cultural and individual behaviors with the systemic barriers to quality health care.

African American older persons, on average, have lower educational levels than their white counterparts. It is speculated that this may lead to lower levels of health literacy among an already vulnerable population. For example, Cagney, et.al. (2005) found that socio-economic status, as manifested in education and income was strongly predictive of self reported health by African American older persons. Health literacy has been defined as "the degree to which individuals have the capacity to obtain, process, and understand basic health information and services needed to make appropriate health decisions "(Institute of Medicine, 2004). Sudore, et.al. (2006) concluded in their study of 3,075 community dwelling older persons that health literacy rates are higher among the more "traditionally disadvantaged groups, including African American men." Although many studies of health disparities, when controlling for education and literacy, still report differences, education and health literacy may be very important factors in reducing these differences.

Cagney et.al. also discovered that in their secondary analysis of large data sets, that marital status and insurance coverage were not predictive of self reported health status discrepancies between African American and white older persons. However, weight problems were associated with lower self ratings of health status among African American older persons. They also found a relationship between neighborhood affluence and health status as self reported by African Americans. This information has to be considered along with the facts that older persons in general prefer to remain in their homes, or at least in their own neighborhoods.

Relationships with others may impact the overall health of African American older persons. In many situations, the informal networks available to the older persons have great significance for health status and maintenance in the community. Studies have shown that moving an older person from the community into institutional care places him/her at greater risk for degeneration and death (National Long Term Care Survey, 2004). Additionally, other people may contribute to an individual's health through providing social support (Bulatao & Anderson, 2004). Studies have shown that African American Families are less likely to admit their impaired older relatives into nursing homes (Hargrave, 2006). The expectation is that this part of the character of the African American family would be a protective factor. However, it is not strong enough to reduce the disparities.

Cultural factors present as two-way streets. On the one hand, cultural norms and traditions may promote healthy living by encouraging positive behaviors and discouraging unhealthy behaviors. However, some contribute to the behavioral risks for disease and injury pointed out by Anderson (1995) and discussed above. Norms and traditions that promote unhealthy lifestyles, including poor diet and alcohol use can greatly contribute to the health disparities among the African-American elderly. Religious involvement can promote positive health behaviors in several ways. Positive religious leaders will prompt their congregations to adopt healthy lifestyles. Also, faith often acts as a protective factor, impacting attitude towards health and the future.

Cultural and social factors can also impact the way that the consumer of health services reacts to the delivery system. If the health care practitioner and other staff are not welcoming either because of individual prejudice and discrimination, or institutional racism, the patient may not want to attend a delivery point, or may not trust the health care system. In either of these cases, the patient may be non-compliant, affecting his/her prognosis, or even an early diagnosis.

King (2003) has suggested that a response to the evidence of a possible a lower level of trust of health care providers among African-Americans might be found in solutions such as cultural competency curricula in medical and other health care educational settings, sensitivity training, and increasing the number of African-American physicians.

Recently, the issue of under-representation by African Americans in research studies has resulted in insufficient knowledge about the causes of disparities, as well as the understanding of the variations in the natural courses of diseases among African Americans, and their reactions to interventions, including drugs and other therapies. Some speculate that in the absence of this information, the disparities cannot be fully addressed.

Access to care involves not only transportation and convenience of location, although these are very important and can sometimes affect whether a person receives health care services. Access includes the consumer's impression about whether he/she belongs in the environment. This includes assessments on the part of the consumer such as: "Do the staff and practitioners understand and welcome me?" "Are there at least some people here who look like me?" "Do the staff and practitioners understand that I need to be able to communicate my needs and ask questions?" All of these questions may not be on the minds of the consumers, but many of the African American consumers will have at least one of these questions. If the consumer does not feel that the services are accessible, he/she will not attempt to use them.

Special Issues

These authors chose to feature two special issues of concern for the elderly as they are not in the limelight of discussion about minority health issues. These are oral health and immunization. Both of these are gaining recent attention as research reveals their importance in the quality of life and health status of African American older persons. Studies have shown that these two issues are often neglected by African American older persons, yet minor efforts to comply with recommended interventions could yield large results in terms of prevention and treatment for this population.

Oral Health

Oral health's overall importance to health is recognized among the top 12 leading health indicators in Health People 2020. Poor oral health is associated with various diseases, including diabetes, stroke, and heart disease. There is also recent research suggesting a possible link between tooth loss related to periodontitis and cognitive impairment (Matthews, et.al., 2011).

Loss of teeth and dental caries are key indicators of oral health. The percentage of older adults in the general population who have lost all their natural teeth has declined substantially since the 1950s. This decline is the result of major improvements in the field of oral health, including community water fluoridation; advanced dental technology; better oral hygiene and prevention care; more frequent use of dental services, and improved patient attitudes about oral health in general. In spite of this decline, the prevalence of complete loss of teeth is twice as high for older adults (aged 65-74) living below 100% of poverty compared with those living above the poverty line For this age group, 34% of those below the poverty line were edentulous in the United States in 2009. (Dye et.al. 2012b).

In 2009, 20% of adults over the age of 65 had untreated dental caries and 89% had dental restorations. Twice as many non-Hispanic Blacks and Mexican-Americans older adults (36%) had untreated caries. The rate of untreated dental caries was almost three times greater for older adults living in poverty.

Periodontal (gum) diseases are associated with diabetes and possibly with cardiovascular disease and stroke. Prevention of these diseases depends heavily on proactive behaviors and frequent trips to the dentist for routine hygiene services. These and other oral health problems among older adults can also lead to needless pain and suffering; difficulty speaking, chewing, and swallowing; and loss of self-esteem. (Bulatao & Anderson, 2004) The most prevalent oral diseases: dental carriers, periodontal disease and oral cancer have multifactorial etiologies that include systemic factors, local factors, environmental factors and economic factors. Oral diseases are mostly preventable, therefore, assessing risk factors among African-American elderly could reduce the disparities in oral health. (Slaughter, et. al., 2004).

Older adult population groups have differing dental care needs, and thus dental health promoting behaviors vary by culture and class. For example, as the Baby Boomers age and become "Senior Boomers" (Kiyak 2000) many will retain all or most of their natural teeth; access professional dental care on a regular basis, as they did when they were younger, and will continue to demand the emerging innovations in cosmetic dentistry (Kiyak et al. 2002; Ettinger et al., 2006). On the other hand, older African Americans have generally been described as crisis care utilizers, or seeking dental care mostly when experiencing oral pain. They also have been reported to have lower expectations of retaining natural teeth with increasing age as compared to their counterparts in the general population. Therefore, oral health promotion targeted to aging Baby Boomers, in general may not require as much emphasis to the positive benefits of preventive dental care relative to saving natural teeth and annual oral cancer screenings; while these approaches may have more relevance in public health promotion strategies targeted to older African Americans. Small studies have reported success of oral health screening and educational projects targeted to African American older persons (Slaughter, et. al., 2004).

Immunization

The Centers for Disease Control and Prevention recommend that older persons consider getting immunizations against Influenza, Pneumococcal (Pneumonia), Shingles, and Tetanus, Diphtheria, Pertussis (whooping cough). Many older adults believe that vaccines are just for young children. However, many older adults have serious complications from illnesses that can be prevented by immunization.

African American older persons have significantly lower influenza and pneumococcal immunization rates compared to their white counterparts. Studies have not identified any one factor that accounts for this difference. Xakellis (2005) in his analysis of the Medicare Beneficiaries Survey found that blacks were less likely to receive vaccines for influenza. The American Association of Retired Persons (AARP) reported that even though Medicare pays for influenza and Pneumonia vaccines, rates of immunization for these two illnesses are less than optimal among the older population and "even lower rates" have been observed among African American older persons (AARP, 2012). Studies suggest that there are multiple factors including health literacy, educational levels, poor access, less awareness about the benefits of vaccination, and missed opportunities by providers.

It has been suggested that one way of motivating older African Americans to receive vaccines is to point out the importance of protecting their grand children from disease by protecting themselves. The READII (Racial and Ethnic Adult Disparities in Immunization Initiative), an effort of the Centers for Disease Control and Prevention was initiated to address these disparities. This initiative funds multi-year demonstration projects in five geographic areas. The projects target African American and Hispanic older persons to increase the levels of vaccination among these two groups. They focus on both influenza and pneumococcal vaccinations, using evidence based interventions and community partnerships to conduct outreach and education (Centers for Disease Control and Prevention, 2007).

Summary and Recommendations for Public Policy

In summary, African American elders face double jeopardy issues. They are vulnerable because of age and because of health disparities related to race and ethnicity. These disparities have been documented in the literature over the past two-three decades and have been the topic of various deliberations at the federal, state, and local levels. The Healthy People series has addressed these disparities in each of its publications. Federal agencies have initiated efforts to research and address these disparities. Older African

Americans themselves have paid attention to the public health efforts to increase health literacy and improve lifestyle behaviors. All of these efforts have yielded positive results. However, the differences in health status between African Americans and whites may have narrowed, but the gap is still obvious when examining mortality rates and morbidity rates in the top three disease categories.

Addressing this gap is important and we offer recommendations for public policy, communities, and health care providers.

Public Policy

Medicare and Medicaid make coverage for at least basic health care needs possible. Initiatives such as those implemented by the Centers for Disease Control and Prevention, the Institute for Aging, the Administration on Aging, and state and local government programs are actively pursuing knowledge and solutions to the health disparities for ethnic minorities. The next step should be the development of action research projects that implement and evaluate models to address the reduction of risky behaviors, the increase of proactive behaviors such as immunization and preventive oral health, and improve cultural competence in the health care delivery system. Additionally, wide dissemination of study results evaluating federally and locally funded initiatives to address disparities should be a priority.

Communities

Quality of life is affected by health status and having a healthy environment. Studies have shown that the health of the community is strongly associated with the health status of older persons. It is important that communities where African American older persons live adopt an "age friendly" environment. As older African Americans are very likely to "age in place," the community can be the stabilizing force by providing emotional support, offering assistance with instrumental needs, fostering intergenerational activities, including the older person in the community planning activities, and making the community a safe place for everyone.

Health Care Providers

Health care providers are cautioned to provide real access to care and services. African American older persons need to feel comfortable with their providers and in the environment where they receive their care and services. Older patients should be assisted with health literacy issues in a manner that is not demeaning. Staff and practitioners should address older African Americans in a manner that shows respect for them as individuals and as people of color. Health education is important and should be available to all older African Americans. This should not be limited to brochures and commercials, but should include face-to-face discussion, as well as time for and encouragement of questions.

References

American Association of Retired Persons (AARP) Public Policy Institute. Racial and ethnic disparities in influenza and Pneumococcal immunization rates among Medicare. *Brief #83*. Retrieved from website: http://assets.aarp.org/rgcenter/health/ib83_disparities.pdfIssue (Accessed September 30, 2012).

Anderson, N. B. (1995). Behavioral and sociocultural perspectives on ethnicity and health. *Health Psychology, 4*(7), 581-595.

Bulatao, R. A. & Anderson, N. B., Editors, (2004). *Understanding racial and ethnic differences in health in late life: A research agenda*, Washington, DC: National Academies Press.

Cagney, K., Browning, C., & Wen, M. (2005). Racial disparities in self-rated health at older ages: what difference does the neighborhood make? *Journal of Gerontology: Social Sciences, 60B*(4), 181-S190.

Crimmins, E. (2004) Trends in the health of the elderly. *Annual Review of Public Health, 2*, 79-98.

Dye, B., Xiafen, L., & Beltran-Aguilar, E. (2012a). Selected Oral Health Indicators in the United States, 2005-2008. *National Center for Health Statistics Data Brief*, U. S. Department of Health and Human Services, Centers for Disease Control and Prevention. No. 96, May.

Dye, B., Xiafen, L., & Thornton-Evans, G. (2012b). Oral Health Disparities as Determined by Selected Healthy People 2020 Oral Health Objectives for the United States, 2009-2010. *National Center for Health Statistics Data Brief,* U. S. Department of Health and Human Services, Centers for Disease Control and Prevention. No. 104, August.

Ettinger, R. L., 2006. Rational dental care. part 2. A case history. *Journal of Canadian Dental Association, 72*(5), 447-452.

Hargrave, R. (2006). Caregivers of African-American elderly with dementia: a review and analysis, *Annals of Long Term Care: Clinical Care and Aging, 14* (10), 1-3.

Institute of Medicine (2004). *Health literacy: a prescription to end confusion.* Washington, D.C: National Academic Press.

King, W. (2003). Examining African Americans' mistrust of the health care system: Expanding the research question, *Public Health Reports, 18,* 66-367.

Kiyak, H. A. (2000). Successful aging: Implications for oral health. *Journal of Public Health Dentistry, 60*(4), 276-281.

Kiyak, H. A., Kamoh, A., Persson, R. E., & Persson, G.R. (2002). Ethnicity and oral health in community-dwelling older adults. *General Dentistry, 50*(6), 513-518.

Matthews, J. C., You, Z., Wadley, V., Cushman, M., & Howard, G. (2011). The association between self-reported tooth loss and cognitive function in the reasons for geographic and racial differences in stroke study. *The Journal of the American Dental Association, 142*(3), 379-390.

Slaughter, A, Smith, VJ. & Taylor, L. (2004). Progressing toward a more culturally competent approach to dental care for African American elders. *Special Care In Dentistry, 24*(6), 301-307.

Sudore, R., Mebta, K. Simonsick, E., Harris, T., Bewman, A., Satterfield, S., Rosano, C., Rooks, R., Rubin, S., Ayonayon, H., and Yaffe, K. (2006). Limited literacy in older people and disparities in health and healthcare access, *Journal of the American Geriatric Society, 54*(5), 770-776.

U.S. Census Bureau (2008). *Population projection release* (Thursday, August 14, 2008).

U.S. Department of Health and Human Services. *Healthy People 2020.* Retrieved from Website: www.healthypeople.gov (Accessed 9/30/2012).

U.S. Department of Health and Human Services, Centers for Disease Control and Prevention (2007). *State of Aging and Health in America.*

U.S. Department of Health and Human Services, National Center for Health Statistics, Centers for Disease Control and Prevention (2011). Prevalence of complex activity limitations among racial/ethnic groups and Hispanic subgroups of adults: United states 2003-2009. *Data Brief 73.*

Xakellis, G. (2005) Predictors of influenza immunization in persons over age 65. *Journal of the American Board of Family Medicine, 18*(5), 426-433.

CHAPTER FIVE

Corporate Social Responsibility and African-American Health Care: The Case of the Tobacco Industry

William Kwame Dadson
Lincoln University

Abstract

The dominant issue surrounding corporate management today is the concept of corporate social responsibility and profit maximization. The tobacco industry's corporate social responsibility and profit maximization in the African-American community is under scrutiny in this study. The purpose of this research is to answer the question "Was the relationship between the African-American Community and the tobacco industry a business relationship or a genuine effort to bring about economic self sufficiency to the African-American community?" The results of the research indicated that the relationship was both a business relationship and a genuine effort to bring about economic self sufficiency in the African-American community. However, overwhelming evidence indicates that the industry allowed profit greed to overpower its best efforts and made the industry violate laws, disobeyed ethical standards, codes of responsibility and finally, drove it to social disrepute to the demise of the entire industry.

Introduction

The dominant issue confronting corporate management today is corporate profit maximization in relation to corporate social responsibility (CSR). The idea of corporate social responsibility (CSR) is a vision of corporate accountability to an array of stakeholders which includes shareholders, employees, customers, environmental protection, civil society its communities. CSR is intended to be an inbuilt and self-regulating mechanism fostering corporate adherence to laws, international norms, ethical standards and codes of responsibility. Through this mechanism, it is assumed that as a business becomes profitable, it should also accept the impacts of their activities and actively seek to protect, encourage community growth and development, and voluntarily eliminate the practices that harm the public sphere, regardless of legality. Following this positive behavior will go a long way to promote the interest of their stakeholders and the society as a whole (Branco and Rodriguez, 2007).

Branco and Rodriguez consider CSR as one of ethical and moral issues facing corporate decision making, and behavior, and that social issues deserve moral consideration of their own and should lead managers to consider the social impacts of corporate activities. Regardless of any stakeholders' pressures, actions which lead to things such as the conservation of the Earth's natural resources or bio-diversity preservation are morally praiseworthy (Branco and Rodriguez, 2007).

The Purpose of the Chapter

The purpose of this chapter is to review the literature on corporate social responsibility of the Tobacco Industry in the African American community which will enable us to answer the question "Is the relationship between the African American community and the tobacco industry just a business relationship, or is it a genuine effort on the part of the corporations to help bring about economic self sufficiency and, at the same time, promote good health outcomes in the African American community through corporate social responsibility?" Dating back to 1938, the tobacco industry has been the major sponsor of athletic, civil, cultural and entertainment events (Sylvia A. Law, 1992). Studies on cigarette smoking also indicate that African Americans suffer disproportionately from smoking which caused chronic and preventable diseases. An estimated 45,000 African Americans die from a smoking related illness every year (Health and Human Services, 1998).It is estimated that 1.6 million African Americans under the age of 18 today will become regular smokers and about 500,000 of these will die prematurely from tobacco-related diseases (Center for Disease Control, 1998). Further, the tobacco industry disproportionately targets African America communities with cigarettes sales. This leads us to the question, "Is the relationship between the African American community and the tobacco industry just a business relationship or a genuine effort on the part of the corporations to help bring economic self sufficiency in the African American community?"

Recent corporate scandals have increased public mistrust of corporations as to their ability to maximize profit and at the same time engage in socially responsible activities. Scandals such as those of Enron, Arthur Anderson, Fannie Mae, Toyota, and AIG have certainly eroded the public trust in corporations. For many years, this has been the concern of the legal community and economists. Both groups have been examining the role of the large corporation in society and the controversy surrounding the model of corporate governance. For the legal scholars, the concern over the corporate role is whether corporate decision makers should also consider the interests of "stakeholders" other than the shareholders. This stems from the fact that the resulting economic, social, and political power inherent in the corporate form enables them to aggregate a large amount of resources (Solomon, 1990).

Literature Review

The literature review the follows surveys the theories of corporate social responsibility (CSR), namely, the concepts of a corporation, the moderate view, classical view, stakeholder view, and the mute stakeholder view.

The Concept of a Corporation

The notion of corporate social responsibility has been a controversial subject for about two thousand years. The word corporation was derived from the Latin word "Universitas" from which the "University" was derived. Under the Roman Laws, the purpose of "Universitas" was to create institutions for social benefit. They were not profit making institutions and were strictly controlled by the Roman Government. During the medieval ages, it was used to describe specialized associations of students and teachers with collective legal rights usually guaranteed by charters issued by princes, prelates, or the towns in which they were located (Colish, 1997).

The concept of a corporation as an individual entity began in the 14th century. However, the full recognition under the law as major individual entity, which could be sued was fully developed within the 18th and 19th centuries. By the early 20th century the question of corporate social responsibly has began to attract the attention of legal and economic scholars. One of the pioneers of CSR was Professor Maurice Clark. In his essay, "The Socializing of Theoretical Economics," John Maurice Clark criticized orthodox economics. He termed their theories as "Euclidean economics". He emphasized that the treatment of business under orthodox economics which asserted the primacy of individualism, free contract, and laissez-faire—produced an "economics of irresponsibility (Clark 1921; Champlin and Knoedler, 2004). He was of the opinion that the stress on business is excessive individualism could lead to a denial of any responsibility for the public interest. He termed it an irresponsible economic notion. In its place, he proposed an "economics of responsibility" in which business recognized and accepted its responsibility for the public interest and in which the rest of society worked toward that same end. Two other professors who joined Professor Clark in the corporate social responsibility debates were Professors Todd and Berle.

In the 1930s, series of articles were published by Professors Adolf Berle, a member of President Franklin Roosevelt Economic Advisors, and Merrick Dodd, a Law Professor, in which they expressed their divergent opinions on CSR. Professor Berle believed that the stockholders' wealth maximization should be the utmost prerogative of a corporation. He stressed that corporate activity should be evaluated in terms of the extent to which it benefits the company's shareholder. In short, he strongly concluded that objective measurement of shareholder benefit is wealth maximization through business activities (Berle, 1931and 1932).Contrary to Berle, Professor Dodd's main concern was the protection of the society. He strongly held the opinion that a corporation operates to serve the public interest by which it furnishes the shareholders with profit maximizing wealth. In other words, a business exists not only for the sole purpose of making profits for their stockholders, but also as an economic institution with social as well as profit maximizing function.(Dodd, 1932). Different models of CSR have evolved from Clark, Belre and Dodd's debates. They are the Moderate View, The Classical View, the Stakeholder View and Mute Stakeholders view.

The Moderate View

The Moderate View also known as the Doctrine of Enlightened Self-Interest states that "since a corporations profit from social activities, it is important that they contribute to the enlargement of the market, improvement of the workforce and helping the disadvantaged." These social actions will lead to reduction in welfare costs, crime, and wasted human potential. Further, they will aid in the combating of the insensitivity to society's changing demands thereby reducing the public pressures for government intervention and regulation (Solomon and Collins, 1987). The proponents of this theory strongly believe that corporations should price their products within the legal norms. They encourage, corporations to obey the law, despite the fact that compliance of this duty could reduce the profits. Especially, if the compliance costs exceeds the expected social value which could render the company unprofitable. Some of the moderate scholars view the legal compliance as irresponsible. They postulate that obeying the law is not the duty of a corporation and may be irresponsible socially if the return from an illegal act, CSR initiatives, will exceed the expected social value, especially in situations where the corporate resources are continuously used for non-profit and socially-maximizing activities. Further, since the objectives of investors, employees, customers and general public often are in conflict with corporate goals, managers must be guided by the shareholder interest. However, they cannot remain insensitive to other constituencies and remain consistent with long run interest of the enterprise. (Small, 1979).

The Classical View

In their dealings with corporate social responsibility, the classical economists separate social functions from economic functions. They are of the opinion that the main obligation of a corporation is to maximize profit for its owners. Carr, a proponent of the classical model asserts that "a company has the legal right to shape its strategy without reference to anything but its profits, so long as it stays within the rules of the game legally set out by law" (Carr 1968).

Milton Friedman, a major proponent of the "Classical view", emphasized that companies should behave honestly and resist from engaging in deception and fraud. However, he also stressed that the purpose of a company is to make profits for its shareholders. Thus, the responsibility of business is to use its resources to engage in profit making activities so long as it stays within the rules of the game. Further, managers are agents of the shareholders and therefore, they have a responsibility to conduct business in accordance with their interest. Under this postulation, he made it clear that shareholders are the owners of the company and therefore the profits belong to them. In his opinion, requiring managers to pursue socially responsible objectives may be unethical, because it obligates managers to spend money that belongs to the shareholders. Hence, requiring a company to engage in social responsibility activities is harmful to the foundations of a free society with a free-enterprise and private-property system. Social problems, therefore, should be left for the state to address. (Friedman, 1970).

Friedman's view on corporate social responsibility was echoed by Levitt in 1958. Levitt believed that companies should be concerned with improving production and increasing profits while abiding by the rules of the game, which include acting honestly and in good faith. For him, social problems should be left for the state to address (Levitt, 1958).

David Henderson, an ex-OECD Chief Economist and a critic of CSR, focused on outside interferences in corporate operations. He believed that CSR could lead to inefficient resource allocation. His concern was that CSR adversely affects a company's performance. However, his case against CSR rests primarily on the contention that it impairs the performance of business enterprises in their primary role as profit making entities. He opposes over-regulation, and views increased legislation in this matter to be harmful, and detrimental to business activities. He sees CSR as a leading contributor to ineffective markets, reduced wealth generation and increased social inequity and poverty (Henderson, 2005).

Although some of the classical theorists were adamant in defending the rights of shareholders' wealth maximization as the sole responsibility of corporate managers, others believed that stakeholders interest must be given due consideration in corporate operations. Carr, a strong defender of the pure profit-making view recognized that if a company wishes to take a long-term view of its profits, it will need to preserve amicable relations with whom it deals. He emphasized that a wise businessman will not seek advantage to the point where he generates dangerous hostility among employees, competitors, customers, government, or the public at large. However, he thought that "decisions in this area are, in the final test, decisions of strategy, not of ethics (Carr, 1968)."

The Stakeholder View

Stakeholder View Theory asserts "that companies have a social responsibility that requires them to consider the interests of all parties affected by their actions." The stakeholder view theory emphatically establishes that beyond shareholders there are several agents with interests in the actions and decisions of a company. The agents whom the corporations benefit from are the creditors, employees, customers, suppliers, and the communities at large. It is wise that management does not only consider the interest of its shareholders in the decision making process, but also the interest of anyone who is affected by business decisions (Freeman, 1998).

In contrast to the classical view, the stakeholder view holds that "the goal of any company should be the flourishing of the company and all its principal stakeholders (Ethane and Freeman, 1999).

As a particular version of stakeholder theory, shareholder view's moral presuppositions can be seen as including "respect for property rights, voluntary cooperation, and individual initiative to improve everyone's circumstances. "These presuppositions provide a good starting point, but not a complete vision of value creation (Werhane and Freeman, 2004)."

Research Question

The main research question is "Is the relationship between the African American community and the tobacco industry just a business relationship or a genuine effort on the part of the corporations to help bring about economic self sufficiency, and, at the same time, promote good health outcomes in the African American community?" In other words, are they likely to undertake corporate social responsibilities while at the same time pursuing profit maximizing goals in the African American communities?

In the United States, the corporate social responsibility of the tobacco industry within the African American community could be traced back to the 1930s.In the 1930s; Tobacco companies had a long-time financial support of educational and cultural organizations within the African American community. When the doors to mainstream society were closed to African Americans, the tobacco companies opened their doors wide, offering substantial contributions of time and money to support positive programs in the African American community (Sutton, 1992).In 1938, William Reynolds, the brother of RJ Reynolds, donated money to build the Kate Bitting Reynolds Hospital for Blacks in the segregated Winston-Salem, North Carolina (Morain, 1993). Approximately, half of all persons employed in manufacturing positions in the tobacco industry in the 1930s were African American (Northrup, 1970). Philip Morris was the first tobacco company to hire black salesmen (Brown, 1953) and RJ Reynolds (RJR) was the first in the industry to desegregate its facilities and integrate production lines (Kluger, 1996).

By the 1950s, the tobacco industry executives had established relationships with black organizations. Weissman volunteered with the National Urban League (NUL) and Cullman was an "active supporter of Urban League, National Association for the Advancement of Colored People(NAACP),United Negro College Fund(UNCF)," Cullman later joined the National Urban League(NUL) board of directors. By the time they became Philip Morris' top executives, Weissman and Cullman had been forming ties within the black community for over 30 years. The industry used its relationships with black organizations to recruit African Americans into its workforce, (which, in turn, intensified tobacco industry presence in black organizations. Many individuals hired by the industry were influential within the African American community. For example, in the 1940s, Phillip Morris hired Herb Wright, a former youth director for the NAACP. Wright worked for Phillip Morris for 30 years, expanding PM's reach into black colleges and black organizations (Yerger and Malone, 2002).

Targeted Market

The African American community has been targeted by the cigarette manufacturing companies for decades. Recognizing a declining consumer base, tobacco companies attempted to protect their profits by increasing smoking among African-Americans. It splashed inducements to smoke on billboards and buses, on subways, and in African-American publications. They sponsored athletic events, outdoor media campaigns, sports/cultural events, and academic scholarships. The tobacco industry developed specially named brands targeted specifically toward African-Americans. They spent a disproportionate amount of their promotional budget in an effort to hook black smokers (Lawrence, 2010).

The tobacco companies drew upon cultural stereotypes and played off their desire to eliminate racial inequalities in the United States of America. They specifically used mentholated cigarettes, as an accessory of necessity for African Americans seeking to maintain their culture and sense of "blackness", but also seeking upward social mobility. Menthol has been used as a medicinal practice for thousands of years (Stain, 2003).Menthol is steamed and distilled from peppermint oil to serve as a mild anesthetic that numbs the throat. Simultaneously, it protects the throat from the harsh elements of tobacco smoke, thus allowing for a deeper and longer inhalation (Stain, 2003).

A market research study conducted by R Davis in 1978 revealed that the cigarette companies knew that most African-American smokers prefer menthol cigarettes, and exploited that fact in their marketing efforts to African Americans in general and to African-American kids in particular, who tobacco companies often refer to as "young adult blacks(Davis,1978)." Menthol cigarettes have higher carbon monoxide concentrations than non-mentholated cigarettes and may be associated with greater absorption of nicotine. Specifically, research indicates that mentholated cigarettes may increase the risk of lung and bronchial cancer by promoting lung permeability and diffusion of smoke particles (Stain, 2010).

Relationships with African American Organizations

To ingratiate themselves with the African American community, powerful members of the tobacco industry strategized and sought out Black opinion leaders in order to enhance their corporate image, and to improve their market position within African

American communities (JRH, 1990). The industry also established a strong association with the public service efforts of African American organizations (Yerger and Malone, 2002). In 1989, Philip Morris sponsored a symposium organized in collaboration between the Joint Center for Political and Economic Studies, an African American, public policy think-tank, and the Smithsonian Institution. The symposium consisted of eight half-hour programs airing during Black History Month. The series was aired on over 200 radio stations in 50 countries (Knox, 1989). It was estimated that about three million listeners heard the broadcasts; each opened and closed with credits for Philip Morris, as well as the highlights of the tobacco industry's association with African American accomplishments.

RJ Reynolds, for example, associated the corporation with a highly regarded civil rights organization when it placed its corporate logo on billboards promoting the National Urban League's community service campaigns (RJ Reynolds, 1990). In addition, the tobacco industry financially supported African American civil, educational, social, and political organizations and community leaders elected on local, state and federal levels (Ruffin, 1991). Some of the events sponsored during the Congressional Black Caucus Foundation's Annual Legislative Weekend attracted up to 50,000 of the most influential black leaders in politics, government, business, education, and law (Smith, 1990).

The industry was very determined that its relationship with African American political organizations would achieve political and policy goals of the African American organizations. Its relationship with the Congressional Black Caucus Foundation (CBCF) became very important. It intensified its support for CBCF fund raising efforts and CBC's political activities. CBCF administers fellowship, internship, and scholarship programs for aspiring African American leaders. The tobacco industry supported the CBC and CBCF, including at least $125,000 in 1985, $45,000-$50,000 in 1986, and $155,000 in 1993 (Yerger and Malone, 2002; Scotts, 1987). For the tobacco industry, their involvement in these programs provided opportunities for the industry to link with individuals deemed likely to become future policy leaders and eventual allies (RJ Reynolds, 1983).

Answers to the Research Question

The results of this literature review indicate that the tobacco industry pursued an ambivalent relationship with the African American community. Yes, they were committed to corporate social responsibility through their financial support and association with African American organizations, political leaderships and socio-political causes. Their relations appear to have been established on genuine grounds. They were there to hire African Americans, put some of them in corporate leadership positions and fund their organizations when other industries had deprived them of all employment and economic opportunities. However, their subsequent behavior makes one question their motives for all the economic support they had been given by the African American communities since the 1930s. Were these supports just intended to gain major market access into the African American Community? Or was it purely a business relationship? If it was a genuine CSR, why did they ignore the cigarette related, detrimental impact on health outcomes in the African American Community? Why did they fight to hold on to their profit-maximizing interests? In other words, were they likely to pursue their marketing hold on the African American Community shrouded in corporate social responsibility or philanthropic initiatives mode regardless of the health problems emanating from cigarette smoking? For example the industry was clearly aware that smoking related diseases were devastating the African American Community. However, they adamantly opposed any legislation that could reduce cigarette smoking. For example in the 1980s, the Federal Government felt that by increasing the excise tax on tobacco, it could reduce tobacco use, especially among African Americans and Spanish speaking communities. Unfortunately, the tobacco industry came out heavily against it. A Philip Morris, 1987 memo expressed the industry's objection to such legislation as follows:

> You may recall that the 1982-83 rounds of price increases caused two million adults to quit smoking and prevented 600,000 teenagers from starting to smoke. Those teenagers are now 18-21 years old, and since about 70 percent of 18-21 year-olds and 35 percent

of older smokers smoke a PM brand; this means that 700,000 of those adult quitters had been PM smokers and 420,000 of the non-smokers would have been PM smokers . . . . [we] don't need to have that happen again (Johnston, 1987).

Unfortunately, the industry turned to the major African American organizations in opposing the excise tax on tobacco. According to the Tobacco Institute memo, released on June 27, 1985, they gained the support of major African American Organizations in their effort to defeat the excise tax:

Philip Morris staff has reported that the following groups have, or will submit statements in support of our position [on the excise tax]: NAACP, National Urban League, National Association of Black County Officials, National Coalition of 100 Black Women, National Black Police Association, West Coast Black Publishers Association and the Georgia Association of Black Elected Officials (Chilcote, 1985).

Owing to their major advertisement in black publications, the industry was also able to gain the support of some black media leaders. The back drop of this support even the Congressional Black Caucus was convinced that the increase in the excise tax was unfair, regressive, and disproportionately affected low income families, blacks and other minorities (Yerger and Malone, 2002).The industry representatives conducted press conferences and placed op-eds in Black new papers. Spearheading this effort was Congressman Mervyn Dynally, (Democrat California) who was the chair of the Congressional Black Caucus. By December 1987, the tobacco industry, convinced of Dynally's support, began to promote Rep. Dynally's report:

[Dynally] will conduct a press conference next week to release His report on excise tax regressivity . . . [The Tobacco Institute] is coordinating the press event and coverage . . ."92 "By the end of December [1987], twenty black publications had published op-eds prepared by . . . Dymally opposing increased federal excise taxes. We [the Tobacco Institute] coordinated the project (Sparber, 1988).

Opposition from the African American Community

As the tobacco industry and its allies were protecting their interest, the opposition to their activities was growing in the African American Community. The protest was led by Benjamin Hooks of the NAACP. His anti-targeting protest was heard very loudly by the tobacco industry. For Hooks, the NAACP, as an organization, was established to protect the interest of the African American community has the responsibility to lead this protest. Ben. Hooks, in his opposition to the tobacco industry, especially against RJ Reynolds, attempted to introduce a new cigarette, called *Uptown*, targeting the African American community. He said:

> As an organization deeply rooted in the black community, we at the NAACP are aware that the decision of the RJ Reynolds Company to single out this community as the target of its marketing efforts on behalf of . . . . *Uptown*, is being broadly perceived in a negative manner; the NAACP will seek a meeting to express our concerns with company officials (Hooks, 1990; Yerger and Malone, 2002).

The Action taken by the NAACP put the tobacco industry on notice that some of the black leadership would no longer stand aside to allow the negative impact of cigarette smoking on the health of the African American community. The African American opposition to the tobacco industry came to a head in Philadelphia in 1994, when a coalition of tobacco control activists accused the industry of targeting the African American community with a deadly product (Robinson and Sutton, 1994; Sutton, 2001).

Discussion of the Answers to the Research Question

It is an open secret that during the 1960s and 1970s, African American organizations, including the NAACP, National Urban

League, and several others received financial contributions from the tobacco industry (Gardiner,2004). In the 1950s and 1960s, when most US Corporations refused to support African American issues, the tobacco industry was willingly supporting education and cultural events in the African American community. It was also the tobacco industry which was willing to hire and promote African American employees even to the executive level, when other industries refused to do so. It was not by accident that the tobacco industry was considered a major ally in the struggle for racial equality by the African American community. For example, in the 1930's almost half of the people working in the tobacco manufacturing industry were African Americans. It was the only industry that was willing to provide some of the only industrial jobs at that time to African Americans (Yerger and Malone, 2002). At that time, Philip Morris and RJ Reynolds competed to see who could provide "equality" for African Americans (Center for Multicultural Health, Fall, 2006).

> It appears that the tobacco industry developed ties with virtually every African American leadership organization for three specific business reasons:
>
> i.   To increase use of tobacco among African Americans;
> ii. To use African Americans as a frontline force to defend the industry's policy positions; and
> iii. To defuse tobacco control efforts
>   (Yerger & Malone, 2002, Gardiner, 2004).

Consequently, the African American community, a marginalized group of people, sought financial help in their struggle for civil rights and economic self-sufficiency from its long term "ally", the tobacco industry which provided about $25 million yearly (Gardiner, 2001).

Limitations

This chapter was not intended to discuss all the problems associated with the relationship between the tobacco industry, the African American community and all anti-smoking legislatives. Neither was it the intention to discuss all the diseases associated with mentholated cigarettes and all the cigarettes smoked or used in the African American community. The main aim of the chapter was to find an answer to the research question: "Is the relationship between the African American community and the tobacco industry just a business relationship or a genuine effort on the part of the corporations to help bring economic self sufficiency, and, at the same time, promote good health outcomes in the African American community through corporate social responsibility?" The research was based on a review of the literature focusing on the tobacco industry and its relationship with the African American community.

Conclusion

The relationship between the tobacco industry and the African American community creates a philosophical dilemma among the competing theories regarding corporate social responsibility. The findings indicate that corporations can be profit maximizing and, at the same time, engage in corporate social responsibility initiatives. This was apparent in the tobacco industry's philanthropic and marketing initiatives in the African American organizations and community.

We can safely conclude that, as a corporate entity, the tobacco industry maximized profit, and, concurrently, engaged in a corporate social responsible policy which financially benefited the African American organizations and community in general. The hiring records of the industry of African Americans, when other industries refused to do so, provide evidence of a genuine effort on the part of the tobacco industry to help bring some semblance of economic self sufficiency to the African American community. It became obvious in our research that through its philanthropic activities, the industry found a lucrative market in the African American community. At the same time, however, through the establishment of a niche market in the African American community, the industry targeted that community with copious advertizing of menthol cigarettes, thereby influencing negative health outcomes.

The research results contradicted a part of the Classical View that states requiring managers to pursue socially responsible objectives may be unethical because the money belongs to the shareholders. In other words, requiring a company to engage in socially responsible activities is harmful to the foundations of a free society with a free-enterprise and private-property system. According to Friedman and Levitt, social problems should be left for the state to address. In the case of the African American, civil right organizations, some of the state laws were staged against the social and racial equality of the African American. It is obvious that without undertaking serious corporate social responsibility initiatives by the tobacco industry, it is possible that some of the African American civil rights organizations might have not been able to obtain the financial support required to accomplish some of their goals and objectives.

David Henderson of the Classical View was also wrong when he contended (or argued) that CSR adversely affects a company's performance and that that it impairs the performance of business enterprises in their primary role, and would make people in general poorer. For instance, the tobacco industry remained prosperous while, at the same time, gave financial support to African American organizations. Through the industry's financial support to their advertisements, African American media became strong companies. Unfortunately, African American media eventually became the strong supporters of the tobacco industry's product marketing in the African American community. Unwittingly, they became part of the industry's efforts to promote negative health outcomes.

The industry's financial support for African American organizations and leadership bolstered their market grip on the community, and it received the support of the African American leadership in the 1980s in its fight against excise tax legislation which was intended to decrease cigarette smoking especially in the African American community. The tobacco companies, through their internal research, knew that menthol cigarettes, including *Kools* were contributing to the cancer epidemic and other respiratory diseases in the African American community. The industry ignored findings by outside scientists, and negated their own negative findings. Bolstered by their own findings, the industry continued advertising mentholated products to the African American community. Studies have found that more cigarette advertisements were placed in African American magazines such as *Ebony* and *Jet* than mainstream magazines like *Time* and *People* (Jain, 2010) A study conducted in 2002, indicated that there more exterior and interior tobacco advertisements within the poor environments that had a greater number of African Americans than in predominantly white Americans and middle and upper class communities (Jain, 2010). This corporate profit, maximization resulting in major detrimental, health outcomes in the African American community, ignored human suffering, and, should be viewed as unethical and certainly inhumane. Although we cannot ignore the decades of the industry's philanthropic activities in the African American communities, we can only ask the industry this question "Was the profit maximization efforts in the African American community more important than the human suffering resulting from cigarette smoking?" Did not the negative, health outcomes make it questionable or overshadow the decades of the industry's philanthropic efforts in the African American Community?"

Based on the review in this chapter, we can conclude that both the Moderate View and the Stakeholders View have prevailed. This is especially the case with the Moderate View that stresses a corporation profits from social activities; therefore, it is important that they contribute to the enlargement of the market, improvement of the workforce and helping the disadvantaged. These social actions will help to reduce the costs of welfare, crime, and wasted human potential. The tobacco industry's continued employment of African Americans underscores the Moderate View. The Moderate View is fully supported by the Stakeholders View which correctly characterizes the single-objective view of the shareholder advocates, as "a narrow view that cannot possibly do justice to the panoply of human activity that is value creation and trade, i.e., business."

It is our opinion that the relationship between the African American community and the tobacco industry was both a business relationship and a genuine effort on the part of the industry to help foster economic self sufficiency in the African American community and in its fight for civil rights. In this chapter, CSR was intended to be an inbuilt and self-regulating mechanism fostering the tobacco industry's adherence to laws, ethical standards, and codes of responsibility in their operation in the African American community. However, the resulting evidence has shown that the industry allowed economic greed to overpower its best efforts in corporate social responsibility by violating laws and ethical standards, codes of responsibility and driving itself to social disrepute. In the current dynamic global economy and its environments, corporations cannot afford to ignore the interest of other stakeholders and embark on the objective of pushing for wealth maximization policy alone for its traditional stockholders. The wealth maximization policy must be concurrently executed with sound, corporate, responsible policy to ensure the interest of the other stakeholders and the company's long term survival. This principle was ignored by the tobacco industry and this, eventually, has contributed to their demise in the 1990s through court cases brought against them by the states. In the meantime, the policy has led to increasingly poorer health outcomes for such groups as African Americans.

References

Abbot, W.F., and R.J. Monsen (1979). On the measurement of corporate social responsibility self reported disclosures and method of measuring corporate social involvement. *Academy of Management Journal, 2* (3); 501-555.

Alexander, G.J., and R.A. Buchholz, (1978). Corporate social responsibility and stock market performance. *Academy of Management Journal 21*(3); 479-486.

Belkaoui. A. (1976). *The impact of the disclosure of the environmental effects* of *organizational behavior on the* market. Financial Management, Winter: 26-3 1.

Bragdon, J.H., and T.T. Marlin, (1972). Is pollution profitable? *Risk Management 19*(2), 9-19.

Buchholz, R.A. (2004), The natural environment: Does it count? *Academy of Management Executive 18*(2), 130-133.

Berle, Adolf, (1931). Corporate powers in trust. *Harvard Law Review 44,* (1049).

Branco, E.C., and Rodriguez, L.L. (2007). Issues in corporate social responsibility and environmental reporting research: An overview. *Issues in Social Accounting1* (1), 72-90.

Brown, G, F., (1953). *Philip Morris' Human Relations Program Sets Pace for Industry.* Philip Morris Companies Inc. 17 October 1953. Access date: 12 December 2001. Bates No. 2041942541-2544. URL:http://legacy.library.ucsf.edu/tid/nqe45d00.

Capron, M. (2003). *Economie Ethique Privee: La Responsibilite' de Enteprese L'Preuve de L'humanisation de la Mondialisation.* United Nations Scientific and Cultural Organization, Paris: 15.

Carr, A. (1968). Is business bluffing ethical? *Harvard Business Review, 46* (January-February); 143-153.

Center for Disease Control, (1998). *African Americans and Tobacco.* http://www.cdc.gov/tobacco/data statistics/sgr/sgr 1998/sgr-min-afr.htm.

Center for Multicultural Health, (2006). *Searching for Answers, Volume 1*, Issue 1, Fall 2006.

Champling, D.P. and J.T. Knoedler, (2004). J.M Clark and the economics of responsibility. *Journal of Economic Issues, 38* (2), (June 4), 545-552.

Chen, K.H., and R.W. Metcalf, (1980). The relationship between pollution control record and financial indicators revisited. *The Accounting Review 55*(1), 168-177.

Chilocote, S. (1985). *Memo to Executive Committee. Tobacco Institute.27 June 1985.* Access date 6 August 2001.Bates NO.85694277-4279. http//www.legacy.library.ucsf.edu/tid/fci31e00.

Clark, J.M. (1921). The socializing of theoretical economics. *Journal of Economic Issues 132,* 132-147.

Coolish, M.L. (1997). Medieval foundations of western intellectual tradition, AD 400-1400. Yale University Press: New Haven, CT, 26.

Davidson, W. N., and D.C.Worrell, (1988). The impact of corporate illegalities on shareholder returns. *Academy of Management Journal 31*(1); 195-200.

Davis, R. (1978), *Black marketing: Research-findings and recommendations to date, Lorillard.* June 9. Bates NO.84274935/4944. Http://www.legacyforhealth.org/PDF/FDA_Testimony-Dr. CherylHealton.

Freeman, M. and B. Jaggi, (1986). An analysis of the impact of corporate pollution included in annual financial statement on investment decisions", in M. Neimark (Ed) *Advances in public interest accounting.* New Haven CT: JAI. 193-212.

Freeman, R. E., A.C. Wicks, and R. Parmar, (2004). Stakeholder theory and corporate objectives. Revisited. *Organization Science 15*(3), May-June; 364-369.

Friedman, M. (1970). The social responsibility of business is to increase its profits. *New York Times Magazine* (November 13); 126.

Gardiner, Phillip S., (2004). The African Americanization of menthol cigarette use in the United States. *Nicotine & Tobacco Research, Volume 6,* Supplement 1, February, 2004, 55-65.

Gardiner, Phillip, S. (2001). Tobacco industry philanthropy in the black community. *Burning Issues; Tobacco Related Disease Research Program Newsletter,* July 2001; 4:1-3.

Griffin,J.,and J.F.Mahon, (1997). The corporate social performance and corporate financial performance debate. *Business and Society 36*(1), 5-31.

Hardie, A., (2009). Wal-Mart supports Communities around the globe with $423 million in charitable contributions. *CSR Wire,* (April 2).

Health and Human Services, (1998). *Tobacco use in racial/ethnic minority neighborhoods; A report of the Surgeon General,* URL, http://www.cdc.gov/tobacco/data statistics/sgr 1998/index.htm

Henderson,D. (2005). Misguided virtue: False notions of corporate social responsibility. The good company. *Economist* (January 22). London Institute of Economic Affairs, 171.

Holman, W.R., J.R. New, and D. Singer,(1990). The impact of corporate social responsiveness on shareholder wealth. In E. Preston (Ed), *Corporation and society research studies in theory and measurement.* Greenwich, CT: JAI, 265-279.

Hooks, B. (1990). Letter to RJ Reynolds: President James Johnston. *NAACP.19 January 1990.* Access date: July 2001. BatesNO507777182. URL:http://www.rjrdocs.com/rjrdocs

Ingram, R.W. and K.B. Frazier, (1983). A narrative disclosure. *Journal of Business Research, Vol.11,* 49-60.

Jacob, M., (1997). The environment as a stakeholder. *Business Strategy Review, 6*(2), 25-28.

Jain, S.L., (2010). Tobacco company markets marketing to African Americans. *Foster Folly News.* Chipley, Florida. Online Newspaper: 22 February, Web 29 April 2010. http://www.fosterfollynews.com/news

Jerrell, G. and S. Peltman, (1985). The impact of product recalls on the wealth of sellers. *Journal of Political Economy 93*(3), 512-536.

Johnson, RA and D W Greening,(1994). Relationship between corporate social performance, financial performance, and firm governance. In *Proceedings of the Academy of Management,* 314-318.

Johnston, M., (1987). Handling on excise tax increase. *Philip Morris, USA. 3 September 1987.*

Access date: 23 July 2001. Bates NO2022216179-6180. URL, Http://www.legacy. library.ucsf.edu/tid/uvk71f00

Jorgenson, H.B., J. Pruzon, M. Junck, and A. Cramer, (2003), Strengthening implementation of corporate social responsibility in the global supply chain. *The World Bank,* (October), 1-1-119.

JRH Marketing Services Inc. (1990). Summary Report of Qualitative Research on Corporate Image Advertising Among African American Opinion Leaders. Prepared for RJ Nabisco,

May 1990. Access date: 25 January 2002. Bates No507712740-2759, URL, http://www. legacy.library.ucsf.edu/tid/dux I4d00

Kedia,B. and E.C. Kuntz,(1981). The context of social performance: An empirical study of Texas banks. In L E Preston (Ed), *Research in corporate social performance and policy, Vol.3,* Greenwich, CT: JAI, 133-154.

Kluger R. (2001). Ashes to Ashes: America's Hundred Years Cigarette, 12 December 2001. Bates No. 2041942541-2544. http://legacy.library.ucsf.edu/tid/nqe45d00

Knox, G. (1989). African Americans and the evolution of a living constitution. *Philip Morris Companies Inc.3 May 1989.* Access date 23 September 200. Bates No2023277409-7410. http://www. legacy.library.ucsf.edu/tid/nsw36e00

Law, S. A., (1992). Addiction, autonomy and advertising, 77 *Iowa L. Review,* 909-913.

Lawrence,D, (2010). Tobacco Industry Targeting of the African-American Community. http://www.blackhealthzone. com/tobacco-industry-targeting.

Lerner,L.D., and G.E Fryxell, (1988). An empirical study of predictors of corporate social performance: A multi-dimensional analysis. *Journal of Business Ethics, 7,* 951-959.

Levitt, T. (1998). The danger of social responsibility. *Harvard Business Review 36*; 41-50.

Marcus, A.A., and R.S. Goodman,(1986), Compliance and performance: Towards a Contingency Theory. In L.E. Preston and JE Post (Eds), *Research in Corporate Social Performance and Policy, Vol.8*, Greenwich, CT: JAI, 193-221.

Morain, Claudia, (1993). Kiss of death: African-Americans and the tobacco industry. *Am. Med. News, November 15*, 13

Moskowwitz, M. (1972). Choosing socially responsible stocks. *Business and Society 10*, 71-75.

Moskowwitz, M. (1975). Profiles in corporate responsibility: The ten worst and the ten best. *Business and Society Review 13*: 28-42

Newgren, K. E., A. A. Rasher, M. E. LaRoe, and M. R. Szabo (1985). Environmental assessment and corporate performance: A longitudinal analysis using a market-determined performance measure. *Research in Corporate Social Performance and Policy, 7*: 153-164.

Northrup H.(1970), Ash R. The Racial Policies of American Industry: The Negro in the Tobacco Industry: Report No. 13. Wharton School of Finance and Commerce, Department of Industry, Industrial Research Unit, University of Pennsylvania.

Phillips, R.A. and J. Reichart, (2000). The environment as a stakeholder? A fairness-based approach. *Journal of Business Ethics, 23*(2); 185-197.

Power, J. (2010). Corporate social responsibility: Profile of United Nations global compact. *CSR Wire,* August 12;(www. unglobalcompact.org).

Preston J. (ed) *Research in corporate social performance and policy, Vol 7*, Greenwich, CT: JAI RJ Reynolds.(1990). Black Market Corporate Creative Strategy.18 January 1990. Access date.10 January 2002. Bates No. O.507234461. http:edu/tid/xsr15d00.

Reynolds, R. J. (1983). Minority Affairs Publicity Programs. Access date:4 march 2002. Bates NO.505478647-8675. http. library. ucsf.edu/tid/xsr15d00.

Robinson,R.G.and Sutton, C.,(1994). The coalition against the *Uptown* cigarette. In D. Jennigan and P.A. Wright (Eds), *Making news, changing policy: Case studies of media advocacy on alcohol and tobacco Issues.* Rockville, MD: University Research. Corporation and Martin Institute for Prevention of Alcohol and Other Drug Problems, Center for Substance Abuse Prevention.

Ruffin, B. (1991). Public Service Billboard Ads: RJ Reynolds Tobacco Co.16 September 1991. Access date: 20 August 2001. Bates NO.507763484-3485. http//www.legacy. library.ucsf.edu/ tid/afs14d00.

Schmeitz, K.E., and M. Epstein, (1990). Does corporate social responsibility pay: evidence from failed 1990 WTO meeting in Seattle. *Graziadio Business Report, 7,* (2), 1-7.

Scot, S., (1987). Congressional Black Caucus Foundation Fashion Shows. Philip Morris Companies Inc. Access date:13 March 2001. Bates No. 204900443. URL, Http://www.legacy.library. ucsf/tid/dew83e00.

Shane, P.B. and B.H. Spicer, (1983). Market responses to environmental information product outside the firma. *The Accounting Review 58*(3); 521-538.

Small, M. L., (1979). Evolving role of the director in corporate governance. *Hastings Law Journal,* 1353-1368.

Smith, G.(1990).,September Report of Public Affairs. Philip Morris Companies Inc.11 October 1990. Access date: 7 February 2001. Bates NO.2047572404-2409.URL: Http://www. legacy.library. ucsf.edu/tid/uqb72e00.

Sparber P. and Ross J, et al, (1988). Public Affairs Progress Report. Tobacco Institute.28 January 1988. Access date:17 April 2001. Bates NO. atidN0018389-8431.URL, Http://www legacy. Library.ucsf.edu/tid/gyh91f00.

Spencer, B.A. and Taylor, G.S., (1987). A within and between analysis of the relationship between corporate social responsibility and financial performance. *Akron Business and Economic Review 18*(3); 7-18.

Solomon, L. D. and Kathleen J. Collins, (1987). Humanistic economics: A new model for the corporate social responsibility debate. *Journal of Corporate Law*, 332-351.

Stain, S.L (2003). Come up to Kool taste: African American upward mobility and the semiotics of smoking menthols. *Public Culture*, 295-322.

Stain, S.L.(2010). Tobacco company marketing to African Americans. *Foster Folly News*—Chipley, Florida: Online Newspaper, 22 February 2010.

Studivant, F.D. and J.L. Ginter, (1977). Corporate social responsiveness: Management attitudes and economic performance. *California Management Review 19*(3), 30-39.

Sutton, C.D. (1992). Tobacco Companies: Targeting the African American Community. The Onyx Group. URL,Http://onyx-gropup.com.

Sutton, C.D.,(2001). The Coalition Against *Uptown* Cigarettes: Marketing Practices and Community Mobilization. Retrieved October 30,2003 from URL,Http://onyx.group. uptown1.html

Vance, S.C., (1975). Are socially responsible corporations good investment risks? Academy of *Management Review 19*; 450-477.

Waddock, SA and S B Graves, (1994). The Corporate Social Performance: Financial Link Paper Presented at the National Meeting of the Academy of Management, Dallas, TX. (August)

Werhane, P.H., and R.E. Freeman, (1999). Business ethics: The state of the art", *IJMR*, (March), 8.

Yerger, VB and Malone, RE., (2002). African American leadership groups: Smoking with the enemy. *Tobacco Control, 11*, 336-345.

CHAPTER SIX

Assessing the Mental Health Concerns of the Hip-Hop Generation for Culturally Competent Health Care

Charles Pinckney
University of North Carolina at Charlotte

Elizabeth Alston-Pinckney
Livingstone College

Abstract

Assessing the mental health affairs of this generation is critical to their overall development. Failure to adequately address the mental health needs of the hip-hop generation will have adverse effects on this population and future generations. The mental health of this population continues to be a hot-button topic. African Americans from this generation are more likely to suffer from one or more mental health disorders. The lack of a comprehensive database focusing on mental health and the hip-hop generation makes working with this population very difficult. It should not come as a surprise that this generation continues to experience an array of emotional struggles. Their concerns are many; the lack of economic opportunities, education, housing, employment, safety and welfare has increased the opportunity for mental challenges not seen in earlier generations. This chapter explores the mental health and cultural realities of this generation, ranging from substance-related disorder, posttraumatic stress disorder, antisocial personality disorders and lack of access to health care that is culturally sensitive to their needs.

Introduction

I think it's time I made a song for niggaz who don't know me.
I think it's time I made a song for niggaz who don't know me.
I graduated out the streets, I'm a real O.G. I been trappin', shootin' pistols since I stood 4 feet.
So all you niggaz actin' bad, you gon have to show me.
You gon make me bring this Chevy to a real slow creep.
My niggaz hangin' out the window, mouth fulla gold teeth (T.I., 2004).

As evident through this short excerpt from the rapper T.I., many older African Americans are clueless and even more fearful of interfacing with members of the hip-hop generation. This is particularly true for many health care providers. It is important to note that many hip-hoppers represent a different set of generational values that are connected to the streets, denoting a mental attitude that is closely related to the preceding verse by T.I. For the purpose of this discussion, the hip-hop generation is defined as those individuals born after 1965. In particular, young African Americans from the hip-hop generation between the ages of 13 and 24 today are twice as likely to carry around with them daily a mixture of emotional baggage.

The hip-hop culture represents the expression of relationships between youth and their environment. It represents the deep rooted culture of Black and Latino people. Other aspects of their culture such as language, styles of dress and politics are of great importance. The hip-hop culture is commonly recognized by its main elements: Graffiti, Djing, Break Dancing, B-Boying, Mcing (Rapping), and Beat Boxing (Kitwana, 2002)). The origins of hip-hop culture can be traced back to New York City, during the mid to late 1970's. The hip-hop culture represents the expression of relationships between youth and their environment. It represents the deep rooted culture of Black and Latinos people. Other aspects of their culture such as language, styles of dress and politics are of great importance. The hip-hop culture is fundamentally an "oppositional culture," which is categorized as a youth subculture, protesting the cultural values and norms of the mainstream. The culture is distinguished by its language, style, fashion, culture, values, beliefs, and mental orientation.

The origins of hip-hop culture can be traced back to New York City during the mid to late 1970's. The culture is so much more than mere art and entertainment, as seen on television or heard on radio, or on internet broadcasts. It is constantly evolving in the form of sprit and consciousness. The culture keeps recreating itself in a never ending cycle of culture realities. From a therapeutic standpoint, hip-hop culture, through its music and various multi-media outlets has presented moments of joy, pleasure, sorrow, pain, victory, defeat, confusion, anger, humor, and even life and death. In its truest form, the spirit of hip-hop culture connects the past to the present and lays the forward path towards future mental scrutiny. The hip-hop culture should not be assimilated, diluted or watered—down; it should be valued and used according to the mental liberation of this generation.

The many forms of emotional baggage that this generation has been confronted with have become a major concern for both health care and human services providers. If members of the hip-hop generation are going to be successful, they must first and foremost be in total control of their emotions. This generation cannot afford to allow their emotions to control their every action. The emotional intelligence of this generation is definitely worthy of investigation. Many of these young people have no clue as to how to manage their emotional intelligence, not to mention their attempts to define emotional intelligence. Emotional intelligence is characterized by a person's social and emotional skills; it also encompasses self-insight and self-control (Salovey, Stroud, Woolery, & Epel, 2002). It is important to note that the life experiences of this generation have reshaped the level and lack of emotional intelligence, as it relates to life challenges and events. Many from this generation continue to demonstrate poor self-control and self-insight. Furthermore, many non-hip hoppers believe that this generation lacks the ability to control their social and emotional feelings. Emotional behaviors ranging from substance use and abuse, posttraumatic stress disorder (PTSD), and antisocial disorders have become very problematic, not to mention a public health concern, among mental health professionals. These and other behaviors are keeping the mental health and counseling professionals extremely busy.

The hip-hop generation is that sub-group within the African-American community that mental health service agencies have the hardest time reaching, because of the cultural gap between the service providers and the people in need of services. This is due in part to inherent mistrust on both sides resulting from the level of cultural difference and misunderstanding. As a result the mistrust they are most likely to be negatively impacted by the influence of the culture and lack of mental health education. Service providers should employ a non-culturally relevant approach to addressing the mental health needs of the hip-hop generation. The primary mental health issues facing the hip-hop generation are wellness and mental health issues. Other common diagnosable mental health illnesses among this generation include bi-polar disorder, schizophrenia and depression. It is estimated that 15 million people suffer with serious mental disorders. Among these risk factors, violence, incarceration, and unemployment also play a significant role. The hip-hop community continues to struggle with mental health issues, because they are often hesitant to seek treatment or openly speak about their problems.

Figure 1 illustrates some of the major social realities associated with the hip-hop culture. This generation embraces thrill seeking and seeks instance gratification. Violence, aggression negative behaviors and challenging lifestyle modeling are all too common with this population. The social realities clearly show that disproportionately members of the hip-hop generation continue to struggle with substance-related disorders, posttraumatic stress disorder, and antisocial disorders. Individuals who experience Posttraumatic Stress Disorder (PTSD) are persons who have recently experienced large amounts of social unrest and community conflict. Specific cultural assessments about the traumatic events are needed by therapists to know the best way to proceed when serving this population. Some of the associated features of PTSD include environmental violence, sexual assault, physical abuse, death, serious injury, natural disasters, incarceration, and life threatening events. It is important to note that interpersonal stressors may also foster negative feelings of hopelessness, and despair among its members.

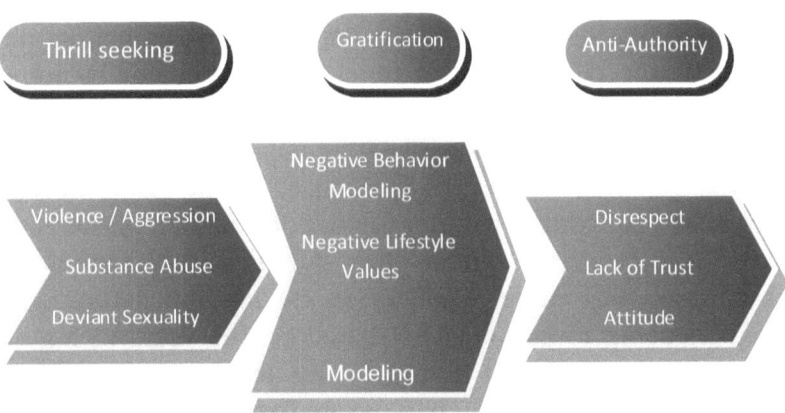

Figure 1. **Understanding the social realities of the Hip Hop generation**

Posttraumatic Stress Disorder

Posttraumatic stress disorder (PTSD) among members of the hip-hop generation has been largely ignored by the larger community. The correlation between the hip-hop generation and PTSD can no longer be overlooked. PTSD symptoms include outbursts of anger, trouble sleeping, inability to concentrate, and heightened anxiety. PTSD, as with many other mental disorders, if left untreated can interfere with this generation's overall success and functioning. The newest group to become victims of PTSD is the hip-hop generation population. Some potential causes of PTSD observed in the hip-hop generation population include poverty, violence, and drug abuse that result in a constant reminder of the negative aspects of life, not to mention personal negative life experiences. It is estimated that one third of all children in the United States are living in urban war zones and have experienced some form of PTSD. Personal experiences including environmental incarceration, abusive relationships, drug addiction, and violence are sure to play tricks on the minds of young African Americans who represent the hip-hop generation.

Many individuals who represent the hip-hop generation that have been directly exposed to violence, substance abuse, physical and inappropriate sexual behaviors are twice as likely to experience problems. The high prevalence of traumatic life events has the potential to increase the number of PTSD outbreaks among members of this generation. It should not come as a surprise that so many young hip-hoppers are suffering from serious traumatic community and social ills. This generation brings with them a unique set of challenges for health care and human service professionals to address. These challenges are based upon their childhood experiences, including, but not limited to abuse, abandonment, poverty, and violence within their families and communities. It is amazing that more members of the hip-hop generation are not experiencing forms of PTSD based on the years of rage and pent-up emotions resulting from the daily negative experiences and stressors of life. More research in the area of PTSD and the hip-hop generation is needed in order to help service providers to better serve this generation.

Substance Use Disorder

The second disorder is substance use disorder, which refers to the use of drugs or abuse of alcohol. The continued use of chemical substances can lead to the development of substance-use disorder. Substance use disorder is divided into eleven substance sub-groups: alcohol, amphetamine, caffeine, cannabis, cocaine, hallucinogens, inhalants, and nicotine, opioids, phencyclidine, and sedatives hypnotics.

Substance use and abuse among the hip-hop population continues to be very problematic, and a major public health problem (Kitwana, 2002). There appears to be a correlation between substance use and the hip-hop generation population (Morgan, 1999). The constant referencing and modeling of alcohol and drugs in hip-hop music lyrics and videos appears to be a form of endorsement or sanctioning. Furthermore, product placement by several alcohol beverage companies has also increased the visibility of alcohol consumption among the hip-hop culture (Ogunnaike, 2005). Rap artists Petey Pablo, Busta Rhymes, and Jay-Z all endorse alcoholic beverages. In addition, Lil Wayne and T-Pain have been tagged for the *Nuvo Black Label Liqueur*. These artists have all helped to reshape and promote alcohol consumption among the hip-hop generation. Many of these companies are getting free advertisement by attaching and marketing their products to hip-hop generation artists (Ogunnaike, 2005). Today, many rap musicians make constant reference to one of the most popular and addictive illegal drugs to surface since crack cocaine. Ecstasy appears to be the drug of choice for the hip-hop generation (Brown, 2000). It is not uncommon to hear Eminem or Jay-Z rapping about Ecstasy (Brown, 2000). Even the late Notorious B.I.G. made reference to Ecstasy in his first album, Life After Death, on which his lyrics include "some say that the X makes the sex spectacular" (Brown, 2000).

In 1992, Dr. Dre released an album entitled *The Chronic*. After the release of the CD, the use of marijuana seemingly increased within the hip-hop generation culture. This CD introduced thousands of African Americans to an array of inappropriate lifestyle modeling. Even today, the term, "the chronic," continues to be a popular term among college students and particularly African Americans.

The term, "the chronic," refers to a high grade of marijuana that is heavily consumed by members of the hip-hop generation. A Dr. Dre video from this album depicts young adults smoking marijuana and consuming alcohol, and the album's lyrics remain fresh in the minds of African American hip-hop generation college students. According to Majors and Billson (1992), many within the hip-hop group use substances as a means of being cool and coping with life's everyday stressors, including depression. It would appear that substance use and abuse is a way of life for some African Americans. Despite the fact that researchers suggest that African Americans drink less alcohol and consume less illegal drugs than their European American counterparts, the issue remains that any alcohol and drug use is problematic within the hip-hop generation population (Kapner, 2003). More empirical research is needed to assess the alcohol and drug consumption habits among members of the hip-hop generation.

Antisocial Personality Disorder

Antisocial personality disorder is the third disorder discussed. This disorder represents a pervasive pattern of disregard for, and violation of, the rights of others. For this diagnosis to be given to an individual, that person must be at least 18 years of age or older. Individuals with antisocial personality disorder fail to obey social norms; they repeatedly engage in unlawful behaviors often resulting in arrest. They also frequently engage in deceitful maladaptive manipulative behavior aimed at gaining some form of pleasure. In addition, they often lie or steal. Most importantly, antisocial personality disorder appears to be associated with low socioeconomic status and urban setting, which is highly represented of the hip-hop culture generation.

Deviant sexual behaviors, violence, and aggression among members of the hip-hop generation are problematic concerns classified in the category of antisocial disorders. Sexual promiscuity is more prevalent today than ever. Sexual references in songs and music videos are very appealing to the hip-hop generation. African American women continue to be exploited in music videos as unfiltered sexual images by artists and music producers to help market and sell hip-hop music (Morgan, 1999). These powerful images and values can easily be learned and modeled, thus causing damaging consequences (Franklin & Franklin, 2001).

Some music videos challenge the perceptions and values of this generation because they have the ability to model and teach new sexual experiences. The musician, Ludacris, for example, raps about a sexual fantasy with a woman vividly illustrated in the song and video entitled, *What's Your Fantasy*.

> I wanna, li-li-li-lick you from yo' head to yo toe and I wanna, move from the bed down to down to the flo'. Then I wanna, ahh ahh, you make it so good I don't wanna leave. But I gotta, kn-kn-kn-know what's your fantasy. (Ludacris, 2000).

In the video, partially nude women dance provocatively as male and female rappers describe their gender-specific sexual fantasies. Many of the women who appear in music videos are often considered sexual play toys for males (Rose, 1994). Music videos that offer suggestive innuendo and half-naked girls are appealing to viewers. The modeling of this type of sexual experience has the ability to challenge cognitive perceptions about appropriate and inappropriate sexual behaviors (Truglio, 1998). According to Truglio (1998), this results in poor social cognitive constructs of reality. Brown (1985) suggested that the types of sexual stimuli found in music videos send conflicting messages, leave viewers overwhelmed and confused about what is appropriate and inappropriate. This type of media exposure has desensitized viewers, thus increasing the risk of irresponsible thoughts and behaviors and resulting in negative consequences such as STDs including HIV/AIDS, sexual assault, and pregnancy. It is equally important to note that the hip-hop generation has one of the highest rates of HIV infection among African Americans.

In 2002, Ward found that hip-hop music videos have the ability to influence sexual politics by promoting and sanctioning irresponsible sexual behavior. Today, historically Black college and university communities are witnessing the very same sexual politics played in music videos being acted out on their campuses. In addition to music videos, the hip-hop generation population continues to be exposed to a variety of sexual stimuli ranging from magazines to daily television and radio programming (Ooms, 1981). Violence and aggression have also become very problematic for the hip-hop culture generation. In the early days of hip-hop, rap musicians rapped about deterring violence; today, they are rapping openly about violence. In fact, their microphones can be compared to weapons, and rap lyrics are similar to gunshots (Kelley, 1997). For example, Fifty Cent raps about alcohol consumption, drugs, sexual behavior, and violence. His song, *Don't Push Me,* promotes aggression and violence as demonstrated in the following lyrics:

> Right now, I'm on the edge, so don't push me. I am straight
> For your head, so don't push me. Fill your ass up with lead,
> so don't push me. I got somethin' for that ass, keep thinkin'
> I'm pussy (Fifty Cent, 2003).

When artists like Fifty Cent and others use the microphone to rap about aggression and violence, the microphone becomes a dangerous cognitive tool. McCall (1997) explained that these rap lyrics can be psychologically damaging to African Americans. Despite this, Fifty Cent and others are recognized as role models, as noted in Kitwana (2002). It is unfortunate that more and more hip-hop artists are viewed as role models, as many of the explicit forms of their role modeling include selling drugs, pimping women, hustling, and misogyny.

Wade and Gunner's (1993) research suggests that some males who watch repeated sexually violent music videos are more likely to engage in aggressive and criminal sexual behavior. In fact, they found that the attitudes of African American male students toward sexual assault were more likely to be influenced by some forms of rap music—in particular, gangsta rap. Wade and Gunner (1993) believed that criminal sexual behaviors such as gang rape and sexual assault by males are likely to be influenced by some forms of suggested gangsta-related rap music and music videos. The perceptions of many from the hip-hop generation have been psychologically damaged as a result of the violent lyrics and inappropriate modeling found in hip-hop music and videos. According to McCall (1997), the very chants and rhythms in hip-hop music appear to be reshaping the attitudes and values of young African Americans. Rose (1994) believed that lyrics found within hip-hop music today suggest that aggression and violence are normal behaviors. A number of issues today continue to challenge health care and human service professionals as they attempt to monitor the pulse of this generation in an attempt to provide competent quality care and service for them.

Counselors or therapists who seek to address the concerns of the hip-hop generation must understand the need for offering a social menu that includes the development of service planning that is connected to the hip-hop culture generation. Disproportionately, this generation has fallen victim to their social environments and stressful circumstances. Counselors who serve this generation cannot afford the luxury of prolonging or possibly confusing the client about the nature and role of the counselor/therapist. Service providers must alter their current strategies in order to enhance the mental health care for the hip-hop generation.

Culturally Competent Strategies

To better understand the impact of hip-hop culture and the roles that society plays in providing mental health services, one must understand that the key to developing effective mental health services includes being more responsive to, and accepting of, the cultural and social context of the hip-hop culture population. Valuing, not de-valuing hip-hop culture is most important, because it bears upon what the client will bring into the clinical setting. This is extremely true in terms of the culture; hip-hop has a tremendous amount of influencing power. The health and mental health care industry in the United States are embedded in Western science and medicine, which places little or no emphasis on hip-hop culture. What follows are four examples, which depict how hip-hop culture has influenced the way that mental health services are being offered:

Example One

Dr. Catherine Sori, Associate Professor of Counseling at Governors State University has been using hip-hop in her counseling sessions for several years. According to Dr. Sori, hip-hop works as a counseling technique because it offers the client the opportunity to utilize a culturally relevant approach to solving their underlining problems. It also allows clients to share relevant stories and themes about their lives in their own words. Within the therapeutic community, hip-hop culture can be used to gain insight about multiple sensory experiences that incorporate illustrations of lifestyle behaviors and interactions (Sori and Hecker 2008). Specific application of using hip-hop in therapy could include allowing the clients to write and perform a mini rap songs telling about their lives, daily struggles, and even hope for the future. The use of various forms of hip-hop culture in the counseling session is a great way to promote positive feelings about oneself and others, thus enhancing the therapeutic experience.

Example Two

The incorporation of hip-hop culture into local community-based mental health centers has proven to be effective. Important messages pertaining to HIV/AIDS, substance abuse, teen pregnancy, violence and other antisocial behaviors can be communicated through the medium of hip-hop culture (Kitwana, 2002). Traditional mental health prevention efforts have failed to reach this generation because of inadequate methods of reaching out to this population (McLaurin & Juzang, 1993). According to (McLaurin & Juzang, 1993), the mental health community can address behaviors such as sexual promiscuity, substance abuse and HIV/AID prevention through the use of hip-hop culture. Mental health professionals must be able to identify specific lifestyles, behavioral clues and social values of this generation This identification could be the music, attitudes, cultural values, fashion, language, and /or the ability to be expressive, or not. One of the more recent campaigns targeting HIV/AIDS was the BET "Rap It Up" campaign. This campaign was co-sponsored by the Kaiser Family Foundation and BET. This campaign featured a number of popular rap artists discussing the importance of safe sex. These campaigns were intended to reach, teach, and re-direct casual sexual behavior of this generation. The "Rap It Up" campaign was an example of the industry becoming more socially responsible, thus promoting social change. Rap musicians have the ability to articulate critical messages about sexuality and sexual politics, through their music and music videos (Ward, 2002).

Example Three

In a study published in the *American Journal of Public Health* in 2003, an important finding was that adolescents who watched excessive amounts of negative rap videos were more likely to engage in anti-social behaviors such as violence against teachers or to have been arrested (Kirchheimer, 2003). They were also found more likely to have contracted a sexually-transmitted disease or have used alcohol and drugs. On the opposite side of the coin, mental health professionals can use positive lyrics, as an attempt to engage their clients and offer them positive alternatives. If a client shows an interest in hip-hop culture, counselors/therapists should consider engaging their clients in assignments associated with hip-hop culture. Linking modern-day mental health issues to hip-hop culture will help to foster a stronger bond between this generation and community mental health centers, whereby the clients can use their creative talent to express their emotions in a control setting. Hip-hop culture has demonstrated that it has the ability to promote a public policy agenda capable of focusing on the reduction of aggression and violence in poor underclass communities (Kitwana, 2002). The powerful voice of hip-hop culture has the ability to reach and articulate critical messages to this generation (Boyd 2003; Kitwana 2002). Utilizing hip-hop culture to increase awareness among this generation about mental health, and public health issues can be an effective weapon. Through various forms of hip-hop culture, critical social issues can be addressed. More importantly, if properly used, it can be an effective communication tool for promoting positive change. Hip-hop culture has significantly increased the awareness of this generation about the horrific social conditions facing this most unstable population. Hip-hop culture can be an effective tool in addressing a number of public health concerns including mental health, substance abuse and behavioral issues impacting this generation.

Example Four

Rha Goddess created the **"Hip Hop Mental Health Project"** after a close friend committed suicide in 2002. He was largely silent about his depression and life struggles. The Hip Hop Mental Health Project was created because there was a lack of safe outlets for those who are struggling with mental health issues. Goddess realized that mental illnesses were having a disproportionate impact within the hip-hop community, and it wasn't being directly addressed at all (Newton, 2009). The Hip Hop Mental Health Project was created to break the silence in the hip-hop generation about mental health and wellness, by providing a culturally relevant, artistic and social justice approach to supporting individuals and groups in being well. The project approaches wellness from the perspectives of hip-hop culture and social justice (Newton, 2009). According to Goddess, the Mental Health Project's use of hip-hop culture as a vehicle for healing and resiliency made their approach and their work within the hip-hop community a natural fit. Other risk factors, including violence, incarceration, and unemployment, also disproportionately impact the hip-hop community, as well as contribute to the overall wellness and mental health of this generation.

The culture of the mental health service system is also equally important to the success of services. In order to adequately address the mental health well-being of this generation, providers must embrace and welcome the hip-hop culture generation with diagnostic, treatment, and case management services that are representative of their culture. It is all too easy to not respect the importance of culture. The overall culture of hip-hop, including the social contexts are critical elements when providing services to members of the hip-hop generation. Cultural misunderstandings will bring about serious fragmentation of services, thus discouraging members from this generation from accessing and receiving appropriate mental health care. With respect to the context of mental health services broader social issues such as racism, discrimination, social economic status, and education all affect mental health services. Disproportionately, these interrelating problems are manifested on some members who represent the hip-hop culture generation.

The failure of the health care and human service community to develop strategies aimed at addressing these very experiences will continue to be problematic if service providers do not take the time to study this generation collectively in an attempt to rehabilitate the psyche of this generation. Furthermore, the proliferation of dysfunctional experiences that this generation has witnessed has led to a lack of emotional intelligence and poor decision-making skills. It is important to note that attitudes transcend into values and beliefs for this generation. The lifestyles that are presented by hip-hop culture have afforded many from this generation the opportunity to develop a tough, or thug, mentality. This is particularly true in terms of African American males. Attitudes and values ranging from drug use, alcohol use, sexuality, and violence have been associated with the hip-hop generation and become yet another problem for service providers. Moreover, these attitudes and values are being transmitted, sanctioned, and approved by members from this generation. The sexual politics associated with hip-hop culture, for example, have influenced the attitudes and values of this generation significantly. The same can be said in terms of this generation's attitudes and values regarding alcohol, drugs, and violence. Getting to the root of why this generation feels this way is critical to their very development and survival.

Figure 2 illustrates some of the major challenges that therapists and counselors are facing when it comes to addressing the mental health needs of the hip-hop culture population. Effectively addressing the poor decision making and problematic fixed behaviors of this generation has derailed many of the mental health attempts. As seen in the figure, the challenges confronting counselors and therapists emanate from lifestyles, negative behaviors of others, the valuing of hip-hop culture, widespread substance use and abuse among peers, violence, and poor role models. Consequently, there is poor decision making, fixed behaviors that are resistant to change, and, resulting in anti-social behavior. The figure shows that the counselor or therapist must understand the interrelationships between these cultural factors and, subsequent, individual behavior in order to effectively help individuals from the hip-hop generation

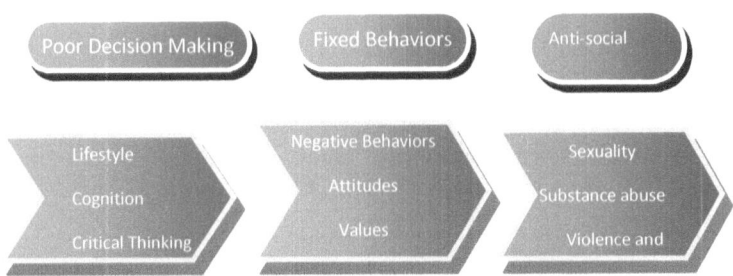

Figure 2. **Major challenges to the therapeutic community**

Summary

The current rates of mental health-related disorders among members of the hip-hop generation cannot be overlooked. One can only imagine the staggering numbers who may be struggling with their emotions. The cultural landscapes have completely changed. Hip-hop culture continues to provide a view into the cultural landscapes of this generation. Many challenging opportunities associated with this generation continues' to broaden their emotional confusion about acceptable and unacceptable behaviors.

An increasing number of hip-hoppers each year now meet the criteria for mental health illness. The trouble is that many more of them are affected by an increased level of stressors. These and genetic risk factors including substance abuse can have serious adverse effects. The inability of some health care and human service providers to adequately deal with the variety of mental affairs of the hip-hop generation population can no longer continue. Service providers must be committed to serving the needs of this generation, despite what mental shortcomings may exist among it. Based on the history of antisocial experiences afforded to the hip-hop generation, it is no wonder that they are suffering emotionally and mentally.

References

American Psychiatric Association. (2001). African-American youngsters inadequately treated for ADHD. *Psychiatric News, 36*(10), 17-24.

Brown, E. (2000). The X factor: Ecstasy has hip-hop heads feeling kinda fuzzy. Can the rap world handle the soft knock life? *Vibe Magazine*, 98-206.

Brown, J. D. (1985). Race and gender in rock video. *Social Science Newsletter (University of North Carolina at Chapel Hill), 70*(2), 82-86.

American Psychiatric Association. (2000). Diagnostic and statistical manual of mental disorders (4th ed., text rev.) Washington, DC: Author.

Fifty Cent. (2002). Don't push me. On *Get rich or die trying* [CD]. Santa Monica, CA: Shady Records/Aftermath Entertainment/ Interscope Records.

Franklin, N. B., & Franklin, A. J. (with Toussaint, P.). (2001). *Boys into men: Raising our African American teenage sons*. New York, NY: Penguin Books.

Johnson, J. D., Jackson, L. A., & Gatto, L. (1995). Violent attitudes and deferred academic aspirations: Deleterious effects of exposure to rap music. *Basic and Applied Social Psychology, 16*(1/2), 27-41.

Kapner, D. A. (2003). *Alcohol and other drug use at historical Black colleges and universities*. Retrieved from http://www. higheredcenter.org/files/product/hbcu.pdf

Kelley, R. E. G. (1997). *Yo mama's dysfunctional! Fighting the culture wars in urban America*. Boston, MA: Beacon Press.

Kirchheimer, Sid (2003). Does Rap Put Teens at Risk? Study: Association Found Between Video Viewing Time and Risky Behaviors, WebMD Health News.

Kitwana, B. (2002). *The hip-hop generation: Young Blacks and the crisis in African-American culture*. New York, NY: Basic Books.

Ludacris. (2000). What's your fantasy. On *Back for the first time* [CD]. New York, NY: Def Jam Recordings.

Majors, R., & Billson, J.-M. (1992). *Cool pose: The dilemmas of Black manhood in America*. New York, NY: Lexington Books.

McCall, N. (1997). *What's going on: Personal essays*. New York, NY: Vintage Books.

Morgan, J. (1999). *When chickenheads come home to roost: A hip-hop feminist breaks it down*. New York, NY: Touchstone.

Newton, Matthew, (2009). *Mental health and the hip-hop generation*: True/Slant

The Notorious BIG. (1994). *Everyday struggles*. On *Ready to die* [CD]. New York, NY: Arista Records.

Ooms, T. (Ed.). (1981). *Teenage pregnancy in the family context: Implications for Policy*.

Ogunnaike, L. (2005). Steve Stouten would like turn into a sneaker. Rolling Stone Magazine, 989, 113-118.

Reber, A. S., & Reber, E. (2001). *The Penguin dictionary of psychology* (3rd ed.). New York, NY: Penguin Books.

Rose, T. (1994). *Black noise: Rap music and Black culture in contemporary America:* Hanover, NH: University Press of New England.

Salovey, P., Stroud, L. R., Woolery, A., & Epel, E. S. (2002). Perceived emotional intelligence, stress reactivity and symptom reports: Further explorations using the trait meta-mood scale. *Psychology & Health, 17*(5), 611-627.

Schoenbach, V., Kaplan, B., Wagner, E., Grimson, R., & Miller, F. (1983). Prevalence of self-reported depression symptoms in young adolescents. *American Journal of Public Health, 73*(11), 1281-1287.

Sori, Catherine and Hecker Lorna. (2008). *The Therapist's Notebook, Volume 3* More Homework, Handouts, and Activities for Use in Psychotherapy, Routledge, New York

T.I. (2004). You don't know me. On *Urban legend* [CD]. New York, NY: Atlantic Records.

Truglio, R. T. (1998). Television as a sex educator. In K. Swaim, C. Meskill, & S. DeMaio (Eds.), *Social learning from broadcast television* (pp. 7-23). Creskill, NJ: Hampton Press.

Wade, B., & Gunner, C. T. (1993). Explicit rap music lyrics and attitudes towards rape: The perceived efforts on African-American college students' attitudes. *Challenge. A Journal of Research on African American Men, 4*(1), 51-60.

Ward, L. M,. (2002). Does television exposure affect emerging adults' attitudes and assumptions about sexual relationships? Correlational and experimental confirmation. *Journal of Youth and Adolescence, 31,* 34-40.

Part II

**Culture in Effective Health Care Delivery:
Assessment and Educational Issues**

CHAPTER SEVEN

The Role of Self-Assessment in Achieving Cultural Competence and Linguistic Competence and its Impact on Addressing Health Care Disparities

Tawara D. Goode
Georgetown
University Medical
Center

Sonja Harris Haywood
Case Western Reserve
University School of
Medicine

Suzanne Bronheim
Georgetown University
School of Medicine

Kristyn Smith
Institute for Health
and Productivity Studies
Emory University
(Washington, D.C.)

Laurie Murphy
Case Western Reserve
University School of
Medicine

Abstract

Self-assessment has an essential role in advancing and sustaining cultural and linguistic competence and reducing health and health care disparities. This chapter provides a discussion of the benefits of cultural and linguistic competence self-assessment processes for patients/consumers, health care organizations, and communities. It provides a comprehensive examination of the extant evidence and the state of the science in cultural and linguistic competence assessment and measurement, and delineates innovations and lessons learned by two academic medical centers, including a new validated measure of cultural and linguistic competence for health care providers. Concludes that there is a critical need for valid instruments and measures of cultural and linguistic competence to improve quality and effectiveness of care, and reduce the burden of health disparities for racially and ethnically diverse communities.

Introduction

Cultural competence and linguistic competence are widely recognized as fundamental aspects of quality in health and mental health care, particularly for culturally diverse patient populations, and as essential approaches for reducing disparities by improving access, utilization, safety, and health status (Betancourt & Green 2010; Goode, Jackson, Bronheim, 2010; Goode, Dunne, & Bronheim, 2006; Betancourt, 2006; Smedley, Stith,& Nelson, 2003 Lavizzo-Mourey,& McKenzie, 1996). An essential element of cultural competence is the capacity to engage in self-assessment at both the individual/provider and organizational levels (Cross, Bazron, Dennis, & Isaacs, 1989; Boutin-Foster, Foster, Konopasek, 2008; Goode, Harris-Haywood, Wells, & Rhee, 2009; LaVeist, Relosa, Sawaya, 2008). Self-assessment is a necessary, effective, and systematic way to plan for and incorporate cultural and linguistic competence within health care systems and organizations (Goode, Mason, & Jones, 2002). Self-assessment can benefit health care providers by heightening awareness, influencing attitudes toward practice, and motivating the development of knowledge and skills (National Center for Cultural Competence, 2002; Goode, Brown, Mason, Sockalingam, 2006; Assemi, Cullander, & Hudmon, 2006). Equally important, self-assessment of cultural and linguistic competence can serve as a catalyst to address the social inequities that contribute to health *and* health care disparities.

The end of the decade (2010) marked increased importance of assessing and measuring cultural and linguistic competence by government, health care organizations, health care accreditation bodies, and organizations focused on health care quality and standards (Association of American Medical Colleges, 2005; Joint Commission Board of Commissioners, 2011; Journal of Transcultural Nursing, 2009; Liaison Committee on Medical Education, 2010; National Quality Forum, 2009; National Standards on Culturally and Linguistically Appropriate Services, 2001). This chapter will explore and describe in detail: (1) conceptual frameworks of cultural competence and linguistic competence; (2) the increasing need for cultural and linguistic competence self-assessment and measurement; (3) need for cultural and linguistic competence assessment and measurement, (4) the benefits and guiding values and principles of cultural and linguistic competence self-assessment for health and mental health care providers and organizations; (5) the extant evidence and state of the science for instruments that assess cultural and linguistic competence in health and mental health care; (6) innovations and lesson learned about self-assessment from a partnership with the National Center for Cultural Competence, Georgetown University Medical Center and Case Western Reserve University, Department of Family Medicine; and (7) future directions for self-assessment and the implications for policy and practice to reduce health care disparities.

Conceptual Framework and Definitions

Cultural Competence. There is no universally agreed upon definition of cultural competence within health care. Definitions have evolved from varied perspectives and interests, are incorporated in state and federal statutes and programs, and have been adopted by health and mental health care organizations, accreditation bodies, and the academic and research communities. In 1989, Cross, Bazron, Dennis and Isaacs created a conceptual framework and definition of cultural competence that established a foundation for health and human services. This framework made a new contribution, as it extended the scope of cultural competence far beyond that of an individual or provider. It posited a comprehensive vision that included an organization's or system's capacity to embed values of cultural competence into policy, structures, attitudes, behaviors, and practices. This vision of cultural competence is highly relevant today as the framework has proven adaptable and universally applicable across multiple systems and domains. A great many of the definitions that have emerged in the past 20 years have their roots in the Cross model; however, they have been adapted for specific disciplines and professional societies in the fields of health and human services (Goode, Dunne, & Broheim, 2006).

This section puts forth a conceptual framework and model of cultural competence adapted from Cross et al. (1989) and embraced by the National Center for Cultural Competence (See Figure 1).

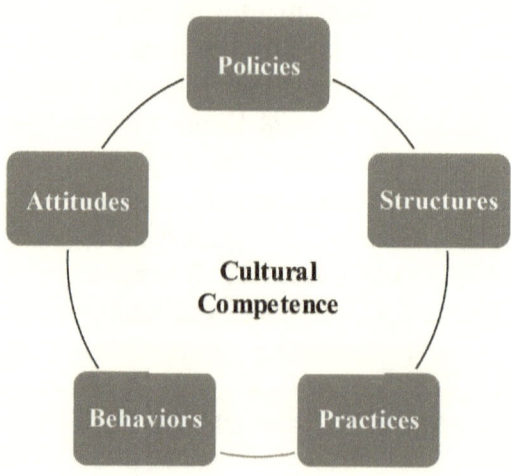

Figure 1. **Cultural Competence Framework**

As Figure 1 shows, cultural competence requires that organizations:

- have a defined set of values and principles, and demonstrate behaviors, attitudes, policies, and structures that enable them to work effectively cross-culturally.
- have the capacity to (1) value diversity, (2) conduct self-assessment, (3) manage the dynamics of difference, (4) acquire and institutionalize cultural knowledge and (5) adapt to diversity and the cultural contexts of the communities they serve.
- incorporate the above in all aspects of policy making, administration, practice, service delivery, and systematically involved consumers, key stakeholders, and communities.

Cultural competence is a developmental process that evolves over an extended period. It is a developmental process that evolves over an extended period. Both individuals and organizations are at various levels of awareness, knowledge, and skills along the cultural competence continuum.

Linguistic Competence. Historically, the term "linguistic competence" has been associated with the scientific study of language. During the past decade, the term has been widely used in the health and mental health care arenas and is often used in conjunction with cultural competence; however the two terms are not synonymous. In the U.S. health care the terms "linguistic competence" and "linguistically appropriate" are primarily used to refer to the communication needs of people who speak languages other than English. They are commonly referred to in federal and state legislation and standards to ensure language access in accordance with statutes. Goode and Jones (2006) developed and refined a conceptual framework and definition of linguistic competence, which will be used for the purposes of this chapter, encompasses a broad range of language needs and preferences and structural supports necessary to ensure optimum communication in health and mental health care setting (See Figure 2).

As Figure 2 shows, linguistic competence is the capacity of an organization and its personnel to communicate effectively, and convey information in manner that is easily understood by diverse groups, including persons of limited English proficiency, those who are not literacy or who have low literacy skills, individuals with disabilities, and those who are deaf or hard of hearing. Linguistic competency requires organizational and provider capacity to respond effectively to the health and mental health literacy needs of populations served. The organization must have policy, structures, practices, procedures, and dedicated resources to support this capacity.

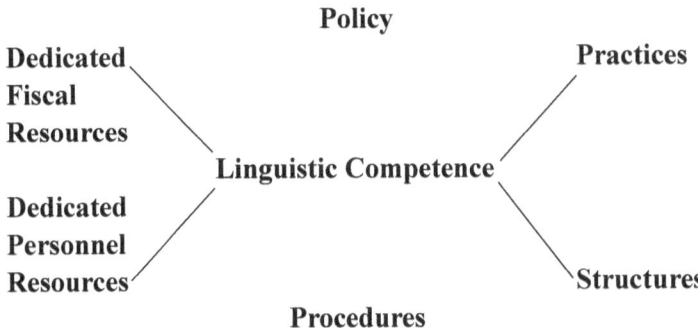

Figure 2. **Linguistic Competence Framework**

Despite compelling evidence of efficacy, many within the health care community continue to struggle with the implementation of cultural and linguistic competency at the individual, organizational, and community levels and measuring and assessing its impact (Kumas-Tan, Z, Beagan, B., Loppie, C., MacLeod, A., Frank, B., 2007).

Increasing the Need for Cultural and Linguistic Competence in Self-Assessment and Measurement

The role of cultural and linguistic competence self-assessment and measurement assumes a greater importance in the current health and mental health care environment. An array of accreditation standards now includes cultural and linguistic competence. The focus on quality of care and quality improvement within the field now embraces cultural and linguistic competence. An upsurge in funding for research to address health disparities and inequities has put a spotlight on assessment and measurement of cultural and linguistic competence. Each of these efforts generates an urgent need for effective self-assessment approaches and measures (Gozu, Beach, Price, Gary, Robinson, Palacio, Smarth, Jenckes, Fuerstein, Bass, Powe, & Cooper, 2007).

Accreditation and Standards. A wide range of accrediting and standard-setting bodies across the spectrum of health and mental health care systems are focusing on cultural and linguistic competence as an essential component in the delivery of quality, safe care and to address health disparities. New standards are being applied to the delivery of care, professional development for the current and preparation of the future health and mental health care workforce, and to the broader assurance of overall national health through public health entities. In 2001, the U.S. Department of Health and Human Services, Office of Minority Health (OMH), promulgated its groundbreaking National Standards for Culturally and Linguistically Appropriate Services in Health Care (CLAS). These fourteen standards provided a framework for the implementation of services and organizational structures to meet the needs of culturally and linguistically diverse populations. Four of the standards are supported by Federal statute to ensure language access for populations with limited English proficiency, and the remainder is recommended for adoption at the state and local levels. The OMH launched the CLAS Standards Enhancement Initiative, a national effort to update and improve the standards after ten years in the forefront of guiding change in this nation's health and mental health care systems.

In the decade that followed the introduction of CLAS, a broad array of organizations added cultural and linguistic competence to their standards and approaches to quality improvement. The Joint Commission moved from placing a minor emphasis on cultural competence to more fully integrating cultural and linguistic competence in its accreditation processes for health care entities. The Joint Commission is advancing standards that support the provision of care, treatment, and services in a manner that is conducive to the communication, cultural, language, health literacy, and spiritual/religious needs of individuals (The Joint Commission, 2009 & 2010). The Commission will issue a new set of standards that address these factors in 2011 with projected compliance in hospital settings in 2012 (The Joint Commission, 2011). The National Committee on Quality Assurance and its HEDIS standards for health and mental health care plans now address cultural and linguistic competence. The recognition of the importance of cultural and linguistic competence in preparing the future health and mental health care workforce is reflected in the adoption of standards for training programs for physicians (e.g. Liaison Committee on Medical Education, Accreditation Council for Graduate Medical Education), for psychologists (American Psychological Association Committee on Accreditation), social workers (Council on Social Work Education),and for occupational therapists (Accreditation Council for Occupational Therapy. Moreover, recent research conducted by the NCCC found a number of states have either introduced and/or enacted legislation that mandates cultural and linguistic competency as a requirement for health professions training and licensure (National Center for Cultural Competence, 2008). Finally, within the public health arena, the Public Health Accreditation Board created a national voluntary accreditation program for state, local, territorial, and tribal public health departments to improve and protect the health of every community by advancing the quality and performance of public health departments. Standards include cultural and linguistic competence and make specific mention of organizational assessment. Within each of these sets of standards is an inherent need for effective self-assessment and measurement.

Quality Improvement. With ever-escalating costs for health and mental health care and less than optimal outcomes including persistent disparities, the focus on quality of services and care has become central. The National Quality Forum (NQF) promotes a three step process to improve health and mental health care that reflects the cultural competence self-assessment process. The first step is defining quality with uniform standards and measures. The second is using that data to determine where patient care falls short. Finally caregivers use this analysis to improve their performance and the quality of the care provided. NQF recognizes the key role of cultural competence in delivering quality care. In 2008, the NQF endorsed a set of national voluntary consensus standards, the Comprehensive Framework and Preferred Practices for Measuring and Reporting Cultural Competency (NQF, 2009). This robust set of standards emphasizes measurement and self-assessment of cultural and linguistic competence within the framework of quality improvement; however they delineate what to assess, not how to conduct assessment. Thus, there is a critical need for effective cultural and linguistic competence self-assessment processes and measurement within the quality improvement movement.

Research and Demonstration Funding. Public funding of research and demonstration projects focused on health disparities is expanding. The National Institutes of Health (NIH) and the Centers for Disease Control (CDC) are the two largest funders of research and public health initiatives that address health disparities. NIH and CDC contribute to an ever-increasing number of studies and project impact evaluations. In September, 2010, the NIH elevated the National Center on Minority Health and Health Disparities (NCMHD) to the National Institute on Minority Health and Health Disparities (NIMHD). This Institute now has responsibility for coordinating the development of the NIH health disparities research agenda. In addition, it expands the eligibility criteria of the NIMHD

Research Endowment program to include active NIMHD Centers of Excellence. The NIMHD, through its predecessor NCMHD, has funded more than 88 centers of excellence around the nation to conduct research on health disparities in many disciplines and on a variety of topics. Among the research priorities for the new Institute are the social determinants of health; patient-centered outcomes research; faith-based approaches to health disparities; and improving the participation of health disparity populations in clinical trials. The CDC provides fiscal and technical support to state and community public health entities to address disparities in an array of health problems through state and local activities. In addition, CDC funded REACH Across the United States, community level programs to eliminate racial and ethnic health disparities. Other public funders also support research and demonstration projects that address health disparities, including the Health Resources and Services Administration, the Substance Abuse and Mental Health Services Administration, and the National Institute of Mental Health's Office for Research on Disparities and Global Mental Health. Foundations and other funders have taken on this issue as well. Given the role of cultural and linguistic competence in addressing health disparities, the need for effective measures of self-assessment becomes increasingly urgent, especially as research and program evaluation expand in the coming years.

Values, Benefits and Outcomes of Cultural and Linguistic Competence and Self-Assessment

Benefits of Self-Assessment. Assessing attitudes, behaviors, practices, structures, and policies is a necessary, effective, and systematic way to plan for and incorporate cultural and linguistic competency within organizations (National Center for Cultural Competence, 2006). The capacity to engage in self-assessment helps organizations to:

- gauge the extent to which they are effectively addressing the preferences, interests, and needs of diverse populations and communities.

- establish partnerships that will meaningfully involve diverse populations, communities, and constituency groups.
- improve patient/consumer access to and utilization of health and mental health care services and supports.
- increase patient/consumer satisfaction with health and mental health care and supportive services.
- plan for and embed culturally and linguistically competent policies, structures, and practices within its core functions.
- allocate personnel and fiscal resources to improve the quality and safety of health and mental health care and services.
- ascertain individual and collective strengths and areas for programmatic growth.
- Self-assessment can provide a vehicle to measure outcomes for health and mental health care organizations, their personnel, and the populations and communities they serve. All of these benefits can have a direct impact in reducing disparities in care provided by health and health care organizations and systems, and in the health and mental health status of culturally and linguistically diverse populations.

Self-assessment at the individual level enables health and mental health care providers to address their own cultural values and belief systems and how these may contribute to disparate care and/or the provision of related services and supports (Goode, Haywood, Wells, & Rhee, 2009). It also provides an approach for others within these fields to engage in self-reflection and probe the extent to which the principles and core components of cultural and linguistic competence are embedded in all aspects of their work.

Guiding Values and Principles of Self-Assessment. For the past 14 years, the NCCC has used the following set of values and guiding principles to conduct and/or assist organizations to engage in self-assessment. Undoubtedly new values and guiding principles will be adopted as the evidence on assessment and measurement of cultural and linguistic competence increases and as the impact of that evidence on reducing both health care and health disparities continues to emerge.

Self-assessment is strengths based. The purpose of self-assessment is to identify and promote growth among individuals and organizations, enhancing their capacity to deliver culturally and linguistically competent care and services. The process allows organizations to identify and acknowledge internal assets that may be inadvertently overlooked.

A safe and non-judgmental environment is essential to the self-assessment process. Self-assessment is most productive when conducted in an environment that: (1) offers participants a forum to give honest statements of their levels of awareness, knowledge, skills about cultural and linguistic competency; (2)allows participants to explore their values, belief systems, and attitudes about diverse populations; (3) provides safeguards to prevent any negative consequences for participation; (4) ensures that results will be used to promote and sustain meaningful change within the organization and communities and constituents served.

Self-assessment ensures the meaningful involvement of consumers, patients and their families, communities, and key constituents. Consistent with principles of self-determination and cultural competence, consumers /patients and their families, and communities are integrally involved in processes to plan, deliver, and evaluate the services they receive.

The results of self-assessment are used to enhance and build capacity. The intent of self-assessment is neither to render a score/ranking nor label an individual or an organization. Rather, self-assessment is intended to provide a snapshot in time in the life of an individual or organization. Results should be used to address disparities in the delivery of care, quality improvement, and to facilitate organizational change. They can also be used at the individual level for professional growth and development, mentoring, coaching, and to set personal goals. The NCCC's experience with self-assessment demonstrates that comparisons between individuals or organizations are of little benefit. Greater benefit is derived from individual and organizational self-comparison over time.

Diverse dissemination strategies are essential to the process of self-assessment. Results should be shared with participants, patients/consumers and their families, communities, and key constituents. Culturally tailored dissemination approaches assist each audience to receive information in the manner that is most useful to them and which will facilitate partnership in change.

Four Phase Approach to Organizational Self-Assessment and Lessons Learned

Self-assessment can yield a wealth of information, including but not limited to, the extent to which cultural and linguistic competence is embedded in such areas as: organizational mission, policies, structures, and procedures; staffing patterns; position descriptions and personnel performance measures; clinical practice, services, and other supports; partnerships with patients and their families; quality improvement; community engagement, outreach, and dissemination approaches; composition of advisory boards and committees; professional development and in-service training; and the conduct of or participation in research. The purpose and outcomes of the self-assessment process should be clearly established, as this will impact who participates, the type of instrument/tool that will be used, and data to be collected. As seen in Figure 3, the NCCC has successfully used a four-step approach to lead and/or provide consultation to organizations interested in conducting self-assessment (Goode, Brown, Mason, & Sockalingam, 2006), and has identified six key lessons learned to facilitate such processes. The six key lessons are described below.

Self-assessment is time and resource intensive. Determine the scope of the organization's self-assessment process. Allow ample time and devote sufficient personnel and fiscal resources to conduct the process.

Gauge organizational readiness. Determine how well positioned the organization is to engage in self-assessment (e.g. buy-in from staff and key constituents, fiscal and personnel resources available). Devote time to conveying the reasons why the organization could benefit from such a process (e.g. how it relates to the mission, business model, or strategic plan; quality improvement, patient/consumer health, and mental health outcomes).

Anticipate resistance. Resistance is natural in any organizational change process. It is important to identify the nature and scope of resistance. Unless staff and key constituents see the self-assessment process as relevant to their day-to-day work, they may resist, undermine, or ignore it, or put forth only halfhearted efforts. Use varied approaches to address fears and concerns by emphasizing the benefits to the organization, its personnel, and most importantly to the patient/consumer populations served. It may be necessary to reassure staff that the self-assessment process is not a test, that their positions are not at stake, or that the outcomes can help to reduce disparities in care.

Remember that the process is as important as the outcomes. To be effective, a self-assessment process should be inclusive and well planned and executed. This requires: (1) paying close attention to the details of the process (e.g. logistics, attitudes of staff and other participants, resources); and (2) addressing concerns when they arise timely and with integrity.

Leadership buy-in is essential. Self-assessment requires shared leadership and ownership, not only executives but throughout the organization as a whole (i.e. front desk, clinicians, and support staff, community advisory boards). Self-assessment processes that lack leadership buy-in and commitment flounder and are often unsuccessful.

Involve communities and key constituents. In any self-assessment process, those individuals and communities that receive services and supports must be involved in a meaningful way. Key principles of cultural competence state "Community members are full partners in decision-making" and "Cultural competence involves working in conjunction with natural, informal support and helping networks within culturally diverse communities" (NCCC, 2011).

PHASE 1
Establish a Structure
To Guide the Work

PHASE 2
Create a Shared
Vision & Shared
Ownership

PHASE 3
Collect, Analyze &
Disseminate Data

PHASE 4
Develop &
Implement a Plan
of Action

Phases to Conduct an Organizational Self-Assessment

▪ **Establish a structure to guide the work**
Assemble a work group, committee, or task force with the responsibility of coordinating the organizational self-assessment. The group can plan, implement, and provide oversight to the process. *Be inclusive.* This group should include representation from all levels of the organization, patients/consumers and their families, volunteers, board members, community partners, stakeholders, and allies.

▪ **Create a shared vision & shared ownership**
Convene forums to explore and define cultural competence and linguistic competence and their value and relevance for your organization. *Ensure diverse participation.* Include representation from staff, volunteers, patients/consumers and their families, community-based organizations in the service area, and other invested constituency groups.

▪ **Collect, analyze, and disseminate data**
Many data sources can be tapped for the self-assessment process including those from any instrument and tool administered, focus groups, interviews, census and other demographic data, and the organization's own records. These data should be carefully reviewed and analyzed. Use these data to develop a report that delineates organizational strengths and areas of growth and details areas for change. Ensure that report findings can be adapted for dissemination to diverse audiences (e.g. patients/consumers, partners, and other invested parties.

▪ **Develop and implement a plan of action**
Create a plan of action using the results of the organizational self-assessment. Identify priorities. Determine the strategies, activities, partners, resources, timetables, and responsible parties to achieve desired goals. Establish benchmarks to monitor and assess progress.

Figure 3. **Four phase approach to self assessment**

The Extant Evidence and State of the Science for Instruments that Assess Cultural and Linguistic Competence in Health and Mental Health Care

While there is a great need for effective, validated measures to assess cultural and linguistic competence, both the peer reviewed and the grey literature (i.e. a body of materials that is not found through conventional publishers), on this topic continues to reflect a significant gap between what is actually needed and what is currently available. Since evidence suggests that self-assessment can be used to improve quality of care and to meet standards and mandates, then tools, measures, and processes are needed that can effectively assess:

- both the provider and organization/practice setting;
- the total experience of care of patients and their families from a cultural perspective;
- the perceptions of communities, partners, and constituents in the geographic service area;
- the multiple types of health and mental health care providers and settings;
- the developmental nature and differing components of cultural and linguistic competence; and
- specifically defined areas such as professional development/ training interests and needs, unconscious bias about communities and patient/consumer populations, and disparities in approaches to care.

In order to determine the extent to which the current measures of cultural and linguistic competence reflect the above stated need, a systematic review was conducted by Case Western Reserve University, Department of Family Medicine, Research Division of peer-reviewed and grey literature published between 1985 and 2010. This systematic review included those peer-reviewed and grey literature tools that use self-assessment measures of cultural competency and/ or linguistic competency in a health or mental health care setting. A two-pronged approach was employed to identify citations that matched inclusion/exclusion criteria developed by the authors. First a nine-item search template was developed and applied to MEDLINE/PubMed databases to generate viewable abstracts and articles. Google Scholar was then used to identify potentially viable citations by searching based on a list of cultural competency tools recommended from the websites or reports of national organizations. From this list of citations, abstracts and articles were reviewed using selection criteria filters. Given the sparseness of the literature in this evolving field, the forward and backward nature of the two-prong search strategy allowed for the identification of tools that may have been missed. As a result of this process, **16** citations from peer-reviewed publications and **26** grey literature tools were gleaned for review. Table I and Table II depict the search results for articles and grey literature tools, respectively. The authors found that a majority of identified measures and tools had neither been subjected to a rigorous research process nor vetted through a peer review process. Tables III and IV provide details on each of the reviewed measures. (See Appendixes A-D for Tables).

Level of Assessment. Within the peer-reviewed literature, the focus has been on the health professional assessment. Of the 20 measures identified, only one focused on assessment at the organizational level. Interestingly, the need for both organization and health professionals assessment is reflected in the grey literature measures—64% of the 26 tools assess the organization and 7 (28%) assess health professionals. Given the lack of rigor in the development of the grey literature measures, there is a gap in the literature related to organizational assessment that needs to be addressed.

Assessment of Patient/Consumer Perceptions of the Organization and the Professional. Two of the 20 peer-reviewed measures were created to garner patient/consumer perceptions of the providers and services that they receive. One was developed for use in mental health settings for people from diverse racial, ethnic and cultural backgrounds who are in recovery. The second was used to assess perceived physician cultural competency and did not address linguistic competence. Two of the grey literature tools captured patient perceptions as well. Again, review of current literature suggests that measures of patient perception are limited and patient assessment of physician cultural competence remains a significant gap in current knowledge and practice.

Inclusion of Linguistic Competence. Tools were reviewed to determine if they addressed linguistic competence based on the NCCC framework described on pages 2-3. Since current standards and mandates include both cultural and linguistic competence, it was important that measures address both. All of the grey literature measures addressed some aspect of linguistic competence, with the majority focusing on cross-cultural communication skills and language access for individuals who have limited English proficiency. All but two of the peer-reviewed tools did so as well. Thus, the literature reflects an understanding of the importance of addressing both concepts in self-assessment.

Types of Providers and Settings. The study settings for the peer-reviewed tools varied greatly. Several settings were so specific, due to type of patients seen, type of services provided, and type of organization that generalizability may be problematic. For example, one tool was tested in pediatric practices treating Medicaid insured patients, another in clinics with patient populations that were comprised of >75% Latinos, and a third in mental health services on college campuses. While highly specific tools have a role in the self-assessment process, these same studies had such small samples sizes that their utility even in specified settings is questionable. In several tools the populations assessed were both health care organization staff and health care professionals. For tools that defined cultural and linguistic competence as a set of knowledge and skills, what is measured may differ greatly based on the individual's role in the health care arena. For example, the areas of knowledge and skills needed for front desk staff are obviously different from those of a nurse practitioner or certified medical interpreter. The majority of the grey literature tools were developed for use in unspecified healthcare settings. Since none of these tools reported psychometric data, the type of providers for which they were designed was not clearly delineated.

Psychometric Soundness. The most glaring concern identified in the review of current literature is the lack of psychometrically sound measures. None of the grey literature measures reported any studies of validity or reliability, with only two mentioning any validity rationale at all. The peer-reviewed measures all addressed validity in their studies; however for eight of the measures, the reported validity studies were done on previous versions of the tool or longer versions from which the items on the reported tool were samples. All but one provided some form of reliability data, yet again in three cases the reliability data was actually based on an earlier version of the tool. In addition, almost half of the studies had sample sizes so small (under 100 subjects, with as few as 15 subjects) that their findings do not support a generalizable measure. The literature points to the critical need for greater rigor in developing psychometrically sound measures.

Innovations and Lessons Learned about Self-Assessment

Filling the Gap. In 2001, the NCCC, under the leadership of one of the authors of this chapter, and a group nationally recognized experts developed the Cultural Competence Health Practitioner Assessment (CCHPA). The CCHPA is a web-based interactive tool designed to engage health care practitioners in self-assessment and identify areas of awareness, knowledge, and skills for future professional growth and development. The CCHPA provides a list of resources and tools per subscale based on response patterns. The CCHPA was launched as a web-based self-assessment tool in 2005. By June 2011, over 30,000 registrants accessed the tool on-line.

Beginning in 2009, the NCCC partnered with Case Western Reserve University, Department of Family Medicine, Research Division, to study the CCHPA's psychometric properties and the profiles of respondents. A psychometric analysis was completed in October 2010 of the responses from **2504** health care providers, including **1864** nurses (RN, LPN), **341** clinicians (PA/NP), and **299** physicians (MD/DO), who responded to the CCHPA online between 2005 and 2008. A multi-step data analysis was conducted that applied classical factor analysis, Item Response Theory (IRT) using Rasch modeling, and Differential Item Functioning (DIF). Factor analysis determined how the items grouped together to measure the domains of cultural and linguistic competency. IRT evaluated reliability and simultaneously assessed the item difficulty level and respondents' knowledge and skills associated with cultural and linguistic competency. DIF revealed items that were biased based on race, profession and/or gender.

This psychometric analysis demonstrates that the CLCHPA is a reliable measure of health care providers' cultural and linguistic competency and meets two validity criteria, including content and discriminant group validity. Based on this analysis, 67 valid and reliable items with acceptable fit statistics, representing 3 factors, were retained from the original 129 items. Three factors representing three conceptual domains were responsible for 46% of the variance: (factor 1) knowledge of culturally and linguistically diverse populations, (factor 2) adapting practice for culturally and linguistically diverse patient populations, and (factor 3) promoting the health of culturally and linguistically diverse communities. The test content validity is based on the expertise of the instrument developers. Discriminant group validity was established by respondents who never received employer-sponsored training in cultural and linguistic competence having statistically significant lower scores on all three factors than respondents who had received such training.

The level of rigor of this study and the resulting new tool, the Cultural and Linguistic Competence Health Practitioner Assessment (CLCHPA), make an important contribution toward filling the gap. The study established that the CLCHPA is a psychometrically sound instrument for measuring cultural and linguistic competency as key factors in quality care, research, and evaluation. Ultimately, the evidence provided by the CLCHPA can be used in future studies seeking to: (a) establish associations between practitioners' cultural and linguistic competency and health outcomes for racially and ethnically diverse populations; and (b) evaluate interventions to increase provider cultural and linguistic competence.

Future Directions for Cultural and Linguistic Competence in Self-Assessment and Measurement

With the increasing need for self-assessment and measurement comes a parallel need for processes and measures that can effectively meet those needs. Given the current status of the field, there is much work to be done to assure that measures are psychometrically sound. In addition, these measures must address the competencies at both the organizational and individual provider levels which reflect cultural and linguistic competence as a key strategy to address health disparities. In order to advance the field of cultural and linguistic competence, research on self-assessment must focus on the development of measures and tools that address the multiple dimensions and purposes of assessment. There is a need for psychometrically sound measures for providers and organizations tested with larger, broad-based samples. Finally we cannot understate the need to develop measures that elicit patient/ consumer experiences and perspectives on how their cultural and linguistic preferences and needs are being met.

Measurement Construction. Whether for meeting accreditation criteria, gathering data for quality improvement, or supplying tools for research or evaluation methodologies, there is a shared need for measures that are psychometrically sound and valid. Measures designed for individuals need to demonstrate an ability to assess a set of competencies no matter what the background of the provider. Health and mental health care providers from all backgrounds need the knowledge, skills, and behaviors to deliver care in cross-cultural situations. Assessment tools should not assume familiarity through lived experience alone to be a measure of cultural competence. Both organizational and provider measures need to demonstrate stability over time and across diverse settings, because data collected will be used to compare those measured to some standard, or to their own performance over time, or to serve as independent variable measures in research protocols. Given what is at stake, those being assessed deserve no less than reliable and valid measures. In addition, measures must be able to reliably assess change following interventions to improve cultural and linguistic competence if they are to be of use in quality improvement and program evaluation. Finally, measures need to demonstrate concurrent validity with patient reports of their experiences and with direct observation of provider behavior or organizational function.

Content of Measures. Moving forward, measures need to recognize that all patients and all providers have cultures. Non-Hispanic, white, English-speaking providers who work with minority populations are far from the only practitioners who must possess the set of competencies for working cross-culturally (Kumas-Tan, 2007). The diversity reflected in health disparities is deeper and more complex than labels of race and ethnicity alone can reflect. Measures will need to include competencies at the individual and organizational level that address factors such as language, literacy, education, socioeconomic status, age, gender, sexual orientation, gender identity and expression, disability, religion and spirituality, geography (urban, suburban, rural, frontier), acculturation, and a host of other factors. With this perspective, all providers will need the competence to work cross-culturally and all organizations will need to support such efforts. Competencies to be measured for providers must exceed awareness to include knowledge about the populations they serve, the skills to implement that knowledge in varied health and mental health care settings, and an investment in addressing the factors that lead to health disparities and inequities both within the systems in which they practice, and the communities in which they live. Organizational measures will need to not only address the policies, structures, procedures, and practices that support providers in culturally competent practices, but also address the issues of health care access, utilization, and satisfaction with care that are impacted by culture and language.

Focusing Assessment to Impact Disparities. To date, there has been more focus on developing measures of cultural competence, and to some extent linguistic competence, with less attention to the ways in which these measures may be used to address the aspects of the service system that contribute to ongoing disparities and inequities. While broad societal issues such as differential socioeconomic status, bias, and ongoing stresses related to racism and discrimination have been implicated in an array of health and mental health outcomes (Williams and Jackson, 2005), cultural competence and linguistic competence are key components of efforts to eliminate health and health care disparities, because they address the issues within the health and mental health service system that impact health outcomes and status. Measures and self-assessment processes need to focus on those aspects of the service system that contribute to disparities—access and utilization of services. Figure 4 illustrates the relationships among organizational policy, infrastructure and resources, and the complex components of accessibility, utilization of services, and health and mental health outcomes and status. Culture and language impact access to and utilization of services. Therefore, self-assessment of cultural and linguistic competence needs to ask questions about where, specifically within that model, there is opportunity to improve the service system.

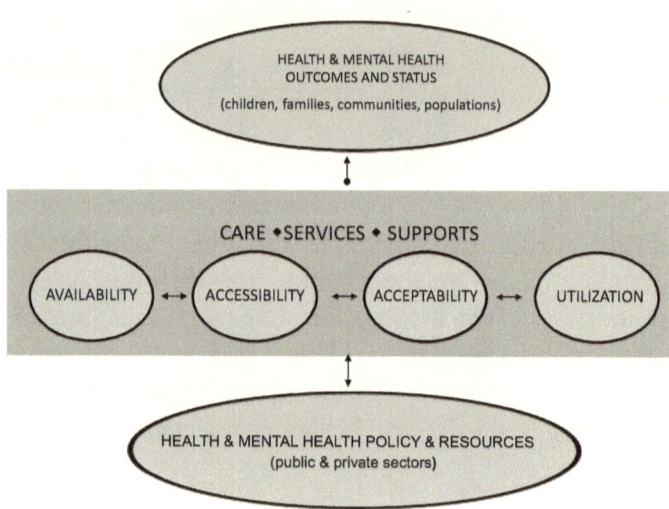

Figure 4. **Health and Mental Health Disparities Framework**

Access to care is a complex concept that embodies five elements. Frequently, approaches to improving access have focused only on the affordability of care. While insurance status and ability to pay do have an impact on access, addressing affordability of care is not the sole solution to impacting disparities in access (Hall, et al, 2008). This premise has been well demonstrated in the failure of providing Medicaid to pregnant women to increase utilization of prenatal care in the hopes of decreasing disparities in infant mortality and poor birth outcomes (Gates-William, et al., 1992; and Sanders-Phillips and Davis 1998 Gonzalez-Calvo, et al., 1998). Sanders-Phillips & Davis (1998) identified a wide range of other types of barriers to accessing care including transportation, lack of childcare, long clinic waits, negative experiences with the health care system and inconvenient clinic hours, as well as, "internal barriers," such as not wanting to get care, or not feeling like getting up to go to the doctor. For women with limited English proficiency, language is also a barrier and may relate to the particularly low levels of prenatal care for most Hispanic women. These findings reflect the more nuanced and complex model of access to care proposed by Perchansky and Thomas (1981) and the interrelationship of access and utilization as put forth by Anderson, et al. (1973). These concepts provide guidance for future development of processes and measures of cultural and linguistic competence that can address the factors presented in Figure 4.

Components of Access to Care and Cultural and Linguistic Competence Self-Assessment. Perchansky and Thomas (1981) describe **availability** of services as the relationship of the volume and type of existing services (and resources) to the patients' volume and types of needs. It refers to the adequacy of the supply of providers, facilities and specialized services. While availability can be interpreted in terms of numbers of services and providers, the concept of matching services to patient needs can be related to cultural and linguistic competence. Measures and processes to assess availability of services to improve health outcomes and status should address the knowledge and skills of providers within the system to provide differential, evidence-based screening, diagnostic and treatment protocols for patients based on factors such as race, ethnicity, gender, language, and sexual orientation, and gender identity.

Accessibility to care has been typically described as the relationship between the location of supply and the location of patients (Perchansky and Thomas, 1981). It relates to issues such as distance to services and transportation. Inequities in geographic location of services are a component of accessibility and its impact on disparities. However, accessibility can also be interpreted in terms on the distance crated by lack of language access within care settings and lack of physical accessibility for individuals with disabilities. Cultural and linguistic competence self-assessment processes and measures need to look at geographic *and* non-geographic factors of accessibility.

Perchanksy and Thomas (1989) describe **accommodation** as the relationship between the manner in which services are organized (hours, walk-in appointments, phone services, home visits, etc.) and the patient's ability to accommodate to these factors. In addition, these researchers note that patient assessment of whether the way services are organized is appropriate is also a component of accommodation. Thus culturally and linguistically competent services are organized based on patient needs and perceptions. For example, patients who are newly emigrated from countries where services are provided on a first-come, first-served basis, may struggle with exact appointment times and policies that penalize lateness or missing appointments. Patients who cannot control their work hours may need flexible or extended service hours to access care. Culturally and linguistically competent organizations address the issue of accommodation within their structures and service models. Self-assessment needs to address this component of accommodation.

Acceptability of care Perchansky and Thomas, 1981) is described as the relationship of what patients want in the personal and practice characteristics of the services they receive and the providers they encounter to the *actual* characteristics of existing services and providers. For example, Tucker, Herman, Pedersen, Higley, Montricahrd, et.al. (2003) reported that low-income minority patients in primary care defined culturally competent care (care that they experienced as sensitive to their needs) as the provider having good "people skills," technical competence, individualized treatment, and effective communication. Cross-cultural communication is a well-documented as a potential impediment to acceptability of care and, thus, to access. Cooper, Gonzales, Gallo, et al.(2003) found that race concordant visits were longer, had higher ratings of patient positive affect, and patients in these visits were more satisfied and rated their providers as more participatory. Language concordance (provider and patient speaking the same language) have been associated with improved adherence to treatment, more interaction during the visit, and better patient recall of recommendations in health care interactions (Manson, 1988; Seijo, Gomez and Friedenberg, 1991). Providers also need to know about and know how to address different values and beliefs about the acceptability of treatment modalities, including the use of alternative or traditional treatments and providers. For example, African Americans have been found to be less likely to find anti-depressants acceptable (Cooper, Gonzales, Gallo, et al., 2003). Culturally competent providers and organizations tailor services to address religious beliefs and practices that impact gender interactions, modesty, diet, and permitted medical interventions. Acceptable services also recognize and adapt to differing family constellations and patient and family preferences about who will be involved in discussions of care and decision-making. Thus to impact disparities in outcomes and health status, processes and measures of cultural and linguistic competence should address issues of accessibility.

Utilization of Care and Cultural Competence. While access to care is focused on characteristics of the services systems and the providers that deliver care, there is an additional set of factors that impact the actual utilization of those services by individuals. Differences in utilization of services also impact health outcomes and status. Anderson, et al., (1973) have identified three types of individual determinants of utilization. The first are predisposing variables, including health beliefs and attitudes about health, health care and how to treat problems, and personal issues that interfere with utilization and assure good health. These include the internal variables noted by Gonzalez-Calvo, et al. (1998). Others may include levels of acculturation, psychosocial problems, drug use, and feelings about the health issue, such as negative feelings about an unwanted pregnancy, (Johnson, et.al., 2007; Weinick, et al 2000; Livingston, et al, 2008; Wells, et. al., 1989). The second variable is resources and this refers to issues such as having health insurance, but also the cost of seeking services in terms of time lost at work, transportation, or loss of time to care for family. For example, lack of childcare has been reported as a barrier to utilization (Johnson, et.al, 2007). Finally, perceived need for services drives utilization. Cultural perspectives that link using health care only to address episodes of serious and acute illness can impact utilization. Livingston, et al., (2008), in a study for the Pew Hispanic Center, reported that when Hispanic respondents were asked why they had no usual source of health care, the primary reason given was that they are seldom sick. Cultural competence within the service system includes identifying such barriers to utilization and creating approaches to change the system and to engage patients in better understanding the relationships between utilization of services and better outcomes and health status. Thus cultural and linguistic competence self-assessment processes and measures need evaluate how providers and organizations engage patients and communities to address utilization of care.

Recommendations for Self-Assessment Processes and Measures

The challenge to health and mental health care systems, organizations, and providers is to utilize self-assessment processes and measures in a nuanced way to identify access and utilization barriers that relate to cultural and linguistic competence to address disparities in outcomes and health and mental health status. Using the model illustrated in Figure 4 provides a framework for honing the self-assessment process to address recognized service system factors that impact outcomes. Assessing and measuring cultural and linguistic competence is not an end unto itself. It provides the information needed to change the service system in ways that can impact health disparities. Thus the following future directions for enhancing cultural and linguistic competence self-assessment are proposed:

1. Create validated measures
2. Create measures to assess the multiple facets of health and mental health systems that reflect disparities in care and contribute to disparities in outcomes and health status.
3. Create self-assessment processes and measures that tap patient and community perspectives on their experiences with the system.
4. Create measures tailored for the specific roles and responsibilities of the array of personnel that make up health and mental health care systems—from organizational executives to clinicians to support and administrative staff.
5. Assure that measures and processes for self-assessment, and the analysis and reporting of such, recognize that cultural and linguistic competence occurs along a continuum. Therefore, such measures and assessment processes must have the ability to discriminate the unique set of

observable benchmarks of progress for each organization and/or provider, rather than a gold standard that must be immediately attained by all. Self-assessment provides the framework for identifying where to start and how to document progress over time.

Summary

This chapter offers a comprehensive discussion on the role of self-assessment in achieving cultural and linguistic competence and reducing health and health care disparities. It clearly articulates the benefits of cultural and linguistic competence self-assessment processes for patients/consumers, health care organizations, and communities. It examines the extant evidence and the state of the science in cultural and linguistic competence assessment and measurement, and delineates innovations and lessons learned by two academic medical centers. Lastly, this chapter puts forth a charge to the health and mental health fields to respond to the immediate need for valid instruments and measures of cultural and linguistic competence to improve quality and effectiveness of care and reduce the burden of health disparities for racially and ethnically diverse communities.

References

American Speech, Language, & Hearing Association (2010). *Cultural competence checklists: Service delivery, personal reflection, and policies & procedures* http://www.asha.org/NR/rdonlyres/07693109-C4F6-48EA-BFC3-58874C8998F9/0/service_delivery.pdf

Amherst H. Wilder Foundation (2002). *Cultural competence: A program self-assessment* Amherst H. Wilder Foundation Services to Children, Elderly, and Families.

Anderson, C. C. (2002). *Linguistically appropriate access and services: An evaluation and review for healthcare organizations*: The National Council on Interpreting in Health Care.

Anderson, R. & Newman, J. (1973). Societal and individual determinants of medical care utilization in the United States. *Milbank Memorial Fund Quarterly, 51*, 95-124.

Andrulis, D., Delbanco, T., Avakian, L., & Shaw-Taylor, Y. *Conducting a cultural competence self-assessment.*

Thomas, J. & Penchansky, R. (1894). Relating satisfaction with access to utilization of services. *Medical Care, 22*(6), 553-568.

Tirado, M. (1996a). *Patient Satisfaction Survey*: California State University—Monterey Bay.

Tirado, M. (1996b). *Provider Self-Assessment Survey*: California State University—Monterey Bay.

Tucker, C., Herman, K., Pedersen, T., Higley, B., Montricahrd, M., & Ivery, P. (2003). Cultural sensitivity in physician-patient relationships: perspectives of an ethnically diverse sample of low-income primary care patients. *Medical Care, 41*(7), 859-870.

Unknown (Unknown). *Questionnaire: Validation of Hospital Data Collection of Patients' Race and Ethnicity and Primary Language.*

Weinick,R., & Jacobs, E. (2000). Hispanic health care utilization: The role of ancestry, language, and duration of residence in the United States. Abstract of the Academy of Health Services Research Health Policy Meeting, 17.

Weiss, C., & Minsky, S. (1996). *Program Self-Assessment Survey for Cultural Competence: A Manual.* Trenton, N.J.: New Jersey Division of Mental Health and Hospitals.

Wells, K., Golding, J., Hough, R., Burnam, M. & Karno, M. (1989). Acculturation and probability of use of health services by Mexican Americans. *Health Services Research, 24*, 237-257.

Williams, D. and Jackson, P. (2005). Social sources of racial disparities in health. *Health Affairs, 24*(2), 325-34.

Appendix A
Table I: *Summary of Peer-Reviewed Studies Utilizing Cultural Competence Self-Assessment Tools (N=16)*

	N	%
INTENDED SETTINGS	**N**	**%**
Mental Health	3	19
Public Health/Other	1	6
Pediatric Primary Care	2	13
Adult Primary Care	2	13
Hospitals/Hospital Systems	4	25
Other/ Misc Settings	4	25
ASSESSMENT LEVEL	**N**	**%**
Organization	1	6
Provider	13	81
Patient	2	13
LINGUISTIC COMPETENCE ITEMS	**N**	**%**
Yes	11	69
No	5	31
SAMPLE SIZE	**N**	**%**
N < 100	7	44
$100 \leq N \leq 200$	5	31
N > 200	4	25
VALIDITY	**N**	**%**
Yes	16	100
No	0	
RELIABILITY	**N**	**%**
Yes	16	100
No	0	

Appendix B
Table II: *Summary of Grey Literature Utilizing Cultural Competence Self-Assessment Tools (N=24)*

INTENDED SETTINGS	N	%
Mental/ Behavioral Health	3	13
Public Health/ Community Health Organizations	2	8
Linguistically Diverse Populations	3	13
Hospitals/ Hospital Systems	1	4
Unspecified Healthcare Organizations	1	58
Pediatric	1	4
ASSESSMENT LEVEL	**N**	**%**
Organization	15	63
Provider	7	29
Patient/Client/Consumer	2	8
LINGUISTIC COMPETENCE ITEMS	**N**	**%**
Yes	24	100
No	0	
SAMPLE SIZE	**N**	**%**
N < 100	NA	
100 ≤ N ≤ 200	NA	
N > 200	NA	
VALIDITY	**N**	**%**
Yes	4	17
No	20	83
RELIABILITY	**N**	**%**
Yes	2	8
No	22	92

Appendix C
Table III. *Analysis of Peer-Reviewed Studies Utilizing Cultural Competence Self-Assessment Tools*

Tool Used to Assess Cultural and/or Linguistic Competence	# of Items	Assessed Linguistic Competence	Article Title	Study Sample (N)	Study Settings	Validity	Reliability
ORGANIZATIONAL LEVEL TOOLS							
Cultural Competence Section of the Practice Site Survey	6 Cultural Competence Practice Policy Questions	Yes	Cultural Competence Policies and Other Predictors of Asthma Care Quality for Medicaid-Insured Children (Lieu, et al., 2004)	83 Practices	Pediatric Practices	Content FA[+]	Cronbach $\alpha = .85$
PROVIDER-LEVEL TOOLS							
Cultural Competence Question	1	Yes	Clinician Ratings of Interpreter Mediated Visits in Primary Care Settings with Ad hoc, In-person Professional and Video Conferencing Models (Napoles, et al., 2010)	26 Physicians, 3rd year Residents, Nurse Practitioners, and Physician Assistants	1 Hospital and 3 Community Clinics	Content	Not Assessed
Cultural Competence Assessment (CCA)	25	Yes	Self-Reported Cultural Competence of Public Health Nurses in a Southeastern U.S. Public Health Department (Starr & Wallace, 2009)	31 Public Health Nurses	Public Health Clinics	Content Construct	Cronbach $\alpha = .90$
	26	Yes	Cultural Competence Among Ontario and Michigan Healthcare Providers (Schim, Doorenbos, & Borse, 2005)	45 Nurses, Clerical Staff, Nutritionists, Therapists, and Other Healthcare Providers	4 Urban Hospitals in Michigan & 3 Urban Hospitals in Canada	Content Construct Face	Cronbach $\alpha = .89$

Tool Used to Assess Cultural and/or Linguistic Competence	# of Items	Assessed Linguistic Competence	Article Title	Study Sample (N)	Study Settings	Validity	Reliability
Cultural Competence Assessment (CCA-Continued)	27	Yes	Psychometric Evaluation of the Cultural Competence Assessment Instrument Among Healthcare Providers (Doorenbos, Myers Schim, Benkert, & Borse, 2005)	Study 1: N_{total} = 51 Hospice Workers	Study 1: Hospice Settings	Study 1: Content,* Face,* Construct, FA+ Criterion-Related by Correlation with the IAPCC* Contrasted Groups* (Dillman, 1999) (Schim, Doorenbos, Miller, &Benkert2003)	Study 1: 4-Month Test-Retest Reliability for the CCA in Hospice Providers; r=.85, p=.002
				Study 2: N_{total} = 405 Healthcare Providers	Study 2: Non-Hospice Settings	Study 2: Construct, FA+	Study 2: Cronbach α for Non-Hospice Healthcare Providers = .89
	25	Yes	Development of a Cultural Competence Assessment (Schim, et al., 2003)	113 Hospice Staff and Providers	Hospice	Content, Face, Construct, FA+ Criterion, Contrasted Groups	Cronbach α = .92
Provider Cultural Competence Measure Attitudes and Behaviors Items from the: 1) Cultural Awareness Questionnaire 2) Modified-Cultural Competence Assessment Questionnaire 3) Cultural Competence Assessment Instrument (CCA)	11	Yes	Provider and Clinic Cultural Competence in a Primary Care Setting (Paez, Allen, Carson, & Cooper, 2008)	49 Internal Medicine Physicians, Family Medicine Physicians, and Nurse Practitioners	23 Primary Care Clinics	Provider Cultural Competence Measure Attitudes and Behaviors Items: Content, Face, Predictive Construct FA+	Provider Cultural Competence Measure Attitudes and Behaviors Items: Cronbach α = .5-.64

Tool Used to Assess Cultural and/or Linguistic Competence	# of Items	Assessed Linguistic Competence	Article Title	Study Sample (N)	Study Settings	Validity	Reliability
Inventory for Assessing the Process of Cultural Competence Among HealthCare Professionals-Revised (IAPCC-R) Scale	25	No	Cultural Competence of Healthcare Professionals Caring for Breastfeeding Mothers in Urban Areas (Noble, Noble, & Hand, 2009)	128 Nurses, Physicians, and Other Allied Health Professionals	General	Content,* Construct* (Campinha-Bacote, 2003)	Cronbach $\alpha = .84$
	25	No	The Effects of Nurse Practitioner Cultural Competence on Latina Patient Satisfaction (Castro & Ruiz, 2009)	15 Nurse Practitioners whose Patient Population was ≥75% Latino	Clinics with a Patient Population of ≥75% Hispanic or Latino	Content, Construct* (Campinha-Bacote, 2003)	Cronbach $\alpha = .88$
Cross-Cultural Counseling Inventory-Revised (CCCI-R)	20	No	Therapist Multicultural Competency: A Study of Therapy Dyads (Fuertes, et al., 2006)	51 Clients, 51 Counselors	Mental Health Settings	Content,* Construct,* Criterion-Related* (LaFrom-boise, Coleman & Hernandez, 1991)	Cronbach $\alpha = 0.93$ for client population Cronbach $\alpha = 0.90$ for counselor population
Cross-Cultural Counseling Inventory-Revised (CCCI-R) (cont.)	20	No	Predictors of Satisfaction with Counseling: Racial and Ethnic Minority Clients Attitudes Toward Counseling and Ratings of Their Counselor's General and Multicultural Counseling Competence (Constantine, 2002)	112 Clients, 37 Counselors	Mental Health Services at College Campuses	Content,* Construct,* Criterion-Related* (LaFrom-boise, T.D., 1991); (Sabnani & Ponterotto, 1992)	Cronbach $\alpha = 0.90$
Ethnic Attitude Scale (EAS)	20	Yes	Cultural Attitudes, Knowledge, and Skills of a Health Workforce (Jones, Cason, & Bond, 2004)	409 Hospital and Outpatient Staff & Providers	General	Content* (Bonaparte, 1979) (Rooda, 1993) Construct FA⁻	Cronbach $\alpha = .57-.72$ for the 3 Different Vignettes* (Rooda, 1993)

Tool Used to Assess Cultural and/or Linguistic Competence	# of Items	Assessed Linguistic Competence	Article Title	Study Sample (N)	Study Settings	Validity	Reliability
Cultural Self-Efficacy Scale (CSES)	30					Content* (Bernal & Froman, 1987)	Cronbach's α= .99* (Bernal & Froman, 1987)
Unnamed Hospital System's Cultural Competency Assessment	137	Yes	Assessing Cultural Competence at a Local Hospital System in the United States (Polacek & Martinez, 2009)	156 Hospital Employees	General	Content, Construct FA+	Not Assessed
Language-Cultural Competence Summary Score Survey	3	Yes	Associations of Providers' Language and Cultural Skills with Latino Parents' Perceptions of Well-Child Care (Arauz Boudreau, et al., 2010)	22 Pediatric Providers who Serve Latino and/or Limited English Proficiency Patients	Community Health Centers	Content* (Fernandez, et al., 2004)	Cronbach α = .75* (Fernandez, et al., 2004)

PATIENT-LEVEL TOOLS

Tool Used to Assess Cultural and/or Linguistic Competence	# of Items	Assessed Linguistic Competence	Article Title	Study Sample (N)	Study Settings	Validity	Reliability
The MHA/MPA Cultural Advisory Group (CCAG) Tool	52	Yes	Developing a Cultural Competence Assessment Tool For People In Recovery From Racial, Ethnic, and Cultural Backgrounds: The Journey, Challenges, and Lessons Learned (Arthur, et al., 2005)	238 Adults	Mental Health	Content, Construct, Criterion FA+	Cronbach α= .92
Measure of Perceived Physician Cultural Competency	9	No	Healthcare provider cultural competency: development and initial validation of a patient report measure (Lucas, et al, 2008)	310 Predominantly Low-income and/or Black Patients	Medical Clinics in Detroit, MI	Content, Construct, FA+ Discriminant, Convergent, incremental	Cronbach α =.68-.89 for each of the 9 Items

*Validity and/or reliability provided from a preceding study

+FA is our abbreviation for factor analysis

References for Appendix C

Arauz Boudreau, A. D., Fluet, C. F., Reuland, C. P., Delahaye, J., Perrin, J. M., & Kuhlthau, K. (2010). Associations of Providers' Language and Cultural Skills with Latino Parents' Perceptions of Well-child Care. *Academic Pediatrics, 10*(3), 172-178.

Arthur, T. E., Reeves, I., Morgan, O., Cornelius, L. J., Booker, N. C., Brathwaite, J., et al. (2005). Developing a cultural competence assessment tool for people in recovery from racial, ethnic and cultural backgrounds: the journey, challenges and lessons learned. *Psychiatric Rehabilitation Journal, 28*(3), 243-250.

Bernal, H., & Froman, R. (1987). The Confidence of Community Health Nurses in Caring for Ethnically Diverse Populations. *Image—Journal of Nursing Scholarship, 19*, 201-203.

Bonaparte, B. (1979). Ego, Defensiveness, Open-closed Mindedness, and Nurses' Attitudes Toward Culturally Different Patients. *Nursing Research, 28*, 166-172.

Campinha-Bacote, J. (2003). *The Process of Cultural Competence in the Delivery Healthcare Services: A Culturally Competent Model of Care* (4th ed.). Cincinnati, OH: Transcultural C.A.R.E. Associates.

Castro, A., & Ruiz, E. (2009). The Effect of Nurse Practitioner Cultural Competence on Latina Patient Satisfaction *Journal of the American Academy of Nurse Practitioners, 21*(5), 278-286.

Constantine, M. (2002). Predictors of Satisfaction with Counseling: Racial and Ethnic Minority Clients' Attitudes toward Counseling and Ratings of their Counselors' General and Multicultural Counseling Competence. *Journal of Counseling Psychology, 49*(2), 255-263.

Dillman, D. (1999). *Mail and Internet Surveys: The Tailored Design Method* (2nd Ed. ed.). New York: Wiley.

Doorenbos, A., Myers Schim, S., Benkert, R., & Borse, N. N. (2005). Psychometric evaluation of the Cultural Competence Assessment instrument among healthcare providers. *Nursing Research 54*(4), 324-331.

Fernandez, A., Schillinger, D., Grumbach, K., Rosenthal, A., Stewart, A. L., Wang, F., et al. (2004). Physician language ability and cultural competence. An exploratory study of communication with Spanish-speaking patients. *J Gen Intern Med, 19*(2), 167-174.

Fuertes, J. N., Stracuzzi, T. I., Bennett, J., Scheinholtz, J., Mislowack, A., Hersh, M., et al. (2006). Therapist Multicultural Competency: A study of therapy dyads. *Psychotherapy: Theory/Research/Practice/Training* </science/journal/00333204>*43*(4), 480-490.

Jones, M. E., Cason, C. L., & Bond, M. L. (2004). Cultural attitudes, knowledge, and skills of a health workforce. *Journal of Transcultural Nursing, 15*(4), 283-290.

LaFromboise T.D., C. H. L. K., and Hernandez A. (1991). Development and Factor Structure of the Cross-Cultural Inventory—Revised. *Professional Psychology: Research and Practice, 22,* 380-388.

LaFromboise, T. D., Coleman, H. L. K., & Hernandez, A. (1991). Development and Factor Analysis of the Cross-cultural Counseling Inventory—Revised. *Professional Psychology: Research and Practice, 22,* 380-388.

Lieu, T. A., Finkelstein, J. A., Lozano, P., Capra, A. M., Chi, F. W., Jensvold, N., et al. (2004). Cultural competence policies and other predictors of asthma care quality for Medicaid-insured children. *Pediatrics, 114*(1), e102-110.

Lucas, T., Michalopoulou, G., Falzarano, P., Menon, S., & Cunningham, W. (2008). Healthcare provider cultural competency: development and initial validation of a patient report measure. *Health Psychology, 27*(2), 185-193.

Napoles, A. M., Sanntoyo-Olssom, J., L.S., K., O'Brien, H., S.E., G., & Perez-Stable, E. (2010). Clinician Ratings of Interpreter Mediated Visits in Underserved Primary Care Settings with Ad hoc, In-person Professional, and Video Conferencing Modes. *Journal of Health Care for the Poor and Underserved 21*(1), 301-317.

Noble, L. M., Noble, A., & Hand, I. L. (2009). Cultural competence of healthcare professionals caring for breastfeeding mothers in urban areas. *Breastfeeding Medicine 4*(4), 221-224.

Paez, K. A., Allen, J. K., Carson, K. A., & Cooper, L. A. (2008). Provider and clinic cultural competence in a primary care setting. *Social Science & Medicine 66*(5), 1204-1216.

Polacek, G., & Martinez, R. (2009). Assessing Cultural Competence at a Local Hospital System in the United States. *Health Care Management, 28*(2), 98-110.

Rooda, L. (1993). Knowledge and Attitudes of Nurses Toward Culturally Different Patients: Implications for Nursing Education. *Journal of Nursing Education, 32*, 209-213.

Sabnani, H., & Ponterotto, J. (1992). Racial/ethnic Minority-specific Instrumentation in Counseling Research: A Review, Critique, and Recommendations. *Measurement and Evaluation in Counseling and Development, 24*, 161-187.

Schim, S. M., Doorenbos, A. Z., & Borse, N. N. (2005). Cultural competence among Ontario and Michigan healthcare providers. *Journal of Nursing Scholarship 37*(4), 354-360.

Schim, S. M., Doorenbos, A. Z., Miller, J., & Benkert, R. (2003). Development of a Cultural Competence Assessment Instrument *Journal of Nursing Measurement 11*(1), 29-40.

Starr, S., & Wallace, D. C. (2009). Self-reported cultural competence of public health nurses in a Southeastern U.S. Public health department. *Public Health Nursing, 26*(1), 48-57.

Appendix D
Table IV. *Analysis of Grey Literature Utilizing Cultural Competence Self-Assessment Tools*

Tool Name	Year Published	# of Items	Assessed Linguistic Competence	Health Care Setting	Validity	Reliability
ORGANIZATIONAL LEVEL TOOLS						
CLAS Standards Assessment Tool (The Office of Minority Health, 2005)	Not Listed	14	Yes	Unspecified	None	None
Conducting a Cultural Competence Self-Assessment (Andrulis, Delbanco, Avakian, & Shaw-Taylor)	Not Listed	122	Yes	Unspecified	None	None
Checklist to Facilitate the Development of Culturally and Linguistically Competent Primary Health Care Policies and Structures (Goode, Cohen, & Dunne, 2003)	Not Listed	14	Yes	Unspecified	None	None
Quality Organizational Self-Assessment (State of Connecticut Department of Developmental Services (DDS), 2008)	2008	56	Yes	Unspecified	None	None
Developing a Multiculturally Competent Service System for an Organization or Program (The Connecticut Department of Children and Families Office of Multicultural Affairs, 2002)	2002	53	Yes	Unspecified	None	None

Tool Name	Year Published	# of Items	Assessed Linguistic Competence	Health Care Setting	Validity	Reliability
Cultural Competency: Measurement as a Strategy for Moving Knowledge into Practice in State Mental Health Systems—Final Report (National Technical Assistance Center for State Mental Health Planning (NTCA) and National Association of State Mental Health Program Directors (NASMHPD), 2004)	2004	55	Yes	Mental Health	None	None
Developing a Self-Assessment Tool for Culturally and Linguistically Appropriate Services in Local Public Health Agencies: Final Report (The Cosmos Corporation, 2003)	2003	108	Yes	Public Health	Content Reported in Preceding Literature (Office of Minority Health)	Reported in Preceding Literature (Office of Minority Health)
Cultural Competence: A Program Self-Assessment (Amherst H. Wilder Foundation, 2002)	2002	171	Yes	Unspecified	Content	None
Linguistically Appropriate Access and Services; An Evaluation and Review for Healthcare Organizations (Anderson, 2002)	2001; Revised 2002	154	Yes	Organizations Serving Linguistically Diverse Populations	None	None
Cultural and Linguistic Competence Policy Assessment (CLCPA) (National Center for Cultural Competence, 2006)	2006	63	Yes	Community Health	None	None

Tool Name	Year Published	# of Items	Assessed Linguistic Competence	Health Care Setting	Validity	Reliability
Cultural Competency Assessment Scale With Instructions (Siegel, Haugland, & Chambers, 2004)	2004	11	Yes	Behavioral Health	None	None
Assessment of Organizational Cultural Competence (Hiranaka, 2004)	2004	23	Yes	Unspecified	None	None
Program Self-Assessment Survey for Cultural Competence (Weiss & Minsky, 1996)	Not Listed	10	Yes	Unspecified	None	None
Cultural Competence Assessment (Evans, 2001)	2001	128	Yes	Unspecified	None	None
Cultural Competence Self-Assessment Questionnaire (CCSAQ) (Mason J & Williams-Murphy T, 1995)	1995	95	Yes	Mental Health	Content	Cronbach $\alpha = .60$ – above .80 for all subscales

PROVIDER-LEVEL TOOLS

Tool Name	Year Published	# of Items	Assessed Linguistic Competence	Health Care Setting	Validity	Reliability
Provider Self-Assessment Survey (Tirado, 1996b)	1996	17	Yes	Organizations serving Linguistically Diverse Populations	None	None
Cultural Competence Checklists: (American Speech, Language, & Hearing Association, 2010)	2002; Rev. 2010	45	Yes	Unspecified	None	None
Clinical Cultural Competency Questionnaire (Pre-Training Version) (Like, 2001b)	2001	56	Yes	Unspecified	None	None

Tool Name	Year Published	# of Items	Assessed Linguistic Competence	Health Care Setting	Validity	Reliability
Clinical Cultural Competency Questionnaire (Post-Training Version) (Like, 2001a)	2001	49	Yes	Unspecified	None	None
Cultural Competence Self-Assessment (Planned Parenthood Federation of America, 2003)	2003	23	Yes	Unspecified	None	None
Promoting Cultural and Linguistic Competency: Self-Assessment Checklist for Personnel Providing Primary Health Care Services (Goode, 2004)	1989; Revised 2004	37	Yes	Organizations serving Linguistically Diverse Populations	None	None
Promoting Cultural and Linguistic Competency: Self-Assessment Checklist for Personnel Providing Services and Supports in Early Intervention and Early Childhood Settings (Goode, 2005)	1989; Revised 2005	49	Yes	Pediatrics	None	None

			PATIENT-LEVEL TOOLS			
Patient Satisfaction Survey (Tirado, 1996a)	1996	50	Yes	Unspecified	Content	None
Questionnaire: Validation of Hospital Data Collection of Patients' Race and Ethnicity and Primary Language (Unknown, Unknown)	Not listed	13	Yes	Hospitals	None	None

References for Appendix D

American Speech, Language, & Hearing Association (2010). *Cultural Competence Checklists: Service Delivery, Personal Reflection, and Policies & Procedures* (http://www.asha.org/NR/rdonlyres/07693109-C4F6-48EA-BFC3-58874C8998F9/0/service_delivery.pdf).

Amherst H. Wilder Foundation (2002). *Cultural Competence: A Program Self-Assessment* Amherst H. Wilder Foundation Services to Children, Elderly, and Families.

Anderson, C. C. (2002). *Linguistically Appropriate Access and Services: An Evaluation and Review for Healthcare Organizations*: The National Council on Interpreting in Health Care.

Andrulis, D., Delbanco, T., Avakian, L., & Shaw-Taylor, Y. Conducting a Cultural Competence Self-Assessment.

Evans, J. (2001). *Cultural Competence Assessment*. The National Maternal and Child Health Resource Center on Cultural Competency for Children with Special Health Care Needs and Their Families; Texas Department of Health.

Goode, T. (2004). *Promoting Cultural and Linguistic Competency Self Assessment Checklist for Personnel Providing Primary Health Care Services*. Georgetown University Center for Child and Human Development

Goode, T. (2005). *Promoting Cultural and Linguistic Competency: Self Assessment Checklist for Personnel Providing Services and Supports in Early Intervention and Early Childhood Settings*. Washington, DC: National Center for Cultural Competence.

Georgetown University Center for Child and Human Development, University Center for Excellence in Developmental Disabilities Education, Research &, Service.

Goode, T., Cohen, E., & Dunne, C. (2003). *Checklist to Facilitate the Development of Culturally and Linguistically Competent Primary Health Care Policies and Structures*. (http://www11.georgetown.edu/research/gucchd/nccc/documents/Policy_Brief_1_2003.pdf). Washington, D.C.: National Center for Cultural Competence— Bureau of Primary Healthcare Project and Georgetown University Center for Child and Human Development.

Hiranaka, C., Richardson, C, Ball, A, Hohlstein, R, Lopez, R, Meaney, F, Parrish, R, Wilson, L (2004) *Assessment of*

Organizational Cultural Competence. (www.aucd.org/councils/ multicultural/Cultural_Competence_Survey.htm): Association of University Centers on Disabilities (AUCD).

Like, R. C. (2001a). *Clinical Cultural Competency Questionnaire (Post-Training Version).* The Center for Health Families and Cultural Diversity, Department of Family Medicine, UMDNJ-Robert Wood Johnson Medical School.

Like, R. C. (2001b). *Clinical Cultural Competency Questionnaire (Pre-Training Version)*: The Center for Health Families and Cultural Diversity, Department of Family Medicine, UMDNJ-Robert Wood Johnson Medical School.

Mason J, & Williams-Murphy T (1995). *Cultural Competence Self-Assessment Questionnaire: A Manual for Users.* Portland: Graduate School of Social Work, Portland State University.

National Center for Cultural Competence (2006). *Cultural and Linguistic Competence Policy Assessment.* (www.georgetown. edu/research/gucchd/nccc/siteindex.html). Washington, DC: National Center for Cultural Competence—Georgetown University Center for Child and Human Development.

National Technical Assistance Center for State Mental Health Planning (NTCA) and National Association of State Mental Health Program Directors (NASMHPD) (2004). *Cultural Competency: Measurement as a Strategy for Moving Knowledge into Practice in State Mental Health Systems (Final Report)* (www.nasmhpd.org/publications.cfm#cultcomp).

Office of Minority Health, D. *National Study of Culturally and Linguistically Appropriate Services in Managed Care Organizations.*

Planned Parenthood Federation of America, I. (2003). *Cultural Competence Self-Assessment* (www.plannedparenthood.org).

Siegel, C., Haugland, G., & Chambers, E. (2004). *Cultural Competency Assessment Scale with Instructions.* (www.csipmh. rfmh.org/projects/id9.shtm). New York: Nathan S. Kline Institute for Psychiatric Research, Center for the Study of Issues in Public Mental Health.

State of Connecticut Department of Developmental Services (DDS) (2008). *Quality Organizational Self-Assessment.*

The Connecticut Department of Children and Families Office of Multicultural Affairs (2002). *Assessment Guidelines for*

Developing a Multiculturally Competent Service System for an Organization or Program. (www.ct.gov/dcf/cwp/view.asp?a=2546&q=314458).

The Cosmos Corporation (2003). *Final Report: Developing a Self-Assessment Tool for Culturally and Linguistically Appropriate Services in Local Public Health Agencies.* (www.cosmoscorp.com/publications.html).

The Office of Minority Health (2005, October). *CLAS Standards Assessment Tool.*

Tirado, M. (1996a). *Patient Satisfaction Survey.* California State University—Monterey Bay.

Tirado, M. (1996b). *Provider Self-Assessment Survey.* California State University—Monterey Bay.

Unknown (Unknown). *Questionnaire: Validation of Hospital Data Collection of Patients' Race and Ethnicity and Primary Language.*

Weiss, C., & Minsky, S. (1996). *Program Self-Assessment Survey for Cultural Competence: A Manual.* Trenton, N.J.: New Jersey Division of Mental Health and Hospitals.

CHAPTER EIGHT

Best Practices in Culturally Appropriate Health Education Approaches

Linda Fleisher
Children's Hospital of
Philadelphia

Sarah Bauerie Bass
Temple University

Evelyn Gonzalez
Fox Chase Cancer
Center

Stacy N. Davis
Fox Chase Cancer
Center

Rachel Slamon
American Diabetes
Association
(Philadelphia)

Stephanie Raivitch
Fox Chase Cancer
Center

Maria Jibaja-Weiss
Baylor College of
Medicine

Luis O. Rustveld
Baylor College of
Medicine

Venk Kandadai
Children's Hospital of
Philadelphia

Michael C. Gibbons
Johns Hopkins Urban
Health Institute

Abstract

The field of health education has evolved resulting in a body of best practices addressing the role of the community and the integration of cultural and linguistic factors. The process of developing effective health education programs requires defining the target audience, their needs, beliefs and outcomes and effective health education programs. They have the potential to reduce health disparities, improve health outcomes and reduce health care costs if developed within the context of culture, community-engagement, health literacy and relevant communication channels. Health education and health communications are vast disciplines and this chapter highlights only a select number of best practices including: a planning framework, key issues related to developing culturally and linguistically appropriate materials and programs, and description of key communication channels that may be most relevant for racial and ethnic minority populations. Three case studies, focusing on cancer prevention and diabetes management, highlight the utilization of these best practices.

Introduction

According to the World Health Organization (WHO), "Health education is any combination of learning experiences designed to help individuals and communities improve their health, by increasing their knowledge or influencing their attitudes". It is important to view health education within an ecological context addressing the individual, organization, community and policy factors (Green & Kreuter, 2004). Within an ecological context, health is the result of a reciprocal relationship between an individual and their environment. Environment includes all of the interpersonal, community, organizational, and policy influences on the individual (Green & Kreuter, 2004). These influences have been established as factors that play a crucial role in interference or adoption of a health behavior. Therefore, effective health education interventions take place within an ecological context (Green & Kreuter, 2004). Moreover, there are multiple, somewhat competing ecological models which are operating for diverse populations in the U.S. and the world. Therefore, for any health education programs, interventions and materials to be successful, they need to be developed within the context of the target populations, the target behaviors and culture.

Developing effective health education programs requires time and preparation. The process usually includes assessment, planning, implementation and evaluation. Part of the assessment process involves defining the target audience, their needs, beliefs and outcomes. With proper planning and implementation a health education program has the ability to change individual behavior, prevent disease and improve quality of life (Glanz, Rimer, & Viswanath, 2008; Green & Kreuter, 2004). At the community level, effective health education programs have the potential to reduce health disparities, improve health outcomes and reduce health care costs.

Emerging evidence suggests that integrating cultural factors into health education interventions may increase the efficacy of

The authors would like to acknowledge the assistance of Ms. Susan Echtermeyer-Fleisher, Administrative Coordinator in the Office of Health Communications and Health Disparities, Fox Chase Cancer Center.

those programs among diverse subpopulations (U.S. Department of Health and Human Services, 2011). Culture has many definitions, but among many scholars culture is broadly defined as a common heritage or learned set of beliefs, norms and values. Specifically, culture can be defined as the customary beliefs, values, and ideas shared by a racial, religious, or social group of people (Arthur & Katkin, 2006). No matter the definition used, culture is a "map" for living that dictates ones interpretation of the world and how one acts in the world. Developing effective health education programs requires time and preparation. The process usually includes assessment, planning, implementation and evaluation. Part of the assessment process involves defining the target audience, their needs, beliefs and outcomes. With proper planning and implementation a health education program has the ability to change individual behavior, prevent disease and improve quality of life (Glanz, Rimer, & Viswanath, 2008; Green & Kreuter, 2004). At the community level, effective health education programs have the potential to reduce health disparities, improve health outcomes and reduce health care costs.

Emerging evidence suggests that integrating cultural factors into health education interventions may increase the efficacy of those programs among diverse subpopulations (U.S. Department of Health and Human Services, 2011). Four racial and ethnic minority groups—African Americans, American Indians and Alaska Natives, Asian Americans and Pacific Islanders, and Hispanic Americans—accounted for approximately 30 percent of the U.S. population in the year 2000 and are expected to account for nearly 40 percent of the U.S. population by 2020 (U.S. Department of Commerce Census Bureau, 2004). Although there are important differences among these four groups, there also is broad diversity within each group. This within group diversity also means that similar racial groups do not always share the same culture. Language also has a clear impact on culture. Language reflects culture and is simultaneously influenced and shaped by it (Torres, 1998). Therefore the impact of language on minority subgroups differs based on social and demographic characteristics. In the United States, about 14% of the population does not speak English (Betancourt & Jacobs, 2000). This lack of understanding of English is a barrier that can cause misunderstandings that lead to inappropriate health decisions (Andrulis & Brach, 2007).

Culture directly affects health by shaping and influencing habits and behaviors related to precursors of health, development of disease, and by influencing the cultural group's physical environment (Arthur & Katkin, 2006; Kreuter & McClure, 2004). Interpretations of health and illness may vary with different cultural groups and ultimately informs why some cultural groups choose to adopt or not adopt preventative health behaviors. Thus health education materials need to be culturally appropriate.

Health education and health communications are vast disciplines and this chapter highlights only a select number of best practices including: a planning approach, key issues related to developing culturally and linguistically appropriate materials and programs, and description of key communication channels that may be most relevant for racial and ethnic minority populations. Three case studies, focusing on cancer prevention and diabetes management, highlight the utilization of these best practices.

Health Education and Communication Best Practices

The goal of a successful health communication program is to promote or improve health. To improve or promote behavior the health communication should be based on the needs and perceptions of the intended audience (National Cancer Institute, 2002). This can only be accomplished through planning and tailoring (Hawkins, Kreuter, Resnicow, Fishbein, & Dijkstra, 2008; Keller & Lehmann, 2008).

Program Planning

The NCI Health Communication Planning Model provides a framework to help plan and develop a successful health communication program that is based on the needs and perceptions of the intended audience (National Cancer Institute, 2002). This model divides the planning process into four stages: planning and strategy development; developing and pretesting concepts, messages, and materials; implementing the program; and assessing effectiveness and making refinements. (See Figure 1).

Stage One is the planning and development stage. Planning is done to provide the foundation for the health communication program and ensures production of meaningful materials. It is therefore crucial that researchers understand the health problem and the role that communication can play in moving towards a solution to the health problem. The planning process includes six steps: assessing the health issue; defining communication objectives; defining and learning the intended audience; exploring the best settings and channels to reach the intended audience; identifying potential partners; and developing and drafting a communication plan for the intended audience. Among diverse target audiences, this step is critical. The target population norms, beliefs, preferences, and preferred communications channels

Figure 1. NCI Health Communication Planning Model

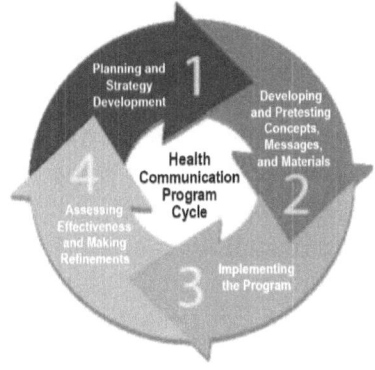

may not be the same as those used by the program developers. Thus, having this information will enable the development of interventions that best meet the objectively identified needs and norms of the target population.

Stage Two is the developing and pretesting of messages and materials stage. During this stage, researchers apply the insight and knowledge gained from stage one to create initial campaign messages and materials. Pre-testing the messages and materials allows the researcher to learn which health messages will resonate with the intended audiences. In addition, pretesting the messages and materials will help to ensure buy-in from the intended audience and partners. This stage includes five steps: review existing materials; develop and test message concepts; decide what materials to develop; develop messages and materials; and pretest messages and materials. As in stage one, this pretesting is essential, particularly when designing interventions for diverse target populations, and can help developers avoid costly mistakes and unintended delays or unexpected failures.

Stage Three is the actual implementation of the program. Before implementing the health communication program, researchers should make a plan for distribution and promotion of the program, the kick-off event, and maintaining media relations after the launch. In addition to reaching out to the intended audience, researchers should track exposure and reactions to the health messages and materials. This will help to ensure that communication messages and materials are being properly distributed and to highlight aspects of the campaign that may need to be adjusted on an ongoing basis.

The Fourth and Final Stage is assessing the effectiveness and making refinements of the health communication program for future use. This stage is crucial to researchers in that it allows researchers to reflect on how close they came to reaching their communication objectives. Conducting outcome evaluations includes the following steps: determine what information the evaluation must provide; decide the data to collect; decide on data collection methods; develop and pre-test data collection instruments; collect data; process data; analyze data to answer the evaluation questions; write an evaluation report, and disseminate the evaluation report.

Culturally and Linguistically Appropriate Interventions

Culturally and linguistically health interventions are those that are respectful of and responsive to cultural and linguistic needs. Cultural and linguistic competence is a set of congruent behaviors, attitudes, and policies that enables effective communication in cross-cultural situations. As noted above 'Culture' refers to integrated patterns of human behavior that include the language, thoughts, communications, actions, customs, beliefs, values, and institutions of racial, ethnic, religious, or social groups. Finally 'Competence' implies having the capacity to function or communicate effectively as an individual within the context of the cultural beliefs, behaviors, and needs presented by individuals and their communities (Cross, Bazron, Dennis, & Isaacs, 1989).

Within the context of these definitions, culturally targeted interventions involve messages that are intended to reach *population subgroups* based on a specific set of *shared characteristics*.

Culturally tailored interventions, involve messages that are intended to reach *an individual* based on specific *characteristics of the individual* as measured in a formal assessment process (Kreuter, Lukwago, Bucholtz, Clark, & Sanders-Thompson, 2003).

Language is an integral part of culture and individuals with limited or no English proficiency are often unable to fully comprehend the information presented, hence jeopardizing good health outcomes. Furthermore, language barriers contribute to a poor exchange of information that compromises the decision-making process. In 2002 the Institute of Medicine (IOM) released *Unequal Treatment: Confronting Racial and Ethnic Disparities in Healthcare* which identified barriers to care for racial and ethnic minorities. The report also produced specific recommendations to address the barriers identified. Targeted intervention to be used in the health care setting stressed the need of supporting interpretation services where community needs exist (Smedley, Stith, & Nelson, 2003). Prior to the IOM report, the Office of Minority Health (OMH) launched an effort to address inequities within the health system and in 2000 produced the national standards on culturally and linguistically appropriate services (CLAS). According to OMH, the standards are especially designed to address the needs of racial, ethnic, and linguistic population groups that experience unequal access to health services (U.S. Department of Health and Human Services Office of Minority Health, 2001). There are 14 standards of which four (4,5,6,7) are mandated and the remainder are guidelines and recommendations. The four mandated standards mandate that health systems, have access to qualified language services, to inform Limited English Proficiency (LEP) patients of their right to language services, qualifications for bilingual and interpreter services and translation of materials (educational and signage) (U.S. Department of Health and Human Services Office of Minority Health, 2001).

Therefore, the development of health education materials should address cultural and linguistic issues for the target population and recognize that both the intervention and the health care exchange or interaction also needs to be culturally and linguistically tailored.

Health Literacy. Health literacy has also been recognized as a key factor related to health disparities (Institute of Medicine, 2004). *Healthy People 2010* defines health literacy as "the degree to which individuals have the capacity to obtain, process and understand basic health information and services they need to make appropriate health decisions." In everyday terms, this means having the ability to understand the directions for giving your baby a new medication, how many hours you need to fast for the blood work your doctor just ordered, or what it means when your doctor tells you that you have hypertension. Sound easy? For 93 million Americans, it's anything but. In 2003, the National Assessment of Adult Literacy found that 43% of adults in this country have either basic or below basic health literacy skills. What does that mean? It means that they lack the critical skills necessary to effectively navigate their way through an often complex healthcare system. The problem of low health literacy is a crisis that affects everyone, but there are particular groups that bear a disproportionate burden: older people, non-whites, immigrants, non-high school graduates and those with low socioeconomic status (Kirsch, Jungeblut, Jenkins, & Kolstad, 1993). Several studies have found that low health literacy was more common among African Americans, persons with lower educational attainment and Spanish-speakers (Institute of Medicine, 2004; Kutner, Greenberg, Jin, & Paulsen, 2006).

Fifty percent of Hispanic Americans and 40% of African Americans have reading problems (Kirsch et al., 1993). The average American reads at the 8th grade level or below, yet over 300 published studies evaluating health-related materials found that most of the materials were written at levels that exceed the reading skills of average high school graduates (Rudd, Moeykens, & Colton, 2000) As a result, people with low health literacy know less about their health problems, are less likely to practice preventive behaviors, are less likely to follow instructions for managing their chronic health conditions, and more likely to have frequent hospitalizations. Recent studies have confirmed that low health literacy is associated with poorer health outcomes and higher mortality rates (Agency for Healthcare Research and Quality, 2010).

Health education materials and approaches should carefully address health literacy issues in the design, content and approach. There are numerous resources and guides that address this important issue (Andrulis & Brach, 2007; Bass, Gallo, Crookes, Berger, & Fleisher, 2008; Doak, Doak, & Root, 1996; National Cancer Institute, 1994; Osborne, 2011).

Community Engagement. Engaging communities for the purpose of addressing an issue that disproportionately affects them, be it one of social justice or health, it is a strategy gaining more recognition. Long before the publication *It Takes a Village,* the practice of community engagement has been utilized worldwide. The formal use of community engagement as a science or practice to address health promotion and research is relatively new (Minkler, Wallerstein, & Wilson, 2008). In 1997, CDC set forth principles of community engagement to facilitate the process for implementation. The working definition provided was:

> . . . the process of working collaboratively with and through groups of people affiliated by geographic proximity, special interest, or similar situations to address issues affecting the wellbeing of those people. It is a powerful vehicle for bringing about environmental and behavioral changes that will improve the health of the community and its members. It often involves partnerships and coalitions that help mobilize resources and influence systems, change relationships among partners, and serve as catalysts for changing policies, programs, and practices (Centers for Disease Control and Prevention, 1997).

For years, practitioners have used surveys, focus groups and interviews to gain knowledge and insight on how specific issues are viewed or how they impact health behaviors with outcomes used to develop interventions. Community engagement can provide similar information however its purpose is to develop a more profound understanding of communities, cultures, partnerships, gaps and assets. Unlike focus groups or other research methods, which tend to be time framed, community engagement is a long term commitment to mutual understanding and respect for one another while finding a solution to a problem (Minkler et al., 2008). By focusing on the relationship and the needs of the community as the priority, a more participatory approach to research and increased relevance of the research emerges. Using principles and frameworks that recognize and honor the insight communities provide will help to ease and eventually overcome negative perceptions regarding research and researchers.

With the broadening use of community-based participatory research (CBPR) we see the use of community engagement as a key function. The nine principles set forth in *Principles of Community Engagement* (Table 1, Appendix A at the end of this chapter) are what are required prior to engagement, during engagement and those necessary for a fruitful outcome (Centers for Disease Control and Prevention, 1997). Successful outcomes of community engagement include shared decision making, shared acknowledgment, stronger relationships and partnerships, better communication, increased trust and commitment to work for a healthy community. With stronger partnerships comes the potential for ongoing opportunities for collaboration, shared resources and expanded networks.

Health Education Channels

Health education approaches can range from efforts to change individual behaviors to much broader systems and/or policy changes formulated to address health disparities. Often, health education is provided as part of a community-based intervention and usually includes face-to-face health education with individuals or groups. Healthy People 2020 has a specific goal to "increase the quality, availability, and effectiveness of educational and community-based programs designed to prevent disease and injury, improve health, and enhance quality of life" (U.S. Department of Health and Human Services). Offered in a variety of community-based settings, organizers have a responsibility to engage the community in the development of the program. The Institute of Medicine (2003) notes that realizing the vision of healthy people in healthy communities is possible only if the community, in its full cultural, social, and economic diversity, is an authentic partner in changing the conditions for health. Engaging the community, as discussed earlier, is a significant strategy to ensure success. It is also important that the health messages used in a large health education intervention are culturally relevant and appropriate and are developed through accessible communication channels. This differentiates the role of health education from the broader strategies of public health interventions.

The foundation of health communication strategies to provide health education and promote health-related behavior change have most often used traditional methods such as printed materials, telephone counseling, and campaigns using broadcast media outlets (Owen, Fotheringham, & Marcus, 2002). The availability of new communication and information technologies, however, has opened a wide range of strategies for health behavior change educational programs and research. The use of health communication channels such as computer-based tutorials, Web 2.0 and cell phones, as interventions have been successfully utilized in a variety of locations (i.e. managed care settings, public areas through the use of kiosks) as well as with a variety of health topics (i.e. cancer screening promotion, smoking cessation, cancer survivorship, diabetes management, exercise, nutrition, sexual health education, STD prevention, emergency preparedness, and even in the psychosocial realm such as anxiety and stress reduction) (Gibbons et al., 2011; Hesse et al., 2005). The Pew Internet and American Life Project defines web 2.0 as, "an umbrella term that is used to refer to a new era of Web-enabled applications that are built around user-generated or user-manipulated content, such as wikis, blogs, podcasts, and social networking sites" (2011b). Here, we further describe traditional types of health education channels (print and telephonic), the newly developing channels (computer based, Web 2.0 communication, cell phones) and examine the evidence and practical uses and implications for addressing health disparities in minority populations.

Print Materials. Print materials such as brochures, pamphlets, and fact sheets have been adopted by the healthcare world for delivering health education to a broad population since the 1970s (Glanz et al., 2008). The body of evidence suggests that these types of channels are an effective way to deliver health education across different populations, especially if they are tailored to a specific audience (Noar, Benac, & Harris, 2007). The provision of print educational information is considered to be important to encourage consumer participation in health care and effective health decision making (Currie, Rajendran, Spink, Carter, & Anderson, 2001). A number of studies have explored the effectiveness of print materials such as pamphlets, booklets and leaflets as tools for public or patient education (Harris, Smith, & Veale, 2005; Little et al., 2001). One review of the effectiveness of print materials found that pamphlets could be effective in changing knowledge, attitudes and behavior in relation to a wide range of health-related issues (Paul & Redman, 1997), however using print materials alone is limited in their effect on health behavior and impact on health outcomes (Farmer et al., 2008; Paul & Redman, 1997). This is especially true in populations with literacy or language deficiencies. Despite this, it is nonetheless apparent that print materials have been integral to public and patient health education strategies and can be an effective component in a larger health education intervention.

Telephone Interventions. The majority of telephone-based interventions has been conducted using landline telephone lines and has been an effective model for delivering health education and health counseling (Cook, Emiliozzi, El-Hajj, & McCabe, 2010; Kluhsman et al., 2010; Marcus et al., 2010; McBride & Rimer, 1999). Sacco and colleagues (2009) used a brief telephone educational intervention as a tool for type-2 diabetes self-management. The intervention increased the amount of exercise and foot inspection, improved dietary habits, and reduced diabetes medical symptoms. In a pilot study, Kluhsman and colleagues (2010) used a telephone based intervention to counsel rural Appalachia patients on the importance of colorectal cancer screening and to complete a home-based fecal immunochemical test (Graham et al., 2000; Heseltine, 2007). Telephone interventions have also shown effectiveness in minority populations. Basch and colleagues (2006) used a telephone-based outreach intervention to increase colorectal cancer screening among an urban minority population who were not current in screening. The authors concluded that targeted telephone outreach was an effective way to deliver colorectal cancer screening education within an urban population. The benefit of using the telephone in health education is the ability to tailor messages for the user to better address their needs. This is a benefit to working with diverse populations, especially those with limited literacy or who speak a language other than English. This main detriment to relying on telephonic channels is the growing number of people who do not have a landline in their house and rely on cell phones for communication or use call screening technologies and do not answer calls on their landlines from numbers they do not recognize (Kempf & Remington, 2007).

Cell Phones. Over the past ten years, there has been a growing trend from a landline-based population to a mobile phone-only population (Smith, 2010b), providing an opportunity to extend evidence-based telephone interventions to a much larger group. Interventions for mobile phone technology are not only limited to traditional telephone calling but also to an ever increasing texting population. Recent reviews have concluded that cell phones, specifically text messaging, can be used successfully to promote behavior change (Cole-Lewis & Kershaw, 2010), including smoking (Free et al., 2009), diet (Haapala, Barengo, Biggs, Surakka, & Manninen, 2009), physical activity (Newton, Wiltshire, & Elley, 2009) and sexual activity (Lim et al., 2011). These interventions have generally provided participants with information and reminders relevant to the behavior of interest, using texts as a non-intrusive way to reach an audience with repeated and consistent health messages. Approaches to designing and delivering the text messages include relatively simple systems, where the same message is sent out to each participant, as well as systems where broadcasts are individually tailored to participants' characteristics and preferences.

These types of interventions may be especially cogent for minority populations. Although a gap between non-Whites (Black and Latino) and Whites in access to the Internet and broadband at home continues to exist, the gap in cell phone ownership is negligible. African Americans and Latinos actually report higher levels of wireless Internet use (Gibbons et al., 2011; Smith, 2010c). According to the Pew Internet and American Life Project, African Americans and Latinos lead the way in using cell phones and mobile devices to access the Internet, use instant messaging, engage social networking sites, look up health information, and track or manage their health with specialized applications (Smith, 2011). Of those who own a cell phone, 51% of English-speaking Hispanics, 46% of African Americans, and 33% of White non-Hispanics use their phone to access the Internet. A similar pattern is seen for use of phones to access a social networking site (Smith, 2010c), making this another potentially effective method to reach minority populations.

Internet Based Interventions. Worldwide Internet usage is growing rapidly, increasing by 300% since 2008 (Gibbons, 2011). In the United States, 77% of adults report using the Internet (Pew

Internet & American Life Project, 2011a), with more than 80% of these (61% of all adults) seeking health information via the Internet (Gibbons, 2011; Rainie, 2011). A recent study found that, among users, the Internet was second only to healthcare providers as an information source important in their health decisions (Couper et al., 2010). Earlier research had shown that the Internet may empower patients to improve their health behaviors and to take a more active role in their health care (Bass et al., 2006; Horrigan, Rainie, & Fox, 2001). More recent studies have indicated that Internet-based health education interventions have many benefits over static print materials. A recent Cochrane review indicated that interactive, computer-based programs had significant positive effects on knowledge, social support and clinical outcomes. Results also suggest these programs positively affect self-efficacy and health behaviors (Murray, Burns, See, Lai, & Nazareth, 2005).

While minorities use the Internet less frequently and have less access to broadband, studies tailored to minority communities have also shown similar effects. One study with African Americans indicated that computer-tailored and Internet-based interventions are able to produce long-term increases in physical activity (Pekmezi et al., 2010). A similar ongoing study funded by the National Cancer Institute is promoting physical activity via an Internet-based program in Latinas (Marcus et al., 2010). Like other health education strategies, Internet-based programs can be effective in minority populations if they are tailored to the needs of specific communities.

Web 2.0 and Use of Social Media. The use of Web 2.0 technologies is rapidly changing. The November 2010 Pew Internet survey revealed that 61% of American adult Internet users age 18 and older use a social networking site like MySpace, Facebook or LinkedIn (Pew Internet & American Life Project, 2011a) up from 8% in February 2005. The most popular is Facebook, with almost three-fourths of those online having an account, followed by MySpace with 48% having an account. At the present time, it is estimated that about 14% of online adults have a LinkedIn account with smaller percentages having accounts with networking sites including Yahoo, YouTube, Tagged, Flickr and Classmates.com (Smith, 2010a). Chou and colleagues (2009) found that among Internet users, approximately 27% reported using at least one form of social media. Social networking was reported by 23% of survey respondents, followed by blogging (7%) and online support groups (5%).

Among racial and ethnic minority populations, the use of social media tools and the use of these tools on mobile devices have drastically increased from 2000 to 2010. For example, nearly half of African American and 20% of English-speaking Latino internet users use social networking sites such as Facebook and Twitter (Smith, 2011). This has provided an opportunity to reach minority populations with innovative health education programs. One example is GirlTrek: A Challenge to Black Women and Girls (http://www.girltrek.org/#!) which is a nonprofit online community. GirlTrek focuses on getting Black women and girls physically active by joining the GirlTrek walking campaign. The GirlTrek site encourages women to walk with teams or train for 5K races by sharing stories and connecting with other healthy Black women and girls. The site includes real testimonies from and photographs of women who have joined the campaign. The site also includes a way to connect through Facebook, the GirlTrek blog, and Twitter. The GirlTrek, or Healthy Black Women and Girls Facebook page, (http:// www.facebook.com/HealthyBlackWomenandGirls)   has more than 24,000 "likes" and a large number of user-generated comments. Most of the comments from these women relate to their progress with training or physical activity. Social relationships have been shown to be important in managing disease (Gibbons et al., 2011). The example of Healthy Black Women and Girls shows that social media could be a powerful tool in using these relationships to impact disease management and maintain health. Web 2.0 applications have thus provided a promising medium to engage in health education and health promotion among disparate populations (Gibbons et al., 2011).

Examples from the Field

Three case studies presented here provide examples of health education materials developed using best practice approaches, addressing important health disparities issues, and using a broad range of health education channels. Each case study describes: the target audience and behavior; the type of delivery channel used;

the developmental process and how the intervention addressed culturally and linguistically relevant issues; and how best practice approaches were integrated.

Case Study #1: *Stop Now For Your Baby*—Linda Fleisher, Fox Chase Cancer Center

Background: Maternal smoking during pregnancy poses substantial long-term and short-term health risks for the mother, the developing fetus and the newborn. Smoking during pregnancy has been associated with increased risk of spontaneous abortion, still birth, perinatal death and low-birth weight. It has also been associated with increased Sudden Infant Death Syndrome. When this program was designed almost 20 years ago, the smoking rate for women attending public health clinics was 40-50% (U.S. Department of Health and Human Services, 1990) and the smoking cessation rate during pregnancy for those women was estimated at only 9% (Kleinman & Kopstein, 1987). Sadly, there has not been as significant a decline in smoking during pregnancy over the past two decades. Some studies indicate that, in the last decade, smoking rates during pregnancy were about 20% and up to 35% in Medicaid populations (Lumley et al., 2009).

Description of the Program and its Target Audience: This program was designed to facilitate smoking cessation and maintenance among lower income mothers utilizing state and federally funded maternal and child health programs. The program was developed based on three behavioral theories, including the Transtheoretical Model of Behavior Change, Theory of Reasoned Action and the Health Belief Model. The program consisted of brief, tailored counseling provided by the health care provider and a unique self-help guide, called *Stop Now For Your Baby* which was specifically designed for pregnant smokers. The counseling was designed to be conducted in five minutes or less and as part of routine prenatal care. Women were identified through a specially designed Smoking History which was provided to all women at the participating sites. If a woman had smoked at the start of her pregnancy or was currently smoking, the staff assessed women's stage and interest in quitting and provided appropriate tailored messages based on her readiness to quit. A Quit Smoking Counseling Form was used by the staff and included the STOP IT protocol (see box below).

S—Sympathize with difficulty of quitting
T—Take a smoking history
O—Offer a clear quit message
P—Plan for quitting based on readiness to quit
I—Introduce quitting materials, *Stop Now for Your Baby*
T—Track and reinforce at subsequent visits

All evaluation data were collected on the STOP IT form and through follow-up calls. The self-help guide, *Stop Now For Your Baby,* is a 28-page, full color magazine style guide which addresses the unique concern of pregnant smokers. It is written for a racially and ethnically diverse population and designed for women with limited literacy skills. For example, visuals were carefully used to support written text, information was chunked into magazine type articles, and the text was written at a 5th grade reading level. The guide included five sections: addressing reasons for quitting; steps to quitting; staying off cigarettes: health promotions tips; and postpartum relapse and effects of passive smoke. First person vignettes based on real stories were used throughout. The guide was developed based on a comprehensive review of existing materials for pregnant smokers and a literature review. Over 70 women and 15 professionals participated in the first stage of the formative evaluation, including central intercept interviews to gather reactions to graphics, layouts, and photographs. The second stage included structured, in-depth interviews with 20 pregnant smokers who reviewed a complete draft of the guide. Prior to implementation, a four-hour training session was conducted with over 30 maternity service staff at three large maternity care organizations.

Evaluation. The program evaluation focused on the accessibility of implementing this program within ongoing prenatal care and on assessing the effectiveness of the program to change women's smoking behavior. The evaluation utilized a one group pretest-posttest design. A historical control group provided baseline quitting rates. Women who participated in the program were queried about their smoking habits at each prenatal visit and at 6 weeks, 12 weeks and 6 months postpartum. Postpartum evaluations were conducted by telephone using a professional interviewing company. In all three sites, 2,553 women were surveyed and 1,351 were eligible for the program (having been smoking at the time of pregnancy) during the two year accrual period. Of these women, 1,179 received the program and 911 were eligible for follow-up. Overall, the sample was ethnically diverse, consisting of 35% African American, 63% Caucasian, and 1% Hispanic. Additionally, 37% had not obtained a high school education. These women represented a very low income: over 60% reported having a household income of less than $10,000. In terms of feasibility, the program was implemented as intended within the maternal and child health clinics. The nurses were able to counsel 87% of those women who were eligible for the program. Nurses reported it was easier to identify new patients rather than having to identify women who were already in the caseload. In addition, we found a drop off in the number of women counseled over the course of their pregnancy. The nurses developed a confidence in their ability to assess readiness to quit and provided the self-help guide to 97% of the counseled patients. Only 16% of the women were ready to quit which corresponded to the 10% who set a quit date. Women were asked on the follow-up interviews if they had read the guide and 61% reported they did read the guide. Smoking behavior during pregnancy was collected at the 6 and 12 week post-partum follow-up interview. Of the 632 women who participated in these interviews, 25% reported quitting during their pregnancy. Almost 40% said they tried and 37% reported not trying to quit. The 25% quit rate was at least 10% higher than the pre-program quit rates.

Although this project was developed and implemented almost 20 years ago, this "low-tech" approach integrating targeted messages into routine care and using a highly engaging printed guide continues to be disseminated and used in practice. The program was developed with community participation (both providers and pregnant smokers) which has been important to its long-lasting relevancy. The self-help guide has been updated with current information (pharmacotherapies, placement of baby while sleeping) and is in its third edition. Similar approaches to brief provider counseling are still in practice.

Case Study #2: Web-based Intervention for Colorectal Cancer Screening—Sarah Bass, Temple University

Background. The feasibility of using computer touch-screen technology to foster behavior change in low adherence populations has been demonstrated as an effective health communication strategy. Computer touch-screens (CTS) can be connected to any computer to allow users to touch the screen as the program directs instead of using a mouse. A special driver translates the touch into something the operating system can understand, much as a computer mouse driver translates a mouse's movements into a click or drag. This can be especially useful for addressing sensitive topics such as CRC screening because an intervention can be administered privately. Generally preferred over pamphlets and leaflets by users (Graham et al., 2000), research utilizing this technology has found it to be useful in motivating behavior change and influencing treatment decisions, as well as increasing knowledge, self-efficacy, and adherence, particularly in primary care settings (Berry et al., 2010; Graham et al., 2000; Lawrence et al., 2010; Lin, Neafsey, & Anderson, 2010). While little research with CTS has been done specifically with low literacy populations, CTS is an ideal tool in that it does not require knowledge of computers and mimics common everyday tasks such as using a bank ATM machine. There is also the ability to provide voice-over via built in speakers, which further alleviates literacy barriers.

Description of Health Education Tool and Target Audience. Our goal was to create a CRC—CST tutorial for low literacy African Americans to strengthen the connection between decision aid framing and content with subjects' mental maps of the risks and benefits of CRC screening by utilizing innovative methods. We used a vigorous method to determine message strategy, including: (Committee on Assuring the Health of the Public in the 21st Century) Focus groups conducted with low-literacy African American patients (Bass et al., 2011); (Committee on Assuring the Health of the Public in the 21st Century) In-depth interviews with

30 third-year medical residents in internal medicine (Ruggieri et al., 2011; Ward et al., 2010) (3) An extensive review of the available research literature on CRC screening (Ward et al., 2008); (4) Perceptual Mapping and vector analysis of surveys with 100 low-literacy African Americans at a general internal medicine clinic of a large urban medical center; and, (5) Extensive statistical analysis, including factor and cluster analysis resulting in a specific typology of respondents. These methods and resulting analyses indicated key message strategies to address patients' perceptions of the barriers and facilitators of CRC screening. Specifically, we focused on the messages presented below.

> **Importance of going to the doctor and getting a recommendation**
> **Importance of having a colonoscopy and its accuracy**
> **That it is better to know if you have cancer and not to fear it**
> **That family is important and would want you to be tested**

Application of Best Practices. Using these messages as the focus of the tutorial, we worked with The Patient Education Institute, whose mission is to develop, implement, and evaluate interactive patient education tutorials. Their *X-Plain* tutorial series consists of the largest library of theory-based interactive multimedia tutorial programs available for patient education (http://www. patient-education.com/). Their software, X-Plain, is the largest library of interactive multimedia software available for patient education. These tutorials are based on learning theory, and are implemented in a variety of settings, including hospitals, physician offices, and corporate wellness departments. They are not, however, tailored to specific populations and require higher levels of literacy. They also focus on medical aspects of a medical decision. For example, the CRC screening tutorial has significant information on what CRC is and how screening tests are done. We thus adapted this existing CRC screening tutorial for use in a CTS format in a clinical setting for low literacy African American patients, as well as revised the tutorial to address the key messages found through our analysis.

The resulting tutorial had significantly different graphics, utilizing culturally appropriate photos, and text was significantly altered not only to address low literacy needs, but also to focus on and address identified concepts. Specifically, we used photographs instead of graphics depicting African American patients, wrote text at a 6th grade reading level, and added "testament" videos that showed actual clinic patients from our study who had had a colonoscopy.

These videos were a significant addition to the tutorial as other X-Plain tutorials do not utilize this feature. We taped and edited these videos to address specific concerns this patient population had with having a colonoscopy, reinforcing key messages and allowing users to see and hear people like them discuss the importance of having a colonoscopy. Text was also significantly altered by deleting much of the medical information about colon cancer and colonoscopy and focusing more on the psycho-social issues found to be more important to our participants when making a decision about colonoscopy (See Figure 2).

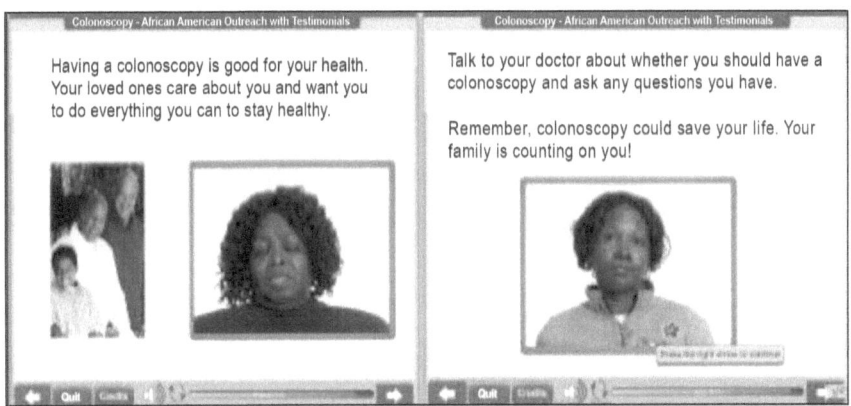

Figure 2. **Sample Screen Shots**

Evaluation Findings and Recommendations. Testing on the effectiveness of the tutorial was done in the General Internal Medicine clinic of a large urban medical system. All participants were over the age of 50 and had low literacy based on testing. They were randomly assigned to either a Usual Care group (n=27) or a CTS Tutorial group (n=33). The "usual care" group received a two-page handout about colonoscopy that is normally provided to patients. Results indicate that the intervention group (CTS) was significantly more willing to have colonoscopy and understood barriers to colonoscopy than the control group (usual care handout). They also liked the tutorial decision aid significantly more than the usual care group liked the handout decision aid. In comparison to the Usual Care print document, the touch screen tutorial was judged to be superior on its length (p=.009), the amount of information it provided (p=.001), the usefulness of the information (p=.005), its balance (p=.001) and its ease of use (p=.000). Users of the tutorial also felt it provided enough information to make a decision about colonoscopy (p=.006) and means on overall attitude about having a colonoscopy (p=.001) and likelihood of having a colonoscopy (p=.002) were significantly higher compared to the usual care group, indicating a tailored decision aid using these methods, and developed specifically for low literacy minority patients, can be extremely effective in encouraging behavior.

This experience illustrated that utilizing a research-based approach is possible when developing low-literacy health education materials as long as the target population is included in all areas of development. It is imperative that materials developed for low literacy populations must be piloted and tested to adequately address the specific needs of the population. It is also important to note that these methods of tailoring to populations are easily adapted to other technologies and forms of health communication, such as web, print and flyers. The main lesson is to create materials that directly address a population's needs.

Case Study #3: *Sugar, Heart and Life—A Guide to Living with Diabetes*—Maria Jibaya-Weiss & Luis Rustveld Baylor School of Medicine

Background. The prevalence of Type 2 Diabetes Mellitus (T2DM) in the U.S. has increased steadily over the past ten years (Centers for Disease Control and Prevention, 2011). In Texas, a combination of increasing obesity, a known risk factor for diabetes, and the projected doubling of the Hispanic population in the next thirty years (Texas State Data Center, 2009), make interventions focusing on prevention and management of diabetes a public health priority. Based on our past experience conducting diabetes studies in Houston's Harris County primary care community clinics, we know that a large proportion of Hispanics who have diabetes have HbA1C levels above 8.0%. To address this high prevalence of uncontrolled Type 2 diabetes in these clinics, our team developed a diabetes education program titled "Sugar, Heart, and Life (SHL)—A Guide to Living with Diabetes." This program utilizes an entertainment education strategy which has been found to be effective with multi-ethnic and multilingual individuals of limited literacy, including English—and Spanish-speaking Hispanics (Jibaja-Weiss & Volk, 2007; Jibaja-Weiss et al., 2011; Jibaja et al., 2000).

Description of the Diabetes Education Program and its Target Audience. Our primary objective from the outset was to develop a culturally and linguistically appropriate diabetes education program. The SHL program is a web-based, user-friendly and fun interactive diabetes education tool to help English—and Spanish-speaking Hispanics with T2DM make lifelong changes needed for glycemic control and to prevent diabetes complications. This program was specifically designed to meet the needs of individuals with limited literacy and/or those who are novice computer users.

During initial stages of SHL program development, focus groups were conducted with 72 primary care English—and Spanish-speaking men and women with T2DM to get a better understanding of their knowledge and attitudes about diabetes management and prevention (Rustveld et al., 2009). We were also interested in learning the format in which they preferred to receive health education messages. The majority preferred diabetes education messages packaged in a "story" format, rather than through printed materials.

In addition, content for the SHL program was informed by a comprehensive review of the literature on diabetes care and self-management as well as consultation with a Content Advisory Panel from Baylor College of Medicine, University of Texas (Houston and San Antonio), and primary care providers from the community health clinics. All diabetes management recommendations and educational content presented in the SHL follow standard practice guidelines of the American Diabetes Association. To guide the design and evaluation of the SHL, we utilized Bandura's Social Cognitive Theory, which links the environment, personal factors, and individual behavior to self-efficacy (Bandura, 2004).

Based on findings from the formative phase of the project, the following short—and long-term objectives and messaging related to diabetes self-management were identified and addressed in the SHL application: 1) <u>Short-term objectives</u>: Promote favorable changes in attitude, beliefs, and knowledge about diabetes and its management; 2) <u>Long-term objective</u>: Improve diabetes regimen adherence in adult Hispanic men and women; and, 3) <u>Overall messages in storyline</u> (sprinkled throughout): a) With good diabetes control one can postpone or prevent the development of complications, b) Importance of family support for diabetes management and prevention.

The primary topics covered in the SHL are diet, physical activity, medication adherence, self-care, and family. The short—and long-term objectives, overall messaging, as well as the primary content topics identified were utilized to design the SHL application with two main didactic components: interactive telenovela (dramatization) episodes, and educational games/modules. (See Figure 3.)

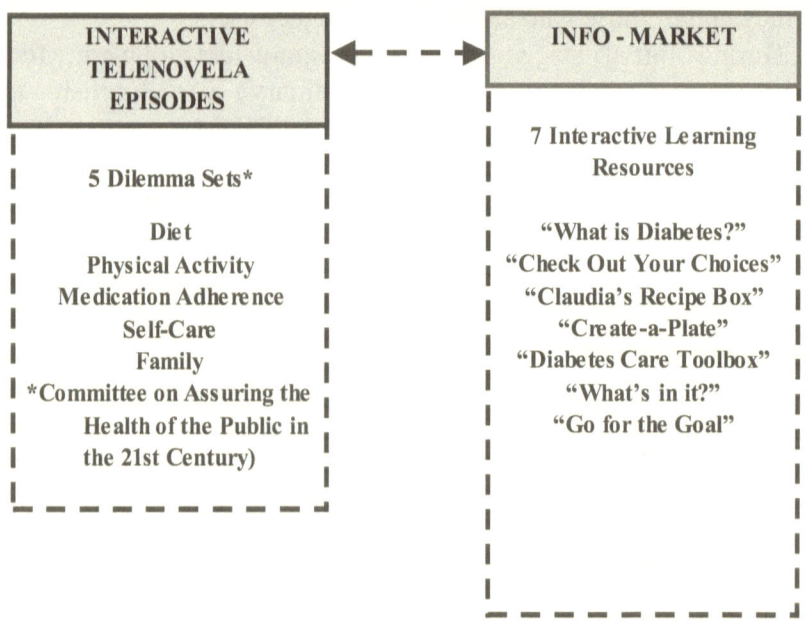

Figure 3. **Content topics.**

The storyline of the interactive telenovela follows a family, who throughout the course of one year learns to deal with the complexities of daily diabetes management. The user may choose to view a particular episode and to follow a particular character (Luis or Victoria).

Then, as the story unfolds, users are presented with decision-points where they may choose between an "appropriate" or "inappropriate" (these terms are used for evaluation purposes only) action for the character selected at the end of each episode. Selections made at each decision-point are unobtrusively tracked in the background and fed into an algorithm to provide feedback (results) to the users based on the choices made throughout the story.

Depending on which "appropriate" or "inappropriate" decisions are chosen for the characters, viewers are presented with one of three "five years later" scenes depicting potential consequences to the Gonzales family; this way users can vicariously experience the outcomes based on the choices made while viewing the storyline.

Evaluation. We conducted a randomized controlled trial to examine the effects of the SHL on diabetes self-management knowledge, and self-care adherence in five local primary care community clinics. A total of 200 adult Hispanic men and women (aged 52.8 ± 10.1 years) with T2DM (mean HbA1c 9.5 ± 1.96) participated in the trial. Intervention patients (N=100) viewed the SHL program in English or Spanish. They were also given a DVD version to take home. Usual care patients (N=100) attended diabetes education classes. Diabetes knowledge and self-care management data were obtained at baseline and at 3 months post-randomization.

Compared to usual care, intervention patients exhibited significant mean improvement in diabetes management knowledge (-0.74 ± 0.14; -0.36 ± 0.13, $p = 0.04$, respectively), and diet adherence approached significance (-0.56 ± 0.11; -0.28 ± 0.09, $p = 0.06$). Further improvement in diabetes management knowledge was observed with additional home viewing of the SHL program (mean, -0.93 ± 0.17, $p = 0.03$).

Findings indicate that this culturally and linguistically appropriate diabetes education program helped increase diabetes management knowledge and diet adherence among Hispanic patients with T2DM. We are currently in the process of obtaining complete three and six month HbA1c data to determine effectiveness of the DVD on glycemic control. The web-based SHL application, as well as other versions that do not require Internet access, are publicly available online at www.bcm.edu/shl.

Summary

Developing effective health education programs requires time and preparation. The process usually includes assessment, planning, implementation and evaluation. Part of the assessment process involves defining the target audience, their needs, beliefs and outcomes. With proper planning and implementation a health education program has the ability to change individual behavior, prevent disease and improve quality of life (Glanz, Rimer, & Viswanath, 2008; Green & Kreuter, 2004). At the community level, effective health education programs have the potential to reduce health disparities, improve health outcomes and reduce health care costs.

Emerging evidence suggests that integrating cultural factors into health education interventions may increase the efficacy of those programs among diverse subpopulations (U.S. Department of Health and Human Services, 2011).

References

Agency for Healthcare Research and Quality. (2010). *The National Healthcare Disparities Report 2009*. Washington DC.

Andrulis, D. P., & Brach, C. (2007). Integrating literacy, culture, and language to improve health care quality for diverse populations. *Am J Health Behav, 31 Suppl 1*, S122-133.

Arthur, C. M., & Katkin, E. S. (2006). Making a case for the examination of ethnicity of Blacks in United States Health Research. *J Health Care Poor Underserved, 17*(1), 25-36.

Bandura, A. (2004). Health promotion by social cognitive means. *Health Educ Behav, 31*(2), 143-164.

Basch, C. E., Wolf, R. L., Brouse, C. H., Shmukler, C., Neugut, A., DeCarlo, L. T., et al. (2006). Telephone outreach to increase colorectal cancer screening in an urban minority population. *Am J Public Health, 96*(12), 2246-2253.

Bass, S. B., Gallo, R., Crookes, D. M., Berger, T., & Fleisher, L. (2008). Your Resource Guide to Health Literacy: Pennsylvania Department of Health and Fox Chase Cancer Center, Health Communications and Public Health Program.

Bass, S. B., Gordon, T. F., Ruzek, S. B., Wolak, C., Ward, S., Paranjape, A., et al. (2011). Perceptions of colorectal cancer screening in urban African American clinic patients: differences by gender and screening status. *J Cancer Educ, 26*(1), 121-128.

Bass, S. B., Ruzek, S. B., Gordon, T. F., Fleisher, L., McKeown-Conn, N., & Moore, D. (2006). Relationship of Internet health information use with patient behavior and self-efficacy: experiences of newly diagnosed cancer patients who contact the National Cancer Institute's Cancer Information Service. *J Health Commun, 11*(2), 219-236.

Berry, D. L., Halpenny, B., Wolpin, S., Davison, B. J., Ellis, W. J., Lober, W. B., et al. (2010). Development and evaluation of the personal patient profile-prostate (P3P), a Web-based decision support system for men newly diagnosed with localized prostate cancer. *J Med Internet Res, 12*(4), e67.

Betancourt, J. R., & Jacobs, E. A. (2000). Language barriers to informed consent and confidentiality: the impact on women's health. *J Am Med Womens Assoc, 55*(5), 294-295.

Centers for Disease Control and Prevention. (1997). *Principles of Community Engagement, Second Edition*. Atlanta, GA: Public Health Practice Program Office.

Centers for Disease Control and Prevention. (2011). National diabetes fact sheet, 2011. Retrieved April 15, 2011, from http://www.cdc.gov/diabetes/pubs/pdf/ndfs_2011.pdf

Chou, W. Y., Hunt, Y. M., Beckjord, E. B., Moser, R. P., & Hesse, B. W. (2009). Social media use in the United States: implications for health communication. *J Med Internet Res, 11*(4), e48.

Cole-Lewis, H., & Kershaw, T. (2010). Text messaging as a tool for behavior change in disease prevention and management. *Epidemiol Rev, 32*(1), 56-69.

Committee on Assuring the Health of the Public in the 21st Century. (2002). *The Future of the Public's Health in the 21st Century*: The National Academies Press.

Cook, P. F., Emiliozzi, S., El-Hajj, D., & McCabe, M. M. (2010). Telephone nurse counseling for medication adherence in ulcerative colitis: a preliminary study. *Patient Educ Couns, 81*(2), 182-186.

Couper, M. P., Singer, E., Levin, C. A., Fowler, F. J., Jr., Fagerlin, A., & Zikmund-Fisher, B. J. (2010). Use of the Internet and ratings of information sources for medical decisions: results from the DECISIONS survey. *Med Decis Making, 30*(5 Suppl), 106S-114S.

Cross, T., Bazron, B. J., Dennis, K. W., & Isaacs, M. R. (1989). *Towards a Culturally Competent System of Care.* Washington, DC: National Center for Technical Assistance Center for Children's Mental Health, Georgetown University Child Development Center.

Currie, K., Rajendran, M., Spink, J., Carter, M., & Anderson, J. (2001). Consumer health information. What the research is telling us. *Aust Fam Physician, 30*(11), 1108-1112.

Doak, C. C., Doak, L. G., & Root, J. H. (1996). *Teaching Patients With Low Literacy Skills* (2 ed.). Philadelphia, PA: JB Lippincott Co.

Farmer, A. P., Legare, F., Turcot, L., Grimshaw, J., Harvey, E., McGowan, J. L., et al. (2008). Printed educational materials: effects on professional practice and health care outcomes. *Cochrane Database Syst Rev* (3), CD004398.

Free, C., Whittaker, R., Knight, R., Abramsky, T., Rodgers, A., & Roberts, I. G. (2009). Txt2stop: a pilot randomized controlled trial of mobile phone-based smoking cessation support. *Tob Control, 18*(2), 88-91.

Gibbons, M. C. (2011). Use of Health Information Technology among Racial and Ethnic Underserved Communities. *Perspectives in Health Information Management, 8*(1f), 1-13.

Gibbons, M. C., Fleisher, L., Slamon, R. E., Bass, S., Kandadai, V., & Beck, J. R. (2011). Exploring the potential of Web 2.0 to address health disparities. *J Health Commun, 16 Suppl 1*, 77-89.

Glanz, K., Rimer, B. K., & Viswanath, K. (Eds.). (2008). *Health Behavior and Health Education: Theory, Research, and Practice* (4 ed.). San Francisco: Jossey-Bass, Inc.

Graham, W., Smith, P., Kamal, A., Fitzmaurice, A., Smith, N., & Hamilton, N. (2000). Randomized controlled trial comparing effectiveness of touch screen system with leaflet for providing women with information on prenatal tests. *BMJ, 320*(7228), 155-160.

Green, L., & Kreuter, M. (2004). *Health promotion planning: An educational and ecological approach* (4 ed.). Columbus, OH: McGraw-Hill.

Haapala, I., Barengo, N. C., Biggs, S., Surakka, L., & Manninen, P. (2009). Weight loss by mobile phone: a 1-year effectiveness study. *Public Health Nutr, 12*(12), 2382-2391.

Harris, M., Smith, B., & Veale, A. (2005). Printed patient education interventions to facilitate shared management of chronic disease: a literature review. *Intern Med J, 35*(12), 711-716.

Hawkins, R. P., Kreuter, M., Resnicow, K., Fishbein, M., & Dijkstra, A. (2008). Understanding tailoring in communicating about health. *Health Educ Res, 23*(3), 454-466.

Heseltine, P. (2007). Fecal Immunochemical Test: Improving Detection of Colorectal Cancer with the New Generation Occult Blood Test. *Clinical Laboratory News* (January 2007), 8-10.

Hesse, B. W., Nelson, D. E., Kreps, G. L., Croyle, R. T., Arora, N. K., Rimer, B. K., et al. (2005). Trust and sources of health information: the impact of the Internet and its implications for health care providers: findings from the first Health Information National Trends Survey. *Arch Intern Med, 165*(22), 2618-2624.

Horrigan, J., Rainie, L., & Fox, S. (2001). *Online Communities: Networks that nurture long-distance relationships and local ties.* Washington, DC: The Pew Charitable Trusts.

Institute of Medicine. (2004). *Health Literacy: A Prescription to End Confusion.* Washington, DC: The National Academy Press.

Jibaja-Weiss, M. L., & Volk, R. J. (2007). Utilizing computerized entertainment education in the development of decision aids for lower literate and naive computer users. *J Health Commun, 12*(7), 681-697.

Jibaja-Weiss, M. L., Volk, R. J., Granchi, T. S., Neff, N. E., Robinson, E. K., Spann, S. J., et al. (2011). Entertainment education for breast cancer surgery decisions: a randomized trial among patients with low health literacy. *Patient Educ Couns, 84*(1), 41-48.

Jibaja, M. L., Kingery, P., Neff, N. E., Smith, Q., Bowman, J., & Holcomb, J. D. (2000). Tailored, interactive soap operas for breast cancer education of high-risk Hispanic women. *J Cancer Educ, 15*(4), 237-242.

Keller, P. A., & Lehmann, D. R. (2008). Designing effective health communications: a meta-analysis. *Journal of Public Policy & Marketing, 27*, 117-130.

Kempf, A. M., & Remington, P. L. (2007). New Challenges for Telephone Survey Research in the Twenty-First Century. *Annual Review of Public Health, 28*(1), 113-126.

Kirsch, I. S., Jungeblut, A., Jenkins, L., & Kolstad, A. (1993). *Adult Literacy in America: a first look at the findings of the National Adult Literacy Survey*: U.S. Department of Education.

Kleinman, J. C., & Kopstein, A. (1987). Smoking during pregnancy, 1967-80. *Am J Public Health, 77*(7), 823-825.

Kluhsman, B. C., Lengerich, E. J., Fleisher, L., Lyle, J., Paskett, E. D., Miller, S. M., et al. (2010). *Telephone Barriers Counseling for Colorectal Cancer Screening in Primary Care: A Feasibility Study for Rural Appalachia*. Oral presentation presented at the Society of Behavioral Medicine 31st Annual Meeting & Scientific Sessions.

Kreuter, M. W., Lukwago, S. N., Bucholtz, R. D., Clark, E. M., & Sanders-Thompson, V. (2003). Achieving cultural appropriateness in health promotion programs: targeted and tailored approaches. *Health Educ Behav, 30*(2), 133-146.

Kreuter, M. W., & McClure, S. M. (2004). The role of culture in health communication. *Annual Rev Public Health, 25*, 439-455.

Kutner, M., Greenberg, E., Jin, Y., & Paulsen, C. (2006). *The Health Literacy of America's Adults: Results From the 2003 National Assessment of Adult Literacy*. Washington, D.C.: National Center for Education Statistics.

Lawrence, S. T., Willig, J. H., Crane, H. M., Ye, J., Aban, I., Lober, W., et al. (2010). Routine, self-administered, touch-screen, computer-based suicidal ideation assessment linked to automated response team notification in an HIV primary care setting. *Clin Infect Dis, 50*(8), 1165-1173.

Lim, M. S., Hocking, J. S., Aitken, C. K., Fairley, C. K., Jordan, L., Lewis, J. A., et al. (2011). Impact of text and email messaging on the sexual health of young people: a randomized controlled trial. *J Epidemiol Community Health*.

Lin, C. A., Neafsey, P. J., & Anderson, E. (2010). Advanced practice registered nurse usability testing of a tailored computer-mediated health communication program. *Comput Inform Nurs, 28*(1), 32-41.

Little, P., Roberts, L., Blowers, H., Garwood, J., Cantrell, T., Langridge, J., et al. (2001). Should we give detailed advice and information booklets to patients with back pain? A randomized controlled factorial trial of a self-management booklet and doctor advice to take exercise for back pain. *Spine (Phila Pa 1976), 26*(19), 2065-2072.

Lumley, J., Chamberlain, C., Dowswell, T., Oliver, S., Oakley, L., & Watson, L. (2009). Interventions for promoting smoking cessation during pregnancy. *Cochrane Database Syst Rev*(3), CD001055.

Marcus, A. C., Garrett, K. M., Cella, D., Wenzel, L., Brady, M. J., Fairclough, D., et al. (2010). Can telephone counseling post-treatment improve psychosocial outcomes among early stage breast cancer survivors? *Psychooncology, 19*(9), 923-932.

McBride, C. M., & Rimer, B. K. (1999). Using the telephone to improve health behavior and health service delivery. *Patient Educ Couns, 37*(1), 3-18.

Minkler, M., Wallerstein, N., & Wilson, N. (2008). Improving health through community organization and community building. In K. Glanz, B. K. Rimer & K. Viswanath (Eds.), *Health behavior and health education: theory, research, and practice* (4 ed.). San Francisco.

Murray, E., Burns, J., See, T. S., Lai, R., & Nazareth, I. (2005). Interactive Health Communication Applications for people with chronic disease. *Cochrane Database Syst Rev*(4), CD004274.

National Cancer Institute. (1994). *Clear & Simple: Developing Effective Print Materials for Low-Literate Readers* (No. NIH Publication No. 95-3594). Rockville, MD.

National Cancer Institute. (2002). *Making Health Communication Programs Work*. Rockville, MD: U.S. Department of Health and Human Services,.

Newton, K. H., Wiltshire, E. J., & Elley, C. R. (2009). Pedometers and text messaging to increase physical activity: randomized controlled trial of adolescents with type 1 diabetes. *Diabetes Care, 32*(5), 813-815.

Noar, S. M., Benac, C. N., & Harris, M. S. (2007). Does tailoring matter? Meta-analytic review of tailored print health behavior change interventions. *Psychol Bull, 133*(4), 673-693.

Osborne, H. (2011). *Health Literacy from A to Z: Practical Ways to Communicate Your Health Message* (2 ed.). Sudbury, MA: Jones and Bartlett Publishers.

Owen, N., Fotheringham, M. J., & Marcus, B. H. (2002). Communication technology and health behavior change. In K. Glanz, B. K. Rimer & F. M. Lewis (Eds.), *Health behavior and health education* (3 ed., pp. 510-529). San Francisco, CA: Jossey-Bass.

Paul, C., & Redman, S. (1997). A review of the effectiveness of print material in changing health-related knowledge, attitudes and behavior. *Health Promotion Journal of Australia, 7*, 91-99.

Pekmezi, D. W., Williams, D. M., Dunsiger, S., Jennings, E. G., Lewis, B. A., Jakicic, J. M., et al. (2010). Feasibility of using computer-tailored and internet-based interventions to promote physical activity in underserved populations. *Telemed J E Health, 16*(4), 498-503.

Pew Internet & American Life Project. (2011a, May 2011). Trend Data. *Pew Internet & American Life Project.* Retrieved May 31, 2011, from http://www.pewinternet.org/Trend-Data/Whos-Online.aspx

Pew Internet & American Life Project. (2011b). Web 2.0. Retrieved May 2011, from http://www.pewinternet.org/topics/Web-20.aspx

Rainie, L. (2011). The Rise of the e-Patient: Understanding Social Networks and Online Health Information-Seeking, *Pew Internet & American Life Project*. Philadelphia, PA: Pew Charitable Trusts.

Rudd, R., Moeykens, B. A., & Colton, T. C. (2000). Health and literacy: A review of medical and public health literature. In J. Comings, B. Garners & C. Smith (Eds.), *Annual Review of Adult Learning and Literacy*. New York: Jossey-Bass.

Ruggieri, D., Bass, S. B., Rovito, M. J., Ward, S., Gordon, T. F., Paranjape, A., et al. (2011). Perceived colonoscopy barriers and facilitators among urban African American patients and their medical residents. *Journal of Health Communication* (In press).

Rustveld, L. O., Pavlik, V. N., Jibaja-Weiss, M. L., Kline, K. N., Gossey, J. T., & Volk, R. J. (2009). Adherence to diabetes self-care behaviors in English—and Spanish-speaking Hispanic men. *Patient Prefer Adherence, 3*, 123-130.

Sacco, W. P., Malone, J. I., Morrison, A. D., Friedman, A., & Wells, K. (2009). Effect of a brief, regular telephone intervention by paraprofessionals for type 2 diabetes. *J Behav Med, 32*(4), 349-359.

Smedley, B. D., Stith, A. Y., & Nelson, A. R. (Eds.). (2003). *Unequal Treatment: Confronting Racial and Ethnic Disparities in Health Care*: The National Academies Press.

Smith, A. (2010a). Home Broadband 2010 [Electronic Version]. *Pew Internet & American Life Project*. Retrieved April 2011 from http://www.pewinternet.org/Reports/2010/Home-Broadband-2010.aspx.

Smith, A. (2010b). Mobile Access 2010 [Electronic Version]. *Pew Internet & American Life Project*. Retrieved April 2011 from http://www.pewinternet.org/Reports/2010/Mobile-Access-2010.aspx.

Smith, A. (2010c). Technology Trends Among People of Color [Electronic Version]. *Pew Internet & American Life Project*. Retrieved April 2011 from http://www.pewinternet.org/Commentary/2010/September/Technology-Trends-Among-People-of-Color.aspx.

Smith, A. (2011). Who's on What: Social Media Trends Among Communities of Color, *Webinar Presentation for California Immunization Coalition on January 25, 2011*.

Spradley, B. W., & Allender, J. A. (1996). *Community Health Nursing: Concepts and Practice* (4 ed.). Philadelphia: Lippincott.

Texas State Data Center. (2009). Projections of the population of Texas and counties in Texas by age, sex and race/ethnicity for 2000-2040. Retrieved April 15, 2011, from http://txsdc.utsa.edu/Data/TPEPP/Projections/2008/Methodology.aspx

Torres, R. E. (1998). The pervading role of language on health. *Journal of Health Care for the Poor and Underserved, 9*(5), S21-S25.

U.S. Department of Commerce Census Bureau. (2004). *Statistical Abstract of the United States: 2004-2005, The National Data Book* (124 ed.). Washington, DC: Commerce Dept., Economics and Statistics Administration, Census Bureau.

U.S. Department of Health and Human Services. Healthy People 2020 (Publication. Retrieved November 1, 2011, from Office of Disease Prevention and Health Promotion: http://www.healthypeople.gov/2020/default.aspx

U.S. Department of Health and Human Services. (1990). *The Health Benefits of Smoking Cessation: A report of the Surgeon General* (No. (CDC) 90-8416). Rockville, MD: DHHS.

U.S. Department of Health and Human Services. (2011). *HHS Action Plan to Reduce Racial and Ethnic Disparities: A Nation Free of Disparities in Health and Health Care*. Washington, D.C.

U.S. Department of Health and Human Services Office of Minority Health. (2001). *National Standards for Culturally and Linguistically Appropriate Services in Health Care*. Washington, D.C.

Ward, S. H., Lin, K., Meyer, B., Bass, S. B., Parameswaran, L., Gordon, T. F., et al. (2008). Increasing colorectal cancer screening among African Americans, linking risk perception to interventions targeting patients, communities and clinicians. *J Natl Med Assoc, 100*(6), 748-758.

Ward, S. H., Parameswaran, L., Bass, S. B., Paranjape, A., Gordon, T. F., & Ruzek, S. B. (2010). Resident physicians' perceptions of barriers and facilitators to colorectal cancer screening for African Americans. *J Natl Med Assoc, 102*(4), 303-311.

Appendix A
Table 1: *Community-Based Participatory Research Principles and Corresponding Health Education Best Practices*

CBPR Principles	Community Engagement	Health Education Best Practices
1. Acknowledges community as a unit of identity	Be clear about the purposes or goals of the engagement effort and the populations and/or communities you want to engage.	• Develop a community advisory committee • Conduct community forums • Include community leader or organization on the project team
2. Builds on strengths and resources within the community.	Become knowledgeable about the community's culture, economic conditions, social networks, political and power structures, norms and values, demographic trends, history and experience with efforts by outside groups.	• Community Assessment and Asset Mapping • Informant Interviews • Historical documents • Community Visits and Interviews
3. Facilitates a collaborative, equitable partnership in all phases of research	Go to the community, establish relationships, build trust, work with the formal and informal leadership, and seek commitment from community organizations and leaders to create processes for mobilizing the community.	• Develop a partnership agreement at the onset • Share resources and staffing • Provide seed funding
4. Fosters co-learning and capacity building among all partners	Remember and accept that collective self-determination is the responsibility and right of all people in a community. No external entity should assume it can bestow on a community the power to act in its own self-interest.	• Provide capacity building training (e.g. grant writing) • Adapt project based on community feedback
5. Integrates and balances knowledge generation and intervention for mutual benefit of all partners	Partnering with the community is necessary to create change and improve health.	• Focus groups and interviews with stakeholders can provide richer insights that go beyond the literature. Quotes and narratives can enhance the relevancy of materials.
6. Focuses on the local relevance of public health problems and on ecological perspectives	All aspects must recognize and respect the diversity of the community. Awareness of the various cultures of a community and other factors affecting diversity are paramount in planning, designing, and implementing approaches to engaging a community.	• Tailor efforts to the address the local issues and provide data that speak to the issue. • Broaden the approach to address areas using the Ecological Model. http://www.cancer.gov/cancertopics/cancerlibrary/theory.pdf

7. Involves systems development using a cyclical and iterative process	Community engagement can only be sustained by identifying and mobilizing community assets and strengths and by developing the community's capacity and resources to make decisions and take action.	• Community Assessments and asset mapping enable communities to identify existing resources to build upon. • Coalition building can be helpful to unite the communities to advocate or champion a mutual cause of interest. • Leadership development will foster stewardship of a project and the associated decision-making process.
8. Disseminates results to all partners and involves them in the wider dissemination of results	Organizations that wish to engage a community as well as individuals seeking to effect change must be prepared to release control of action or interventions to the community and be flexible enough to meet its changing needs.	• Sharing results with communities and partners serves to acknowledge their role and strengthens partnerships. • Partner and community involvement in the analysis phase can greatly enrich the final outcomes of a project while validating contributions from everyone. • Partners and communities are more likely to disseminate results if they are part of the process. • Partners and communities are more likely to collaborate on other project s if they are included in all or most facets of the project.
9. Involves a long-term commitment	Community collaboration requires long-term commitment by the engaging organization and its partners.	• Community engagement must be a commitment that goes beyond a specific project. • Having a long-term commitment to a community or partnership will benefit all parties by expanding ones understanding of each other while building trust.

Sources: Methods in Community-Based Participatory Research for Health, Barbara A. Israel, Eugenia Eng, Amy J. Schultz, Edith A. Parker, Jossey-Bass & Principles of Community Engagement, Second Edition, NIH Publication No. 11-7782, US Govt Printing Office, bookstore.gpo.gov

Part III

Prevention and Intervention Strategies in African American Communities: Selected Examples

CHAPTER NINE

Using a Culturally Responsive Framework for HIV/ AIDS Prevention and Intervention in African American Communities

Dominica F. McBride
HELP Institute, Inc.

Pamela Frazier-Anderson
Frazier-Anderson Research and
Evaluation, LLC

Dayna Campbell
University of South Carolina

Abstract

Persisting health disparities in the US are one of the most ostensible manifestations of lingering racial inequality. The discrepancy in rates of HIV/ AIDS between African American and Euro American communities is one such disparity that represents this current presence of injustice. In addressing this predicament, health professionals and researchers must construct a comprehensive perspective on the problem. This purview must include Black history, contextual issues, and culture. This chapter describes the importance of culture in addressing health issues, the problem of HIV/AIDS in the African American community, how culture can be used in addressing this problem, culturally specific HIV prevention programs, and culturally responsive program evaluation.

Introduction

Culture permeates the life of all human beings, from the language we speak to daily rituals, practices, and behaviors. This comprehensive construct encompasses beliefs, the way we teach, the manner in which we learn, how we relate to one another, our health-related practices, and how we understand and ingest the outside environment. If culture is not considered in addressing any problem that concerns behavior and beliefs, the impact of the solution is likely null or lacking (Kirkhart, 2010). Extricating context and culture from discussions and policy making on HIV, specifically, has shown to be ineffective as demonstrated by the current numbers of Black people infected with HIV. In order to progress, researchers and policy makers must study and respond to culture, including a culture's evolution. Each culture is molded by history and context (i.e., physical and social environment). To understand one's culture, a person must study the context and history of that group. Therefore, this chapter emphasizes using culturally responsive practices that focus on context and culture and their role in the amelioration of HIV/AIDS in the African American community.

The authors will use a culturally responsive platform to examine emerging issues in HIV/AIDS. An electronic search suggests that the term 'culturally responsive' appears most frequently in academic settings to address the professional's inclusion of instructional practices and curricula that are most conducive to the learning styles and needs of the various cultural groups represented in those settings. In the text *Culturally Responsive Teaching: Theory, Research and Practice* (2000), Geneva Gay defines culturally responsive (pedagogy) as "using the cultural knowledge, prior experiences, frames of reference, and performance styles of ethnically diverse students to make learning encounters more relevant to and effective for them" (p.29). Therefore, in order to be culturally responsive, an individual must be knowledgeable about and sensitive to the culture, worldview (both current and historical), as well as verbal and nonverbal styles and patterns of a specific cultural group. Additionally one must be able to incorporate this knowledge and sensitivity into their daily practices in order to optimize targeted outcomes and have the most impact with the population(s) she plans to serve.

As such, this chapter will review the current state of HIV/AIDS in the Black community, and include (from a sociohistorical perspective) the cultural and contextual factors believed to contribute to the current state. Next, this chapter will present the theory, principles and program exemplars shown to prevent risky behaviors leading to HIV infection. Relevant and emerging issues related to HIV/AIDS will be examined. Finally, the authors will introduce how certain elements of Culturally Responsive Evaluation may provide useful tools in the evaluation of HIV/AIDS prevention and treatment programs in U.S. Black communities.

The ability to be culturally responsive and utilize those skills is beneficial to the education, research, prevention and treatment of HIV/AIDS—related services and programs in the Black community. In order to understand HIV/AIDS in African American communities and to be responsive to the needs of those within the community, one must begin by examining the sociohistorical elements that have contributed to the current state of HIV/AIDS in the Black community.

The Problem of HIV/AIDS in the Black Community

The prevalence of HIV/AIDS in the Black community is a quintessential manifestation of racial inequality in the United States (Airhihenbuwa et al., 2002). Black Americans are anywhere from six to 18 times more likely to have or contract the virus than Euro Americans (Center for Disease Control and Prevention, CCS, 2010). The causes of this discrepancy are varied and complex, and the solutions can be equality complicated. While this predicament requires a significant amount of resources and time, confronting this disparity is necessary, not only for the good of the Black community for the complete betterment and health of the nation.

As is well known in American history, African Americans have endured great hardship that has had indelible consequences on life, including health, economic status, and culture. Throughout this history, African Americans and their culture have been degraded and shunned at all levels. On the micro-level, African Americans intercept a myriad of microaggressions (i.e., subtle offenses or insults that are made towards Black people (or people of color) in daily practice, including environment, interactions, language, behavior, etc., e.g., thinking and subsequently treating a black man in a grocery store as an employee when he is actually a customer) throughout their lives. These microaggressions ware on a person's time, space, and energy (Sue et al., 2007), that caused undue stress and angst. On the exo-level (i.e., local community), schools and healthcare facilities, for examples, may disregard the needs of the local African American community (McBride, 2009) or value of cultural integration. Racist historical and current policies (on the macro-level), such as the work policies, segregation, and the "war on drugs" (Blankenship, Smoyer, & Bray, 2005), have also spurred a 'domino effect' resulting in slower progress for African Americans. This slow progress manifests today as disproportionate poverty, morbidity, premature mortality, drop-out rates, and, at times unwarranted, incarceration. Tragically, each of these phenomena has a bidirectional relationship with HIV and its associated behaviors and consequences. In other words, each of these phenomena contributes to the spread of HIV in the Black community, and HIV exacerbates the extant problems. Due to the present situation being rooted in racism and cultural marginalization, the solution must address these ills on multiple societal levels and integrate culture where possible and essential.

Reasons and Contributors to the Current Problem

McBride and Bell (in press) delineate various risk and protective factors that can lead to or preclude the contraction of HIV can be applicable to any group, regardless of ethnicity. These factors include individual factors (e.g., genetics, cognitions), familial/ parental mediators (e.g., lack of parental monitoring, lack of familial connectedness), and community solidarity or dissolution. Since these variables are generally applicable, this section will focus on those risk factors or contributors relatively or especially unique to the Black community.

One of the main reasons for the current HIV problem in the Black community is the disproportionate amount of disadvantaged communities within the general African American community. There are various markers of a disadvantaged or marginalized community but the most prominent is that of poverty. Poverty, in many cases in the United States, has contributed to various problems, including low quality education, incarceration, violence, and single parenthood. According to the US Census Bureau (2010), 25.8 percent of African Americans live below the poverty line compared to 9.4 percent of Euro Americans. This disadvantage has been shown to lead to many behavioral problems and risk factors for Black youth, including premature sexual intercourse, other high risk sexual activity (Baumer & South, 2001; Browning et al., 2008), and increased substance use (Wallace, Neilands, & Sanders-Phillips, 2009).

Airhihenbuwa and colleagues (2002) describe four main reasons for this stark HIV/AIDS disparity: 1) funding and policy, 2) stigma, 3) gender inequality, and 4) implementation language. They reported insufficient funding allocated towards HIV prevention in the African American community. One example they gave was the lack of funds invested around heterosexual men and men on the "down-low" (i.e., men who identify as heterosexual but engage in homosexual intercourse). Since 2002, the Center for Disease Control and Prevention (CDC) has given more money to prevention initiatives in minority communities; however, there remain insufficient funds to address this problem in the Black community.

HIV/AIDS-related stigma is another insidious phenomenon that constitutes a large barrier to alleviating this predicament. HIV is a unique virus because it is both deadly and transmitted through avenues that are seen as "sinful", including sex (both hetero and homosexual) and intravenous drug use. Fear of blame and/or feelings of shame compel many who are living with HIV to hide the fact that they have the virus in order to avoid being stigmatized by their loved ones and others in their community. Many others avoid getting tested for HIV for fear of being rejected, which is a cross-cultural and transnational occurrence (Castro & Farmer, 2005). This stigma-induced silence is a significant cause in the spread of HIV. Airhihenbuwa and colleagues highlighted the stigma around both HIV/AIDS and towards homosexuality, particularly in the African American community. Since unprotected anal intercourse is the easiest way to contract the virus, "down-low" behavior complicates the problem of comprehensively addressing HIV in the Black community. Many of these men on the "down-low" do not admit their bisexual behavior and, thus, continue to have unprotected sex with both genders, potentially spreading HIV (Airhihenbuwa et al., 2002).

This behavior places women at further risk and often overlaps with the problem of gender inequality. The theory of gender and power (see Connell, 1987) elucidates the antecedents of the current gender gap in power in relationships and other areas. The power differential may begin on a societal level and manifest in the micro level, in male-female relationships and the expectations they have of one another (Wingood & DiClemente, 2000). These expectations transcend roles and seep into sexual relationships. These expectations, coupled with fears or discomfort around condom use, can often lead to female acquiescence to have unprotected sex. Airhihenbuwa et al. asserts that the power differential within African American romantic relationships must be considered as it relates to condom use, particularly women asking the man to wear a condom. The context of their relationship must also be considered as it influences the power dynamics within the relationship (e.g., lack of power outside for Black men leads to power hunger inside the relationship). So, again, context affects both relationships and risky behaviors.

The final barrier Airhihenbuwa and colleagues highlighted is the language of implementation (i.e., the language used to guide the implementation or provision of services). This language too often overlooks essential aspects of the problem that must be targeted. They give the example of men on the "down-low." The implementation language may focus on men who have sex with men or MSMs, which does not explicitly include "heterosexual" men who engage in bisexual activity. If a man calls himself heterosexual, he may not receive the necessary services or information. This dilemma excludes a significant portion of the problem of HIV in the Black community, especially when it is unknown just how many men are on the "down-low."

Yet another main contributor to continued transmission in this community is the problem of iatrophobia (i.e., the fear of medical care; Washington, 2006). Due to various historic injustices incited by the healthcare system, many African Americans are now leery of the present services offered. This skepticism has strong roots in history, starting with the period of African enslavement in the United States. In the book, *Medical Apartheid*, Washington (2006) reviews the myriad of medical atrocities experienced by African Americans throughout American history. Enslaved individuals were not only used as "workhorses"; physicians bought and/or used them as subjects in dangerous medical experiments that were seen as not being safe enough for Euro Americans. In surgeries, the enslaved were deprived of anesthesia and were often given subpar medical treatment. Following slavery, medical (both physical and psychological) injustices persisted, such as the deprivation of proper psychological treatment for African Americans. Further, there were few mental hospitals in which they were allowed to be admitted.

Because syphilis is a disease that potentially erodes the body and the mind if left untreated, the Tuskegee Syphilis study is a fitting example of how physical and psychological problems of African Americans were addressed. Beginning in 1932, the US Public Health Service (PHS) in Alabama began an investigation of how syphilis impacted the physiology of the body, particularly among Black men. While their subjects were alive, their study was mere observation, watching the progression of the disease until death. Once they died, the physicians performed autopsies to better study the bacteria. These men were regarded by an impatient PHS as living cadavers, more valuable to American medicine as dead than alive" (p. 164). Although their study was disguised as treatment, PHS's intentions were never to provide treatment but to catalogue the dying process and dissect at death. In their recruitment of subjects, they "offered" treatment. Throughout the study, they pretended to provide treatment, giving vitamins and insufficient doses of medication. Even when penicillin was introduced as an "effective drug" in the treatment of syphilis, the physicians continued their study and their deception. The study was maintained despite the availability of treatment until 1972. Within the span of three decades, over 100 African American men died, 40 of their wives contracted the disease, and nearly 20 children were infected at birth (Washington, 2006).

Although public health services have progressed since 1972, Wells, Klap, Koite, and Sherbourne (2001) reported that, even in recent years, African Americans have a "greater unmet need" in the area of healthcare than their Euro American counterparts. The Agency for Healthcare and Research Quality (2006) described several areas where this group, among others, has not received the level of quality healthcare as their Caucasian peers. According to this study, African Americans were less likely to receive timely and efficient healthcare than Euro Americans. The relationship between healthcare professionals and African Americans was often inadequate, which was likely to have had detrimental impacts on health.

The patient-professional relationship is imperative in patients feeling comfortable and thus, implementing the health education they receive. When compared to Euro Americans, African Americans less frequently reported feeling carefully listened to, given proper explanations, or respected by the healthcare professional. Often, it is thought that these experiences are accounted for by socioeconomic status; however, when compared to their White counterparts, this disparity persisted on all levels of education for African Americans (Agency for Health Care and Research Quality, 2006). African Americans were also shown to have less access to high quality healthcare, specialty medical services, and other clinical resources (Bach, Pham, Schrag, Tate, & Hargraves, 2004). Consequently, a smaller proportion of African Americans compared to Euro Americans, use the healthcare system (Barrio, Yamada, Hough, Hawthorne, Garcia, & Jest, 2003), leaving less opportunities to receive HIV testing or learn of HIV/AIDS (Airhihenbuwa et al., 2002).

Health care policy changes in HIV prevention may also present new emerging concerns for African American communities and other communities of color. Specifically, the 2006 recommendations by the Centers for Disease Control and Prevention (CDC) that encourages HIV testing in adults, adolescents, and pregnant women at all health care encounters (Centers for Disease Control and Prevention, 2006a; Bayer & Fairchild, 2006; Centers for Disease Control and Prevention, 2006b) are not necessarily culturally sensitive or responsive. These changes which are primarily focused on altering current voluntary HIV testing processes and procedures, informed consent and pre-counseling are sparked by the growing domestic HIV/AIDS epidemic, but do not directly address issues of fear, stigma, and cultural beliefs and behaviors. They are, however, rooted in the notion that advances in HIV treatment and testing technologies are compelling enough to encourage people to be tested and know their status (Bartlett, Branson, Fenton, Hauschild, Miller, & Mayer, 2008).

In September 2006, the Centers for Disease Control and Prevention (CDC) published *"Revised Recommendations for HIV Testing of Adults, Adolescents and Pregnant Women in Health-Care Settings"* to make voluntary HIV testing a routine part of medical care for Americans aged 13-64 (CDC5). These recommendations for HIV testing in the United States prefer an "opt-out" strategy, meaning the test will be performed as a routine part of care unless the patient declines (Centers for Disease Control and Prevention, 2006A; Bartlett, et al, 2008). According to the CDC, specific signed consent would no longer be required, because "general consent for medical care is sufficient to encompass consent for HIV testing" (Bayer & Fairchild, 2006). The World Health Organization made similar recommendations in May 2007 (Swamy, 2007).

The 'opt-out' testing procedure is a radical departure from strict voluntary testing and re-conceptualizes notions about the requirements for consent. At the outset of the disease, AIDS activists and public health professionals sought approaches that would respect the autonomy and privacy rights of people with or at risk for HIV infection and protect against measures such as isolation and quarantine, which were so entrenched in public health tradition (Bayer & Fairchild, 2006). More than twenty-five years later, those same fears and stigmas are still present in many African American communities and communities of color and provide disconnection between being tested, knowing your status, changing/adapting risk-taking behaviors and beliefs about mortality.

In order to expand testing to the masses, the health care community had to identify opportunities or situations of "missed opportunities" to offer HIV testing. Settings with high rates of undiagnosed HIV infection include emergency departments (Rothman, 2004; Kelen, Shahan, Quinn, 1999) and inpatient services of general acute care hospitals (Kates & Levi, 2007), as well as traditional screening venues such as sexually transmitted disease clinics, chemical dependency clinics, and correctional facilities (CDC2). Even before the revised CDC recommendations, the highest proportion of new cases of HIV infection were diagnosed in hospital inpatient settings and emergency departments (27%), community clinics (21%), and physician offices (17%)(Fenton 2007).

Emergency departments have become a high priority for testing because they represent a missed opportunity, especially for vulnerable populations, and prior studies have shown high rates of emergency department visits by patients with HIV infection (Rothman, 2004; Kelen, Shahan, Quinn, 1999). But during a perceived emergency situation, a person's judgment to consider the weight of HIV diagnosis, particularly when it is an "opt-out" process and there is little or no pre-counseling, is compromised. This further places the vulnerable person at increased disadvantage.

Since the release of the CDC recommendations, at least 5 barriers to implementation have been identified (Hanssens, 2007; Gostin, 2006; Lifson & Rybicki, 2007; Valdiserri, 2007; Holtgrave, 2007; Gruskin & Ferguson, 2008; Wynia, 2006). These include state and other federal agency laws that conflict with the CDC's recommendations (Hanssens, 2007; Gostin, 2006; Bayer & Fairchild,

2006), concern about absence of mandated counseling for primary HIV prevention, persistent stigma associated with HIV infection (Gostin, 2006; Lifson & Rybicki, 2007; Valdiserri, 2007; Holtgrave, 2007; Gruskin & Ferguson, 2008), fears regarding discrimination, and a perception that risk based testing is more cost-effective (Holtgrave, 2007).

What are most significant to the African American community are stigmatization and discrimination. Many of the cultural and social factors (e.g. poverty, culture, unemployment, lack of insurance) that influence HIV risk-taking behaviors are the same that counteract prevention strategies (Aral, Adimora, & Fenton, 2008) and exacerbate disparities (Wyatt et al, 2008; Wyatt, 2009) in HIV outcomes (see section ___ of this paper). Poverty, for example, influences differential access to treatment and high-quality health care, and, thus contributes to racial and ethnic disparities in many chronic disorders (Smedley, Stith, & Nelson, 2003), including HIV/ AIDS. More importantly, many of these factors create inherent population and personal vulnerabilities (e.g., use of the emergency rooms as primary care; lack of access to higher quality health care; lack of community ecologic features that promote good health) (Smedley, Stith, & Nelson, 2003; Chandra & Skinner, 2003) that should be considered in policy development and prevention programs, but is often not done so. Chandra and Skinner (2003) showed that within hospitals black and white patients are often treated differently, and that African Americans are more likely to reside or seek care in areas in which health-care quality is low for all patients (Chandra & Skinner, 2003). To be culturally sensitive and responsive, recommendations for HIV prevention and treatment should consider the cultural context of the lives of vulnerable populations. For African Americans, the socio-political conditions of HIV have not changed drastically in the last 30+ years of the disease.

Ways to Confront the Problem

McBride and Bell (in press), Bell et al. (2001), and Bell, Flay, & Paikoff, R. (2002) describe seven field principles that have been shown to be effective in HIV prevention: 1) rebuild the village or creating social fabric, 2) provide access to modern technology, 3) build connectedness/relationship on various levels, 4) facilitate improvement of self-esteem, 5) develop social and emotional skills and intelligence, 6) re-establish the adult protective shield, and 7) minimize the effects of trauma. These are guidelines that can be applied in general, to any disadvantaged community regardless of ethnicity or culture. In short, these relate and contribute to *human* dynamics and can be considered universal principles, as shown to be effective in Trinidad (Baptiste et al., 2006), South Africa, and the US (Bhana, McKay, Mellins, Petersen, & Bell, 2010).

Specific to African Americans, and, due to the historical and contextual contributions to the marginalization of the group, the culture of African Americans must be included in solving the problem. As stated previously, culture permeates every aspect of life including how we learn, understand, and relate. Thus, in order to teach life saving information, change risky behaviors, and create an environment ripe for holistic health, culture must be utilized. Cultural competence must be infused in every step of HIV prevention, policy, and programming. If an instrument, teaching style, or bit of information is not culturally competent or delivered in a culturally competent way, the target person/group may not comprehend or apply the knowledge. Further, there are protective factors in every culture that can be used. Employing inherent strengths in solving the problem may be one of the most cost effective and efficient ways of resolution because the necessary tools are often already in place (e.g., human resources—the people). The African American community, in general, has various cultural,-historical protective factors that can, and, are indicated to be used in healing the community: 1) religion/spirituality/the Black church, 2) racial socialization, and 3) extended family (McBride, 2009).

Religion, Spirituality, and the Black Religious Institution

The constructs of religion, spirituality, and the Black religious institution are potent mechanisms in Black culture that, either used altogether or separately, have transformed many lives. Although similar in nature and root, each variable has unique aspects that are used to overcome hardship. For instance, spirituality is often dictated by the individual; the individual decides the spiritual practice or belief. Religion is a more collective experience, where a group decides on the belief and practice, which is then followed by the individual (Elkins, Hedstrom, Hughes, Leaf, & Saunders, 1988). The focus of the Black religious institution is also on the group but places more emphasis on structured institutions and social change.

The trilogy of religion, spirituality, and the Black religious institution has had a tremendous impact on the Black community and in the movement toward racial equality. This combination has provided and continues to provide solace in times of hardship and sustained peace, health, and well-being (Boyd-Franklin, 2003; Taylor, Chatters, & Levin, 2004). However, the individual parts have contributed uniquely to social and individual well-being. The following subsections describe how religion/spirituality and the Black religious institution have influenced the progress of the African American community.

Religion and spirituality. Religion and spirituality are terms that are often confused and have been used interchangeably (Taylor et al., 2004). Elkins et al. (1988) refer to religion as a collection of systematic and ritualistic endeavors that encompass beliefs and practices. They define spirituality as the experience of the essence of life through one's belief system of nature, life, and divinity or spirit. Both religion and spirituality have had individual, collective, and societal benefits for African Americans and have become characteristic of Black culture in general (of course there is variation in every culture and community). Participation in religious activities (e.g., attending church) and spiritual expressions (e.g., meditation, prayer) in the African American community is performed at a higher frequency than the Euro American community (Mattis, 2003; Taylor et al., 2004). Taylor et al. found that 69.9% of African Americans identified with being both religious and spiritual, while 50.2% of White Americans identified with being both religious and spiritual. Participation in both "public and private" religious activities, such as attending church service and maintaining daily devotionals, was reportedly higher for the Black population when analyzing black-white differences. African Americans also reported a higher frequency of positive thoughts and feelings towards religion and religious involvement than their Euro American counterparts (Taylor et al., 2004).

Prayer is an integral part of religious life, especially for those participating in religious activities in the Black community. Through prayer, individuals can cope (Taylor et al., 2004), and hope (Frazier, 1974). This tool has been used as a catalyst for intrinsic emotional change and a path towards happier, freer living in the Black community (Frazier, 1974). Presently, prayer holds a very special place in the religious and spiritual experience, being a part of daily lives and livelihoods especially for many African American women (Gilkes, 2001; Taylor et al., 2004). This was another spiritual activity in which Black individuals reported higher levels of participation when compared to the Euro American community (Taylor et al., 2004). As demonstrated by the above-stated findings, prayer and other religious/spiritual activities are integral in general African American culture and history. Not only do these activities have emotional valence in this community but also impact individuals on other levels.

Through participation in prayer and other religious activities and spiritual experiences, positive change has occurred on many levels. This type of participation is negatively correlated with chronic illness and mental health concerns, meaning that it promotes both physical and mental health (Taylor et al., 2004). Boyd-Franklin (2003) asserts that if religion and spirituality are not incorporated into health treatment for Black families when pertinent, there is less likelihood for therapeutic successes and higher probability of misunderstanding and attrition. Thus, considering religion and spirituality are integral endeavors in striving for Black health.

The Black Church. The Black church is one of the most prominent cultural-historical pieces of the story of the Black community. According to Frazier (1974), slavery disrupted the lives of enslaved Africans. The act of slavery created a barrier between enslaved Blacks and central Africentric values—communal living and collectivism. "Social cohesion" was disrupted and prevented. Following emancipation, the Black church became a means of re-attaining social cohesion. This sacred place provided a space for reunifying an emotionally and physically separated community (Frazier, 1974).

During slavery, the family structure was destroyed. Biological families were torn apart due to the selling of men (Douglas, 1845).

Children were raised by women forced to be single mothers or other women on the plantation. The construction of the Black church ameliorated this tragedy and reconstructed the family. The members became "family" (Frazier, 1974). Here, people were able to rebuild a culture and recreate social system in which they identified and prided themselves. The Black church offered a place for positive shared experiences and an opportunity to enjoy ownership, symbolizing newly found freedom. In a time when racism invaded policy making, distancing Black people from home ownership and job opportunities, the church was one of the few properties they could claim as their own. This institution served as a safe place to express emotions in a world that did not acknowledge their humanity or human existence (Frazier, 1974).

The Black church evolved and realized freedom and leadership. This establishment served as a path to self-reliance. Manifesting the familial African American value of reciprocity (Boyd-Franklin, 2003), the church was a way to provide an opportunity for members to give and obtain economical support within the Black community (Frazier, 1974). The church established colleges, seminaries, and schools (Lincoln, 1974), providing religious and secular education (Frazier, 1974; Lincoln, 1974) in a period when quality education was difficult to obtain.

During these times of overt racism, Black men suffered constant attacks to their egos and "masculinity." Due to high unemployment rates and blatant degradation by American society, the esteem of many Black men declined. The church offered remedies, including an avenue to be leaders (e.g., as deacons, who are leaders in the church and often assist the head minister). It also "became the arena of their political activities . . . [becoming a] nation within a nation" Not only did members have a chance at leadership, they had the freedom to vote for the leaders of the church. This freedom was particularly significant in a period where voting for federal leaders was prohibited and unlawful (Frazier, 1974, p. 48-49).

Playing a lead role in the Civil Rights Movement, the Black religious institution spurred the fight towards racial equality and Black empowerment. Out of the struggle and religiosity came a religious philosophy that added to the hope of the Black community. These sentiments drastically differed from previous religious teachings, void of juxtaposing Biblical ideas with racial equality.

This combination became central to the purposely shaped culture of the Black church and was deemed Black theology:

> Black theology is a theology of black liberation. It seeks to plumb the black condition in the light of God's revelation in Jesus Christ, so that the black community can see that the gospel is commensurate with the achievement of black humanity. Black Theology is a theology of 'blackness.' It is the affirmation of black humanity that emancipates black people from white racism thus providing authentic freedom for both white and black people. It affirms the humanity of white people in that it says No to the encroachment of white oppression (Lincoln, 1974, p. 192).

This religious philosophy is still evident today. Many Black religious leaders continue teaching and advocating for racial equality and Black empowerment. Although the Black family structure has attenuated since the 1970s, the church serves as a cohesive foundation for reconstruction, with church members being perceived as family. The literature supports this notion through the words used. "Church home" is often a term used (Boyd-Franklin, 2003; Mattis, 2003) as well as 'church mother', 'brother', and 'sister' (Mattis, 2003). This entity also functions as a family, providing emotional and economic support. Further, the leaders and members of the church offer guidance to biological families on topics such as marriages and parent/child relations (Mattis, 2003).

The Black religious institution historically and currently serves an important and positive role in the progress and success in African American communities. It continues to be a strong scaffold for Black individuals, families, and communities. Along with religion and spirituality, this is a tool that can and, when applicable, should be an integral part in serving Black families, especially in the area of mental and emotional health (Boyd-Franklin, 2003). As stated previously, it has also been equally potent on a societal level, especially in shifting the connotation of racial socialization. The Black religious institution has targeted negative racial socialization and, in many ways, has been successful in transforming it into positive self-construction.

Racial Socialization

Racial socialization has been at the root of both negative and positive self—concepts and behaviors for many African Americans. It has had both positive and detrimental impacts on general health and wellbeing and has been used to both control and liberate African Americans. This process not only includes cognitive and motivational patterns but also those behaviors that are adopted through participation within a family, community, or social activities (Roof, 1995). Through general socialization, humans learn the rules and norms of their families and communities, which guide their own participation in social activity. Socialization provides models of what to think, how to act, what to value, and how to express oneself. Since this process is embedded in the context of a community, researchers cannot isolate this process from the context. Thus, research must look at the context of the socialization to understand the roots of socializing messages and behaviors.

Racial socialization transposes this process onto the guidance of the development of children of color and what it means to be a particular ethnicity. Peters (1985), with an emphasis on African American socialization, defined racial socialization as:

> The socialization of children in Black families, then, occurs within the mundane extreme environment of real or potential racial discrimination and prejudice. The tasks Black parents share with all parents—providing for and raising children—not only are performed within the mundane extreme environmental stress of racism but include the responsibility of raising physically and emotionally healthy children who are Black in a society in which being Black has negative connotations. This is racial socialization (Peters, 1985, p. 161).

Many African American parents perceive the value and need of racial socialization. These parents employ a set of techniques to guide this process and buffer their children against the negative effects of racism, especially as it relates to self-esteem and coping (Coard, & Sellers, 2005). Caughy, Campo, Randolph, and Nickerson (2002) found that a majority of African American parents infused racial socialization in their parenting practices. These strategies included a focus on Black pride, spirituality, education on racism, and the promotion of racial distrust. These lessons often lead to lower behavior problems with their children. Smith, Atkin, and Connel (2003) found that the cultivation of Black pride was conducive to enhanced academic performance. These parents realized what various scholars have evidenced—strong ethnic identity fuels a sturdy overall identify and self-esteem (Bynum, Burton, & Best, 2007; McAdoo, 1985; Phinney, 1993; Simons et al., 2002; Stevenson, 1995).

Simmons et al. (2002) advocated for the incorporation of racial socialization practices in parenting in order to prepare children for likely confrontations with racial discrimination, which has found to potentially conducive to risky behaviors. Racism is marginalizing for those who are its targets. This marginalization can also lead to substance use, which can lead to other HIV-related risk behaviors (Wallace, Neilands, & Sanders-Phillips, 2009). Therefore, Simmons and colleagues advised a strong positive racial socialization of youth in families and communities (see McBride (in press) for community-informed strategies to address the effects of racism).

Extended Family

The extended family is a cultural-historical and community building tool in African American culture (Sudarkasa, 2007). In general, African American children have greatly benefited from this kin network, gaining more from "a collective or extended family decision-making structure than do White children" (Livingston & McAdoo, 2007, p. 232). Due to a financial and social system that has failed them, many Black families in need use informal adoption (i.e., where someone other than the biological parent becomes the surrogate parent for a child, outside of the formalized, legal process) by extended family (particularly the grandmother; Boyd-Franklin, 2003). Additionally, outside of informal adoption, the extended family network helps to raise children and bolsters child development. Extended family members often help to create a safe and secure environment, as well as to provide financial and educational support (McAdoo, 1993). This piece of cultural capital can be used in providing HIV intervention to African American families, when pertinent. Boyd-Franklin (2003) strongly advocates for the use of this factor in healing African American families and communities.

Each cultural variable discussed above has been shown to be healing in various ways. Policy and programming can use each said cultural-historical factor. For instance, the church can be used as a vessel through which to disseminate knowledge. In abating the negative effects of racism, parents can be trained in positively racially socializing their children (McBride, in press); and the extended family can be trained to train each other (McBride, 2009) in HIV prevention. On a mere programmatic level, each program can strive to infuse cultural aspects, where and when appropriate[1], when targeting the African American community. For instance, learning style has been shown to be different from other groups, in general (Belgrave & Allison, 2010). African American children may learn more effectively in groups (i.e., communal learning) (Rovia, Gallien, & Wighting, 2005). Cole & Boykin (2008) found that African American children, in general, also enhance their academic performance when rhythm is used in teaching. Holistic learning (i.e., learning in relation to social relationship or social consequence and relevance) versus elemental learning (i.e., learning bits of information independent of other information) is more prevalent and relevant for Black versus White Americans. HIV programming can use this knowledge if found relevant for the localized target Black communities and integrate teaching methods that are more culturally competent and congruent. Figure 1 portrays an integrative and culturally responsive model for HIV prevention and healthy Black communities. This model combines the above information, including universal health principles and culture with HIV prevention information. It also shows that all these activities and phenomena are impacted by history and context.

---

[1]   Before any program is implemented, a community assessment or formative evaluation should be completed to ascertain the applicability and relevance of the program activities and cultural facets. There is more variation within communities and groups than between.

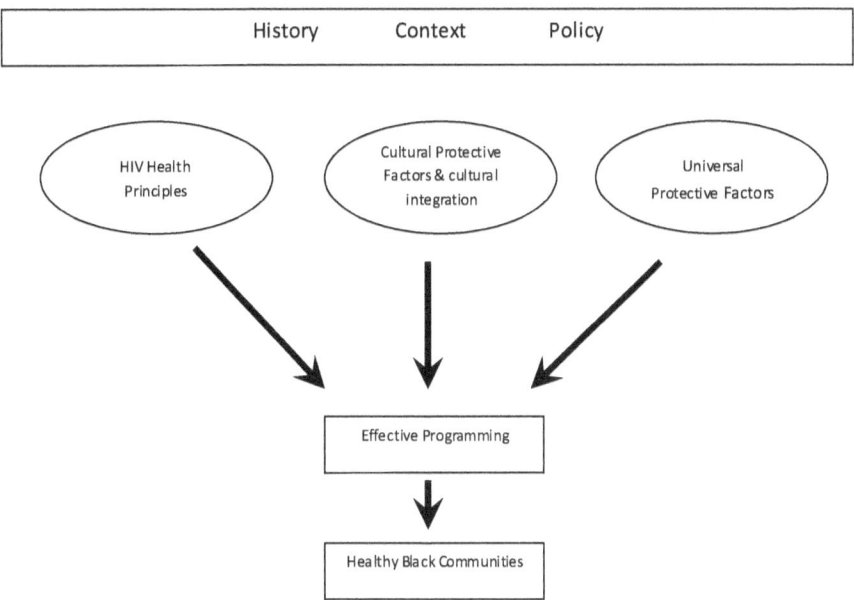

Figure 1. **Conceptual framework for a decreasing HIV disparity**

Albeit few, there are various programs that have been constructed and found effective specifically for African Americans. These programs target African American culture and integrate some of said factors.

Strong African American Families

Brody et al. (2004) created a program based on the Strengthening Families Program, specifically for African Americans in the rural South (i.e., Strong African American Families Program, SAAF). To ensure cultural congruence and appropriateness of program elements, the researchers held focus groups with the target population (i.e., Southern rural families), ascertaining both their families' and children's troubles in the development of this program. The program targets various parental factors that can contribute to drug use and sexual activity in youth, which include parent lack of supervision, communication about sex and drugs, and racial socialization. Some of these parenting issues are especially true for low-income African American youth who may live in potentially pernicious environments. For instance, supervision or "involved-vigilant parenting" (Brody et al., 2004) has been shown to be effective in protecting Black youth living in poverty from dangerous surroundings and often consequent behaviors (Brody et al., 2001). This program was found to be effective in decreasing the occurrence of risky sexual behavior, drug abuse, and antisocial behavior. Further, SAAF addressed and advocated for youth individual protective factors, including goal-directed future orientation, negative perspectives of drinking, resistance efficacy, negative attitudes about alcohol and sex, and acceptance of parental influence. Due to the founded links between racism and risky behaviors such as substance use and the buffering effects of racial socialization, SAAF taught parents how to engage in positive racial socialization with their youth. SAAF significantly increased regulated, communicative parenting and youth protective factors, leading to significant changes in risk behavior, as compared to a control group. The research group asserted that their focus on cultural specificity and ecological considerations was primarily responsible for the success of their family program.

Sisters Informing Sisters about Topics on AIDS (SISTA)

DiClemente and Wingood (1995) created a program for African American women aged 18-29 years. Their program development was guided by the social cognitive theory and the theory of gender of gender and power (see Wingood & DiClemente (2000) for a discussion on how to implement this theory in HIV interventions). Thus, it is facilitated in group format with 10-12 women, guided by an African American woman, and includes discussions on power dynamics within male/female relationships. This focus addresses the previously stated problem of an underlying gender inequality within the Black community. Further, there is an explicit focus on ethnic pride due to the knowledge that racism has led to degraded self-value and can, therefore, lead to self destructive or negligent behavior. The first session focuses on ethnic and gender pride, with discussions on what it means to be an African American woman, positive attributes of being an African American woman, Black women who are personal role models, and values. The facilitator conducts Africentric activities (e.g., the *umoja* (Swahili word for unity) circle), reads poetry by African American women, and spotlights Black women's artwork. The second session provides general HIV education, including transmission and prevention and its impact on African American women. The third session provides assertiveness skills training, focused on assertive versus aggressive and nonassertive behaviors and applying effective communication in self-protection. The forth session trains participants on correct condom use and provides time to role play newly learned skills. The fifth and final session reviews previous material and explores negative (e.g., coping with drug/alcohol use) and positive coping skills, especially as they relate to rejection and negative feedback. Overall, SISTA was found to be effective in significantly increasing condom use, sexual communication, proper assertive communication, and sexual self-control. They conclude that the combination of gender and ethnic specificity and social skills training was conducive to SISTA's success.

An HIV Prevention Program for African American Adolescents

DiClemente et al. (2004) constructed another program devised specifically for African American female adolescents. The program development of this program was also guided by the social cognitive theory and the theory of gender of gender and power. This program was constituted by four sessions. The first session emphasized ethnic and gender pride through focusing on the complex experience of being an African American female, both positive and negative. They supplemented this discussion with poetry, teaching of the achievements, and decorated the room with artwork of African American women. The second through fourth sessions trained on HIV awareness, HIV resistance efficacy (i.e., confidence in negotiating safe sex practices and refusing sex), and healthy relationships. This program was found effective when compared to a control group. Over a 12 month follow-up assessment, the intervention participants were significantly more likely to use a condom and less likely to have a new sexual partner. Again, this group of researchers attributed part of their success to the cultural competence and relevance of the program.

Culturally Responsive Evaluation (CRE)

Although a number of HIV/AIDS programs and services exist, it becomes imperative on many levels to ensure that the programs implemented are effective and beneficial to the African American communities they serve. The programs that purport to be effective must be held accountable, particularly when addressing the needs of populations from traditionally marginalized groups that have a history of participation in programs where the intent has not always been to their benefit.

Each of the previously described programs demonstrated cultural competence in its construction, focus, and/or implementation. CRE carries this trend and more through the evaluation, adaptation, and improvement of programs. One of the strengths of using CRE over other forms of program evaluation is that it recognizes that culture, context, and sociopolitical factors are embedded into every evaluation and cannot be ignored (Frazier-Anderson, Hood & Hopson, in press; Hopson, 2010). Thus, CRE seeks to utilize evaluation methods that consider all of these factors.

Education, research, prevention and treatment strategies on many levels must be culturally responsive and culturally competent in order to be effective. This means incorporating (or sometimes introducing methods what will counter) cultural values, beliefs, and practices of the group(s) when developing programs. In order to distinguish HIV/AIDS programs that are effective from those that are not for various segments of the Black community and to the essential elements that make them effective, it is necessary for an evaluator who undertakes this study to have a thorough understanding of the cultural factors and sociohistorical considerations at work in the community (Hood, Hopson, & Frierson, 2005). Thus, knowledge of the sociohistorical factors presented in this chapter provides an overview of the information a culturally responsive evaluator should possess when evaluating HIV/AIDS programs in Black communities. A culturally responsive evaluator must also simultaneous consider both the similarities and variation within a cultural or ethnic group (Roof & Chavajay, 1995) and be wary of both positive and negative stereotyping a community.

Additionally, the evaluator should possess the ability to view the community from the perspective of the program participants or include someone on the evaluation team who is knowledgeable about and shares the perspective of the cultural group (Hood, Hopson, & Frierson, 2005). It is also important that the evaluator be aware of and sensitive to current HIV/AIDS topics that are relevant to the evaluation or add someone to the team who has this skill set. It is not recommended that a person with no knowledge or limited knowledge of HIV/AIDS attempt to evaluate programs in this area, since there is relevant terminology or other distinctions that only someone with a high degree of familiarity would possess.

As CRE emerges as a method to evaluate HIV/AIDS programs, some of the essential elements of the evaluation may include: 1) an understanding of the history of the community and the cultural groups that are a part of the program or intervention, 2) an understanding of HIV/AIDS and the impact it has had on the community, 3) interviews with all key stakeholder groups (e.g., members of the administration and staff, participants, caregivers) to understand their attitudes and perspectives about the program or intervention, 4) interviews with leaders and representatives from key community groups to also understand some of the community perspectives about the program or service and to gather additional perspectives about HIV/AIDS in their community, and 5) the creation of a panel consisting of representatives from key stakeholder groups that are able to review and respond to the results of the evaluation (Frazier-Anderson, Hood, & Hopson, in press). This collection of evaluation activities indicates one of the primary strengths of CRE—its democratic and inclusive approach to evaluation. This approach ensures representation from all key stakeholder groups, leaving little room for evaluator assumptions when analyzing results or reporting findings. Thus, the process of a CRE bolsters the validity of the findings (Kirkhart, 2010), the credibility of the evaluation, and is conducive to the proper and comprehensive use of the results.

Conclusion

Confronting HIV/AIDS is a multifarious endeavor. Effectively addressing this problem with a historically oppressed group, like African Americans is even more complicated. Due to the necessity of responding to culture, context, and history, comprehensive prevention and intervention with Black communities requires a multifaceted strategic plan. This plan should be inclusive of culturally and contextually responsive assessment, program development and implementation, and program evaluation. Cultural-historical assessment looking at the history, cultural evolution, and contextual issues can provide a cohesive picture of the situation. Culturally responsive program development and implementation can create an intervention path that is conducive to an apt and more potent impact. Finally, culturally responsive evaluation is designed to ensure social justice and lead to equality—the very goal that professionals are striving for in ameliorating the HIV/AIDS disparity.

References

Agency for Health care and Research Quality. (2006). *National Health Disparities Report*. Retrieved July 28, 2008 from http://www.ahrq.gov/qual/nhdr06/report/.

Airhihenbuwa, C. O., Webster, J. D., Okoror, T. O., Shine, R., Smith-Bankhead, N. (2002). HIV/AIDS and the African-American community: Disparities of policy and identity. *Phylon, 50,* 23-46.

Aral, S. O., Adimora, A. A., & Fenton, KA. (2008) Understanding and responding to disparities in HIV and other sexually transmitted infections in African Americans. *Lancet, 372,* 337-40.

Bach, P. B., Pham, H. H., Schrag, D., Tate, R. C., & Hargraves, J. L. (2004). Primary care physicians who treat blacks and whites. *New England Journal of Medicine, 351,* 575-584.

Baptiste, D. R., Bhana, A., Petersen, I., McKay, M., Voisin, D., Bell C., Martinez, D. D. (2006). Community collaborative youth—focused HIV/AIDS prevention in South Africa and Trinidad: Preliminary findings. *Journal of Pediatric Psychology, 31,* 905-916.

Bartlett, JG., Branson, BM., Fenton, K., Hauschild, BC., Miller, V., & Mayer, KH (2008). Opt-out testing for Human Immunodeficiency Virus in the United States: Progress and challenges. *Journal of the American Medical Association, 300,* 945-951.

Baumer, E. P. & South, S. J. (2001) Community effects on youth sexual activity. *Journal of Marriage and Family, 63,* 540-554.

Bayer, R., and Fairchild, A.L. (2006). Changing the paradigm for HIV testing: The end of exceptionalism. *New England Journal of Medicine, 355*, 647-649.

Belgrave, F. Z. & Allison, K. W. (2010) *African American psychology: From Africa to America, 2nd ed.* Thousand Oaks, CA: Sage Publications.

Bell, C. C., Gamm, S., Vallas, P., et al. (2001). Strategies for the prevention of youth violence in Chicago Public Schools. In: Shafii, M. & Shafii, S. F. (Eds.). *School violence: assessment, management, prevention.* (pp. 251-72). Arlington (VA): American Psychiatric Press.

Bell, C. C., Flay, B., Paikoff, R. Strategies for health behavior change. (2002). In: Chunn, J., (Ed.) *The health behavioral change imperative.* (pp. 17-39). New York: Kluwer Academic/ Plenum Publishers.

Bhana, A., McKay, M. M., Mellins, C., Petersen, I. & Bell, C. C. (2010). Family-based HIV prevention and intervention services for youth living in poverty-affected contexts: the CHAMP model of collaborative, evidence-informed programme development. *Journal of the International AIDS Society, 13,* S2-S8.

Blankenship, K. M., Smoyer, A. B., & Bray, S. J. (2005). Black-white disparities in HIV/AIDS: The role of drug policy and the corrections system. *Journal of HealthCare for the Poor and Underserved, 16b*, 140-146.

Boyd-Franklin, N. (2003). *Black families in therapy: Understanding the African American experience.* New York, NY: Gilford Press.

Brody, G.H., Ge, X., Conger, R., Gibbons, F.X., Murray, V.M., Gerrard, M., & Simons, R.L. (2001). The influence of neighborhood disadvantage, collective socialization, and parenting on African American children's affiliation with deviant peers. *Child Development, 72*, 1231-1246.

Brody, G. H., Murray, V. M., Gerrard, M., Gibbons, F. X., Molgaard, V., McNair, L., et al. (2004). The Strong African American Families Program: Translating research into prevention programming. *Child Development, 75*, 900-917.

Browning, C. R., Burrington, L. A., Leventhal T., et al. (2008). Neighborhood structural inequality, collective efficacy, and sexual risk behavior among urban youth. *Journal of Health and Social Behavior, 49*, 269-285.

Bynum, M. S., Burton, E. T., and Best, C. (2007). Racism experiences and psychological functioning in African American college freshmen: Is racial socialization a buffer? *Cultural Diversity and Ethnic Minority Psychology, 13*, 64-71.

Castro, A. & Farmer, P. (2005). Understanding and addressing AIDS-related stigma: from anthropological theory to clinical practice in Haiti. *American Journal of Public Health, 95*, 59-59.

Caughy, M. O., Campo, P. J. O., Randolph, S. M., & Nickerson, K. (2002). The influence of racial socialization practices on the cognitive and behavioral competence of African American preschoolers. *Child Development, 73*, 1611-1625.

Centers for Disease Control and Prevention. (2006). Revised recommendations for HIV testing of adults, adolescents, and pregnant women in health-care settings. *Morbidity and Mortality Weekly Report, 55*,1-14.

Centers for Disease Control and Prevention. (2006). Missed opportunities for earlier diagnosis of HIV infection-South Carolina, 1997-2005. *Morbidity and Mortality Weekly Report, 55*, 1269-1272.

Centers for Disease Control and Prevention. (2007). *CDC HIV Prevention Strategic Plan*—Extended Through 2010. Retrieved on Accessed on January 11, 2011 from http://www.cdc.gov/hiv/resources/reports/psp/pdf/psp.pdf.

Center for Disease Control and Prevention. (2010). *HIV among African Americans.* Retrieved on February 14, 2011 from http://www.cdc.gov/hiv/topics/aa/pdf/aa.pdf.

Chandra, A., and Skinner, JS. (2003). *Geography and Racial Health Disparities.* Retrieved on January 5, 2011 from http://ssrn.com/abstract=382444.

Coard, S. I. & Sellers, R. M. (2005). African American families as a context for racial socialization. In V. C. McLoyd, N. E. Hill, & K. A. Dodge (Eds.). *African American family life.* (pp. 264-284). New York City, NY: The Guilford Press.

Cohen, Y. (1971). The shaping of men's minds: Adaptations to the imperatives of culture, in M. Wax, S. Diamond, and F. Gearing (Eds), *Anthropological perspectives on education,* New York: Basic Books; in Mansemann, V. (1976). Anthropological approaches to comparative education, *Comparative Education Review, 20*, 368-380.

Cole, J. M. & Boykin, A. W. (2008). Examining culturally structured learning environments with different types of music-linked movement opportunity. *Journal of Black Psychology, 34,* 331-355.

Connell, R. W. (1987) *Gender and power.* Stanford, CA: Stanford University Press.

DeNavas-Walt, C., Proctor, B. D., Smith, J. C. (2010). *Income, poverty, and health insurance coverage in the United States: 2009.* US Census Bureau, US Department of Commerce, Economics and Statistics Administration. Retrieved on February 14, 2011 from http://www.census.gov/prod/2010pubs/p60-238.pdf.

DiClemente, R. J. & Wingood, G. M, (1995). A randomized control trial of an HIV risk reduction for young African American women. *Journal of the American Medical Association, 274,* 1271-1276.

DiClemente, R. J., Wingood, G. M., Harrington, K. F., Lang, D. L., Davies, S. L., Hook, E. W., et al. (2004). Efficacy of an HIV prevention intervention for African American adolescent girls: A randomized controlled trial. *Journal of the American Medical Association, 292,* 171-179.

Douglas, F. (1845). *Narrative of the life of Frederick Douglass: An American slave, written by himself.* New York, New York: Oxford University Press.

Elkins, D. N., Hedstrom, L. J., Hughes, L. L., Leaf, J. A., and Saunders, C. (1988). Toward a humanistic-phenomenological spirituality: Definition, description, and measurement. *Journal of Humanistic Psychology, 28,* 5-18.

Fenton, K. A. (2007). Changing epidemiology of HIV/ AIDS in the United States: implications for enhancing and promoting HIV testing strategies. *Clinical Infectious Diseases, 45,* S213.

Frazier, E. F. (1974). *The Negro Church in America/The Black Church since Frazier.* New York, NY: Schocken Books, Inc.

Frazier-Anderson, P. Hood, S. & Hopson, R. (in press). An African American culturally responsive evaluation system. In S. Lapan, M. Quartaroli, & F. Riemer (Eds.) *Qualitative research: An introduction to methods and designs.* San Francisco, CA: Jossey-Bass.

Gay, G. (2000). *Culturally responsive teaching: Theory, research and practice.* New York, NY: Teachers College Press.

Gilkes, C. T. (2001). *If it Wasn't for the Women.* Maryknoll, NY: Orbis Books.

Gostin, L. O. (2006). HIV screening in health care settings: public health and civil liberties in conflict? *Journal of the American Medical Association, 296,* 2023-2025.

Gruskin, S., Ahmed, S., & Ferguson, L. (2008). Provider initiated HIV testing and counseling in health facilities—what does this mean for the health and human rights of pregnant women? *Developing World Bioethics, 8,* 23-32.

Hanssens, C. (2007). Legal and ethical implications of optout testing. *Clinical Infectious Diseases, 45,* S232-S239.

Holtgrave, D. R. (2007). Costs and consequences of the US Centers for Disease Control and Prevention's recommendations for opt-out HIV testing. *PLoS Medicine, 4,* e194.

Hood, S., Hopson, R., & Frierson, H. (Eds). (2005). *The role of culture and cultural context: A mandate for inclusion, the discovery of truth, and understanding in evaluative theory and practice.* Greenwich, CT: Information Age Publishing.

Kates, J. & Levi, J. (2007). Insurance coverage and access to HIV testing and treatment: considerations for individuals at risk for infection and for those with undiagnosed infection. *Clinical Infectious Diseases, 45,* S255-S260.

Kelen, G. D., Shahan, J. B., & Quinn, T. C. (1999). Emergency department-based HIV screening and counseling: experience with rapid and standard serologic testing. *Annals of Emergency Medicine, 33,* 147-155.

Kirkhart, K. (2010). Eyes on the prize: Multicultural validity and evaluation theory. *American Journal of Evaluation, 31,* 400-413.

Lifson, A. R., & Rybicki, S. L. (2007). Routine opt-out HIV testing. *Lancet, 369,* 539-540.

Lincoln, E. C. (1974). *The Negro Church in America/The Black Church Since Frazier.* New York, NY: Schocken Books, Inc.

Livingston, J. N. & McAdoo, J. L. (2007). The roles of African American fathers in the socialization of their children. In H. P. McAdoo (Ed.). *Black Families.* (pp. 219-237). Thousand Oaks, CA: Sage Publications, Inc.

Mattis, J. S. (2005). Religion in African American Life. In V. C. McLoyd, N. E. Hill, & K. A. Dodge (Eds.). *African American family life.* NY, NY: The Guilford Press (pp. 189-210).

McAdoo, H. P. (1985). Racial socialization of young Black children. In H. P. McAdoo. & J. L. McAdoo (Eds.). *Black children: Social, educational, and parental environments.* Sage Publications (pp. 159-162).

McAdoo, J. L. (1993). The role of African American fathers: An ecological perspective. *Families in Society: The Journal of Contemporary Human Services, 74,* 28-35.

McBride, D. F. (2009). Moving towards holistic equity: A process of developing a culturally responsive family health program. Ph.D. dissertation, Arizona State University, United States, Arizona: Dissertations & Theses: Full Text. (Publication No. AAT 3391851).

McBride, D. F. (in press). Manifesting empowerment: How a family health program can address racism. *Journal of Black Psychology.*

McBride, D. F. & Bell, C. C. (in press). Human Immunodeficiency Virus Prevention with youth. *Psychiatric Clinics of North America.*

Phinney, J. S. (1993). A three-stage model of ethnic identity development in adolescence. In M. E. Bernal & G. P. Knight (Eds.), *Ethnic identity: Formation and transmission among Hispanic and other minorities.* Albany, NY: State University of New York Press.

Peters, M. F. (1985). Racial attitude and self-concept of Black children over time In H. P. McAdoo. & J. L. McAdoo (Eds.). *Black children: Social, educational, and parental environments.* Beverly Hills, CA: Sage Publications, (pp. 213-242).

Rogoff, B. (2003). *The cultural nature of human development.* New York, NY: Oxford University Press, Inc.

Rogoff, B. & Chavajay, P. (1995). What's become of research on the cultural basis of cognitive development. *American Psychologist, 50,* 859-877.

Rothman, R. E. (2004). Current Centers for Disease Control and Prevention guidelines for HIV counseling, testing, and referral: critical role of and a call to action for emergency physicians. *Annals of Emergency Medicine, 44,* 31-42.

Rovia, A. P., Gallien, L. B., & Wighting, M. J. (2005). Cultural and interpersonal factors affecting African American academic performance in higher education: A review and synthesis of the research literature. *Journal of Negro Education, 74,* 359-370.

Simons, R. L., Murray, V., McLloyd, V., Lin, K., Cutrona, C., and Conger, R. D. (2002). Discrimination, crime, ethnic identity, and parenting as correlates of depressive symptoms among African American children: A multilevel analysis. *Development and Psychopathology, 14,* 371-393.

Smedley, B. D., Stith, A. Y., & Nelson, A. R., (Eds.) (2003). *Unequal treatment: confronting racial and ethnic disparities in health care*. Washington, DC: National Academies Press.

Smith, E. P., Atkins, J., Connell, C. M. (2003). Family, school, and community factors and relationships to racial-ethnic attitudes and academic achievement. *American Journal of Community Psychology, 32,* 159-173.

Stevenson, H. C., Jr. (1995). Relationship of adolescent perceptions of racial socialization to racial identity. *Journal of Black Psychology, 21,* 49-70.

Sudarkasa, N. (2007). Interpreting the African heritage in African American family organization. In H. P. McAdoo (Ed.). *Black families.* Thousand Oaks, CA: Sage Publications, Inc. (pp.29-47).

Sue, D. W., Capodilupo, C. M., Torino, G. C., Bucceri, J. M. Holder, A. M. Nadal, K. L. & Esquilin, M. (2007) Racial Microaggressions in Everyday Life: *Implications for Clinical Practice, American Psychologist, 62,* 271-286.

Swamy, M. (2007). UN agencies issue new guidelines for HIV testing. *HIV AIDS Policy Law Review,12,* 39-40.

Taylor, R. J., Chatters, L. M., & Levin, J. S. (2004). *Religion in the lives of African Americans: Social, psychological, and health perspectives*. Thousand Oaks, CA: Sage Publications.

Valdiserri, R. O. (2007). Late HIV diagnosis: bad medicine and worse public health. *PLOS Medicine, 4,* e200.

Wallace, S. A., Neilands, T. B., Sanders-Phillips, K. (2009) Neighborhood risks and HIV risk among African American youth. *Journal of Adolescent Health, 44,* s6.

Washington, H. A. (2006). *Medical apartheid: The dark history of medical experimentation on Black Americans from colonial times to the present.* New York, NY: Doubleday.

Wells, K., Klap, R., Koite, A. and Sherbourne, C. (2001). Ethnic disparities in unmet need for alcoholism, drug abuse, and mental health care. *American Journal of Psychiatry, 58,* 2027-2032.

Wingood, G. M. & DiClemente, R. J. (2000). Application of the theory of gender and power to examine HIV-related exposures, risk factors, and effective interventions for women. *Health Education & Behavior, 27,* 539-565.

Wyatt, G. E. (2009). Enhancing cultural and contextual intervention strategies to reduce HIV/AIDS among African Americans. *American Journal of Public Health, 99,* 1941-1945.

Wyatt, G. E., Williams, J. K., & Myers, H. F. (2008). African American sexuality and HIV/AIDS: Recommendations for future research. *Journal of the National Medical Association, 100,* 44-51.

Wynia, M. K. (2006). Routine screening: informed consent, stigma and the waning of HIV exceptionalism. *American Journal of Bioethics, 6,* 5-8.

CHAPTER TEN

Using Community-Based Partnerships to Enhance Prevention Research among African American Youth: A Focus on Child/Adolescent Health

Dionne S. Coker-Appiah
Georgetown U. School
of Medicine

Dawnavan S. Davis
U. of Chicago School
of Medicine

Tiffany G. Townsend.
Georgetown U. School
of Medicine

Abstract

Building community partnerships is one promising strategy in the development and implementation of health disparities research targeting adolescent populations. The evolution of research partnerships requires an understanding of the varying levels of community input as part of the research process. Community-based partnerships grounded in community engagement and collaboration in research has increasingly gained attention, primarily due to the mutual benefits associated with such collaborations. This chapter will describe three community-based research projects. Each project will focus on a different research stage and/or level of community-engagement. The I.S.I.S. project will focus on transitioning from a community cooperative research project to a community collaborative project. Project LOVE will focus on building a collaborative research partnership using community-based participatory research. Finally, The OBGT project will focus on using community engagement and collaboration to inform intervention design and testing.

Introduction

Building community partnerships is one promising strategy in the development and implementation of health disparities research targeting adolescent populations. The evolution of research partnerships requires an understanding of the varying levels of community input as part of the research process. The degree of community input in research exists along a continuum (Winer & Ray, 2000), and the discernment of the extent to which community is involved in the research process is critical to our increased knowledge and application of community-engaged research and practice strategies. Winer & Ray (1995) and Ray (2004) clearly define three levels of community involvement from cooperation to collaboration, reflecting increased formality and intensity across the levels. In addition, it is important to overlay the levels of community involvement in research with the various types of research approaches in order to further elucidate the utility and impact of the intersection between community input, scientific inquiry, and health status and outcomes across various populations.

The first level is *cooperation*. Cooperation, typically seen in basic science research, is defined as two or more entities coming together for a short-term informal relationship in the absence of shared planning by entities in the relationship. At the cornerstone of this level, is a clear separation of resources, authority, and the absence of intention for a sustained relationship beyond a specific task. Power differential and lack of shared benefit or resources may be significant issues at this level.

Example of Cooperation: Researchers want to study smoking behaviors among adolescent boys. Upon funding, researchers contact a local youth community organization to assist in recruiting adolescent boys into the study. After recruitment goals are achieved, the relationship between the community-based organization and researchers is terminated.

Coordination, the next level of engagement, represents a more formal relationship and is characterized by shared mission, planning, and structural processes. Although separation in authority still exists at this level, participating entities begin to share resources to advance the goals of one or more of the participating institutions.

Coordination, the next level of engagement, represents a more formal relationship and is characterized by shared mission, planning, and structural processes. Although separation in authority still exists at this level, participating entities begin to share resources to advance the goals of one or more of the participating institutions.

Example of Coordination. A youth-focused community-based organization and a governmental agency have similar priority areas related to policy research projects aimed to decrease smoking initiation rates among youth. The community-based organization solicits assistance from the government agency to implement their existing project statewide. Both organizations contribute some resources (time, funding etc.) to support this effort.

Third, is *collaboration*. Collaboration is the process in which stakeholders related to a particular problem actively seek a mutually derived solution (Gray, 1989, 1996). Often the impetus for collaboration is motivated by a desire to advance a shared vision or need to positively impact an issue of importance and relevance to all entities. The desired result of collaboration often varies from shared information transference to execution of long-term relationships, and typically is focused on a particular area of mutual interest or concern (Scott-Taplin, 1993; Scott & Thurston, 1997). The hallmark characteristics of this level are: 1) extensive, intensive relationship development; 2) detailed planning and communication; 3) shared creation of partnership mission, goals and objectives; and 4) the collective convening of resources across participating organizations. *Partnership* is a type of collaboration, and occurs when the goal of the collaboration is to advance the mutually determined vision. Partnerships have an expected outcome of the establishment of a joint effort that leads to action-oriented relationships. In research, community-based participatory research or CBPR represents such an approach, where collaboration is the cornerstone. In this approach, collaborative partnerships occur between all entities (for example: community, academic, government institutions), with all partners engaged in all aspects of the research process from inception to dissemination (Israel, Schulz,

Parker, & Becker, 1998; Minkler & Wallerstein, 2002; Minkler, Wallerstein, & Hall, 2008).

Example of Collaboration. A researcher, civic organization, and health insurance company are interested in curbing smoking rates among racial and ethnic minority adolescents. All parties are committed to improving health outcomes in this population. Over a 12-month period, the three organizations work together to build a collaborative partnership focused on the development of a randomized-controlled social marketing research intervention targeting smoking initiation prevention. All partners participate in the generation of the research question, study implementation, evaluation, and dissemination strategies, with funding resources equally distributed across the three participating institutions.

Community Engagement

Community-based partnerships grounded in community engagement (CE) and collaboration in research has increasingly gained attention, primarily due to the mutual benefits associated with such collaborations. It is worth noting that the cornerstone of these levels is community engagement. Over the past two decades, researchers have demonstrated that the social environment, in which people live, as well as their lifestyles and behaviors influence the incidence of illness (Institute of Medicine, 1988). In addition, research has shown that people can achieve long-term health improvements when they become involved in their community and work together to effect change (Hanson, 1988-89). Thus, CE serves as an invaluable tool when it is established with the prerequisite understanding of the culture of a targeted population, as well as a strong alliance with community resources.

Various studies have found that people participate when they feel a sense of community, see their involvement and the issues as relevant and worthy of their time, and view the process and organizational climate of participation as open and supportive of their right to have a voice in the process (Braithwaite, Bianchi, & Taylor, 1994; Thompson & Kinne, 1990). CE strengthens the social fabric of the community, and increases the individual's sense of control and ability to effect change on their own environment Florin & Wandersman, 1990). Furthermore, research that maintains strong community involvement through its development and implementation experiences greater long-term viability and positive results Goodman & Steckler, 1987-1988; Israel, et al, 2005; O'Fallon & Deary, 2002; Putnam, 1995; Shaefer & Bronheim, 2007; Weijer, 2000).

The Centers for Disease Control and Prevention's Committee for Community Engagement describes CE as *"the process of working collaboratively with groups of people who are affiliated by geographic proximity, special interests, or similar situations with respect to issues affecting their well-being,"* which enables environmental and behavioral changes that will improve the health of the community and its members (CDC ATSDR & Committee on Community Engagement, 1997). They assert, and we agree, that the process of CE is both a science and an art that enables the blending of knowledge creation with the appropriate and effective application and adaption of such knowledge in a manner that meets the community's needs, goals, and objectives. The committee established nine principles of community engagement that have been used to guide community-based research. They are:

Before starting a community engagement effort . . .

1. Be clear about the purposes or goals of the engagement effort, and the populations and/or communities you want to engage.
2. Become knowledgeable about the community in terms of its economic conditions, political structures, norms and values, demographic trends, history, and experience with engagement efforts. Learn about the community's perceptions of those initiating the engagement activities.

For engagement to occur, it is necessary to . . .

3. Go into the community, establish relationships, build trust, work with the formal and informal leadership, and seek commitment from community organizations and leaders to create processes for mobilizing the community.
4. Remember and accept that community self-determination is the responsibility and right of all people who comprise a community. No external entity should assume it can bestow on a community the power to act in its own self-interest.

For engagement to succeed . . .

5. Partnering with the community is necessary to create change and improve health.
6. All aspects of community engagement must recognize and respect community diversity. Awareness of the various cultures of a community and other factors of diversity must be paramount in designing and implementing community engagement approaches.
7. Community engagement can only be sustained by identifying and mobilizing community assets, and by developing capacities and resources for community health decisions and action.
8. An engaging organization or individual change agent must be prepared to release control of actions or interventions to the community, and be flexible enough to meet the changing needs of the community.
9. Community collaboration requires long-term commitment by the engaging organization and its partners.

This chapter will describe three community-based research projects. Each project will focus on a different research stage and/ or level of community-engagement, to include: transitioning from a community cooperative research project to a community collaborative project (I.S.I.S); building a collaborative research partnership using community-based participatory research (CBPR) (Project LOVE); and using community engagement and collaboration to inform intervention design and testing (OBGT).

Community-Based Partnerships in Action

Project I: Intelligent Sisters Improving Themselves (ISIS) (P.I. Dr. Tiffany G. Townsend in Collaboration with the Progressive Life Center, Inc. and the ISIS Community Advisory Board)

In the spring of 2002, while on faculty at Penn State University, we decided to develop a partnership with Progressive Life Center, Inc. (PLC), a community-based mental health agency that utilizes a unique Afro-centric approach in the delivery of therapeutic services and psycho-educational programs. Although headquartered in Washington DC., the organization had recently opened a branch in the Philadelphia area. Our partnership represented an opportunity for two entities (the academy and the community) that have not always found common ground to work together to address a mutual goal: risk prevention among African American youth. From this collaboration, the ISIS (Intelligent Sisters Improving Themselves) project was born. ISIS was an integrated HIV/Substance Abuse prevention program that targeted African American girls who lived in Southwest Philadelphia. The program was administered from 2004 to 2008. Initially, it was designed as a 26-week program in which our staff would meet with participating girls for an hour after school on a weekly basis, providing psycho-educational material related to HIV and substance use prevention. Our goal was to instill ISIS participants with the skills necessary to promote healthy behavior and reduce risk. Having been academically "raised" in a traditional psychology setting, I thought that partnering with a community based organization to help implement the program was more than adequate to ensure community involvement and input. However, I quickly learned that working with one community organization was merely a first step. In order to ensure that our program was embraced by the community and tailored to its specific needs, the Southwest Philadelphia community and its residents would need to be involved in the development and implementation of the ISIS project at all levels.

In this section, we will chronicle the transformation that ISIS went through as the community became more involved in the planning process. In many ways, ISIS moved from being a *community cooperative* project to a *community collaborative* project. This transformation dramatically changed the nature of the program and positively impacted program effectiveness. In recounting this conversion, the goal is to highlight practical strategies that can be used to help traditional research make the successful transition into Community Action Research (CAR) and ultimately Community Based Participatory Research (CBPR).

As previously mentioned, the goal of the ISIS project was to help reduce the risk of HIV and substance use among African American girls. But more than that, we hoped to empower this population to make fundamental, lifelong changes regarding healthy attitudes and behaviors. According to Zimmerman (2000), empowerment is the process through which people with limited access to resources gain greater access to and control over those resources. Thus, we knew community outreach would be a necessary component of the program. For true empowerment, ISIS participants, in particular, and the Southwest Philadelphia community, in general, would need to experience a level of ownership of ISIS and the knowledge/ information conveyed. Accordingly, we developed a plan of action that was intended to increase community input, involvement and ultimately buy-in. This constituted the planning phase of the ISIS project, which spanned the 2003 to 2004 academic year.

Phase I: Project Planning and Needs Assessment

During the initial phases of project planning, we knew it would be important to connect with key community members and stakeholders to foster community trust. We soon connected with the Southwest Action Coalition (SWAC). SWAC is a 30-member community advisory board and planning group composed of community members, service providers and community activists dedicated to improving the quality of life for residents in the Southwest Philadelphia area. After providing the mission and goals of the ISIS project, our project director was asked to join SWAC. Forging a relationship with SWAC was an extremely important step to ensure that ISIS' efforts were coordinated with the larger community. It also was a crucial step in obtaining community feedback. Using the connections we developed through SWAC, we set up a community needs assessment.

Our needs assessment included focus groups, workshops and forums designed to increase our understanding of the problems faced by African American girls in the Southwest Philadelphia region. Members of several community organizations based in Southwest Philadelphia were in attendance. In addition to providing basic information on girls, the focus groups and forums served as an opportunity for community members and stakeholders to voice their concerns and provide suggestions on working with adolescent girls in the Southwest Philadelphia community. To obtain feedback from the target population, a pilot administration was conducted during the spring of 2004. The pilot, which lasted 5 weeks, was used to assess implementation and evaluation adequacy. In addition, the pilot gave the project staff an opportunity to fine tune implementation techniques and activities. It also provided an opportunity for the target girls to indicate the topics they wanted to see addressed in the full ISIS implementation.

Every effort was devoted to ensuring that the feedback we received from the community during this planning phase was used to make changes and fine-tune the program. However, it is important to note that at this point, true community ownership of ISIS had not been achieved, primarily because our level of community engagement was limited. As previously mentioned, community involvement in research exists along a continuum (Winer & Ray, 2000), that advances from cooperation to coordination and finally to collaboration. Our initial community efforts hovered at the cooperation side of this continuum. In other words, we were merely cooperating with the community to get their feedback on ideas that were generated from our own research and service agenda. Although our efforts were certainly informed by the community, other than our partnership with PLC, our relationship with the Southwest Philadelphia community was far from being collaborative. To facilitate engagement and community ownership, we realized that we would need to integrate the community more substantively into the planning and implementation process. To this end, an ISIS Community Advisory Board (CAB) was created in the beginning of 2005.

Phase II: Partnership Development and Community Outreach

In developing the Board, we made sure there were members representing different sectors from the community (i.e., faith-based organizations, law enforcement, the school system, etc). Our plan was to develop a diverse community entity that would provide ongoing feedback concerning the progress of the ISIS project. Almost immediately during our first session, the lack of a truly collaborative relationship with the community became quite apparent. One particularly vocal advisory board member indicated that the role of the community seemed marginal to the ISIS planning process. In her opinion, the community was consulted almost as an "after thought." Many of the members questioned the very structure of the CAB. Not only had the community not been fully integrated into the planning process, but the community was not even consulted as to the membership of the CAB. According to these members, the current Board was "top heavy" (i.e., too many organizational representatives and not enough community members who have a direct stake in the program, such as parents, teachers, etc), and the absence of target girls at the planning table was a major oversight in the composition of the Board. This represented the beginning of ISIS' transformation. At the urging of our CAB, the ISIS project began to become much more grounded in the community. The changes that we made to the partnership, the infrastructure and the communication loop pushed us toward a model in which there was shared decision-making and open communication between the community and the project. We hoped this would facilitate community ownership and ultimately improve project outcomes. While not our original plan, we realized that a CBPR approach was warranted to garner the desired project effects. In this approach, research is done collaboratively *with*, rather than *on*, communities, affirming the value of the community's experiential knowledge (Leung et al., 2004). Done properly, CBPR lends itself to the development of culturally appropriate intervention methods (Viswanathan et al., 2004). Therefore, our staff re-conceptualized the project based on these principals, which helped to guide subsequent program changes.

The first changes instituted were changes to the CAB infrastructure. Based on the strong recommendations of the board, we added a Girls Advisory Board (GAB), and we increased the concentration of parents, teachers and community youth service providers on the main CAB. In addition, we met more frequently (from quarterly to monthly) and we developed an email list serve for more efficient communication between meetings. These minor alterations made a noticeable change in the level of CAB participation. By including community members more substantively in the planning and implementation process, we communicated that we valued them as integral members of the ISIS team. Members who feel personally validated and respected are more likely to participate in the group, and feel a sense of ownership (Summit Health Institute for Research and Education, 2004). These changes moved us closer to true community collaboration and engagement, which prompted more dramatic changes to the project infrastructure. For instance, we began incorporating advisory board members into program implementation, which will be described in more detail below, and we hired a community member from the board to serve as a paid Project Coordinator. Although it did not happen immediately, signs of community ownership began to emerge.

For instance, ISIS and our work began to receive media coverage. In March and April of 2005, I was asked to speak about African American adolescent girls' development on *Dialogues* a radio program featured on a local radio station in Philadelphia. In addition, the ISIS project was featured in the Tribune, a local newspaper in Philadelphia that focuses on African American issues. Our emerging community presence prompted other community-based organizations to seek out co-sponsored outreach activities. In 2006, ISIS in partnership with *MEE Productions* and the *Blueprint Project for a Safer Philadelphia* hosted a Community Action Team (CAT) workshop. The goal of the workshop was to help young adults learn ways to combat youth risks, particularly youth violence. During that implementation year, many of our ISIS participants were also participants in the CAT workshop. Slowly ISIS began moving from a narrowly focused after-school program, to a more holistic risk prevention program with broader reach in the community. ISIS was truly becoming tailored to the needs of Southwest Philadelphia.

Phase III: Program Implementation

Program delivery was also altered as a result of our GAB and CAB. CAB representatives from the school system were instrumental in helping to move ISIS from an after-school program, to an in-school activity. The youth requested more contact with the program, so intervention sessions increased from once a week to twice a week. The 26-week program, changed to a 46-week program. This increase in participant contact could have been cost prohibitive, if our CAB had not stepped in. The CAB took the lead in developing the content and administering the program for the second intervention day, which was called the "Culture Day." For several weeks, African American women from the community (many were from the advisory board) served as guest speakers or workshop facilitators. Each workshop covered various topics designed to enhance girls' self-image and self-worth (some of the workshop covered topics such as hair care, jewelry making and quilting). In addition, based on a suggestion from our GAB members, a video project was administered on the "Culture Days" during the spring semesters of the program.

This project consisted of 12 weekly sessions. A video producer from the community met with participants to provide an overview of "what happens behind the making of a video." Participants received a basic understanding of how a video is made from conception to the finished product. Participants also received instructional lessons on how to operate cameras, lights, sound, video dubbing and editing. The girls then developed a music video that conveyed a positive image/message concerning African American girls and women. The finished product was "premiered" to their family, friends and the broader community at the ISIS graduation ceremony, which was held at the end of each ISIS program administration.

Phase IV: Community Collaboration and Program Sustainability

As time progressed, the ISIS CAB served less in the advisory role and began to function more as a true collaborator. In addition to the changes outlined above, the ISIS CAB began sponsoring its own outreach activities. In 2007, they organized a community forum to raise HIV awareness and they hosted a walk-a-thon entitled "Walk for a Teenage Girl", again, to raise awareness concerning the impact of HIV on African American girls, while also raising money for ISIS program activities. However, we noticed that the most consistent and enthusiastic board members were parents of ISIS participants. Given the strength and enthusiasm of our parent board members, we decided to increase the power and input of the parents by developing a Parent Community Council. In the final year, much of the advising from the community was provided by the Parent's Council. In fact, at the urging of the Council, parent led workshops were instituted during the final year to encourage parent participation in the program delivery, and to address topics of concern for interested parents. One workshop even focused on parental stress management techniques. As the parents became more involved in program planning and program implementation, we were encouraged that community ownership had taken place, a key aspect for ensuring that the program would be maintained even after our project funding had expired.

By the final year 2007-2008, it was clear that ISIS had completely transformed from a narrowly focused, academically run after-school risk prevention program to a broad reaching program, deeply grounded in the community. Ownership of the program had shifted from the project staff to enthusiastic community members. In fact, other than curriculum administration many of the ISIS sponsored programs during the final year of the project, were initiated by the Parent Community Council. In the summer of 2008, our project director held a 6-hour training session to teach interested parents, teachers and community members how to administer the ISIS curriculum on their own and the "passing of the baton" was complete. At last report, some ISIS activities were still administered to girls on a limited basis in a Southwest Philadelphia recreation center and one of the CAB members used the principals from ISIS to develop a complementary program for boys, called T.H.E. N.U.B.I.A.N.S. (Teaching, Healing, Empowering—Never Underestimating Brothers' Intelligence, Ambitions & Natural Strengths). Although in altered form, ISIS lives on in Southwest Philadelphia and we credit this longevity and success to the strong involvement of the community.

Lessons Learned

Our experience with the ISIS project was rewarding and certainly taught us many lessons as we continue to work in the community. It is hoped that the information garnered from this process can be used as other scholars begin the journey into community-based research. A few of the more significant points are highlighted below. First, adopt a Community Participatory Model and involve the community early in the process as true partners. This should foster community investment and ownership. Including community members in program development and fundraising is also a good way to foster ownership. Second, develop a training component to ensure sustainability beyond funding. True community coalition building is a long process and often the fruits of your labor are not evident until after the funding period. Developing a sustainability plan will help to ensure that your efforts are not wasted once funding expires. Finally, do not try to recreate the wheel. Use the resources and strengths already present in the community to help run and sustain the program. In addition to conserving resources, it also helps to ensure that the program is relevant and culturally appropriate for the community.

Project II: Project Letting Our Voices Empower (LOVE):
(P.I. Dr. Dionne Smith Coker-Appiah in collaboration with the
Project LOVE Community Advisory Board)

This section will describe how a Community-Based Participatory Research (CBPR) approach was used to build an adolescent dating violence (ADV) prevention partnership and a subsequent research program entitled: Project Letting Our Voices Empower (LOVE). According to the Centers for Disease Control and Prevention (CDC), ADV is defined as the threat or use of physical, sexual or emotional abuse within a dating relationship (Centers for Disease Control and Prevention & National Center for Injury Prevention and Control, 2008). The goal of our partnership is to engage in collaborative research and other community-based activities designed to prevent ADV among rural, African American adolescents. This section will focus primarily on six phases related to partnership development and research design. Our partnership development process and research program most closely matches Winer and Ray's (1995) and Ray's (2004) third level of community involvement, namely, *Collaboration.*

Community-Based Participatory Research

CBPR is a collaborative approach to research that equitably involves all partners in the research process (from conception to dissemination) and recognizes the unique strengths that each brings (Israel, Eng, Schultz, & Parker, 2005a; Israel, Eng, Schultz, & Parker, 2005b; Israel, Schultz, Parker, & Becker, 1998; Minkler & Wallerstein, 2002; Minkler, Wallerstein, & Hall, 2008). Established CBPR principles include building on the strengths of all partners, sharing resources among all partners, basing partnership on mutual trust, respect, and commitment, striving for clear and open communication among partners, and collaborating in all phases of research (Israel, Schultz, Parker, & Becker, 1998; Seifer & Maurana 2000). Not only does it invite important community and academic partners to the table, it ensures that everyone's unique strengths are recognized and voices heard and integrated throughout the research process. Unlike traditional approaches to research, CBPR requires cognition and action on the part of all involved parties. As such, community and academic partnerships are created for the purpose of identifying, addressing, and understanding important community issues, in an effort to promote change by designing, implementing and evaluating culturally appropriate and sustainable interventions (DiClemente, Crosby, & Wingood, 2005). Further, partnerships may guard against what Ingram and colleagues (2008) describe as the possibility of communities resisting the implementation of interventions of which they have little to no ownership. The use of CBPR in research has been found to be effective on multiple levels; particularly as it relates to including youth as partners. For instance, Flicker's (2008) findings show that a CBPR approach increases the chances of research being better conceptualized when conducted with youth (i.e., better questions, recruitment, data collection, analysis, dissemination, and action) and youth stakeholders feel as though they are really listened to and heard. This inclusion increases feelings of belonging to something with which they can make meaningful contributions Ingram, Flannery, Elkavich, & Rotheram-Borus, 2008).

Project LOVE Phase I: Initial Needs Assessment

Project LOVE began in the Spring of 2007 in the mostly rural, Eastern North Carolina. It grew out of a conversation between me (the PI), my community mentor, and one other community member. As the three initial members, we formed the initial Project LOVE community advisory board (CAB), and were all interested in working together to address the needs of local youth. After multiple, lengthy discussions, several youth-related issues emerged. These issues included ADV, education, drugs, and gangs. Due to our collective interests, experience, and expertise, there was a mutual agreement to focus on the prevention of dating violence among rural African American adolescents. After agreeing upon the research focus, we conducted a windshield tour of the county, reviewed existing community documents, and conducted a literature search in peer-reviewed publications. These activities enabled us to better assess community assets and needs that could be used to inform and/or guide the research.

Project LOVE Phase II: Partnership Development for Research Initiatives

Partnership development was initiated to acquire additional partners necessary to carry out our research program. Our initial discussions focused on identifying community partners who could represent all aspects of the research. As such, the initial list consisted of partners from the following sectors: (a) adolescent dating violence, (b) adolescent health, (c) mental health, (d) sexual health, (e) school/family health, and (f) policy. We were able to collaboratively recruit partners from all six sectors, some of whom also served on our CAB. As our research progressed, we realized the need to recruit additional partners deemed necessary to fulfill our current and future research goals. These additional partners were recruited from the following sectors: (a) youth, (b) parents/

guardians, (c) clergy, (d) education, (e) legal/juvenile justice, and (f) law enforcement. To date, we have been successful in recruiting members from the youth, parent/guardian, and legal/juvenile justice sectors. We are actively recruiting additional partners from the remaining sectors.

Community Advisory Board Development. Our CAB was established to carry out all Project LOVE research activities. The CAB is composed of select members of the Partnership. CAB members receive relevant training and participate in annual evaluations and retreats. These activities are in place to ensure that CAB member needs are met and to maintain the integrity of our research. In addition, the CAB is further broken down into four subcommittees. These subcommittees were established to ensure that each Project LOVE activity is carried out effectively and appropriately. The subcommittees and their respective responsibilities are:

1. Membership: This subcommittee is responsible for recruiting new Partnership and CAB members
2. Research: This subcommittee is responsible for the recruitment of research participants, data collection, and data analysis.
3. Dissemination: This subcommittee is responsible for disseminating research findings in both lay and academic publications and venues.
4. Sustainability: This subcommittee is responsible for researching funding opportunities (local, state, federal, etc.) relevant to sustain Project LOVE research activities. This committee is also responsible for coordinating the annual retreats and evaluations.

Our partners currently meet quarterly and our CAB members meet monthly. Our partners and CAB members play active roles in the entire research process. They consistently volunteer their time to serve on the advisory board and are all committed to Project LOVE, to building community capacity, and to empowering youth to develop healthy dating relationships.

Project LOVE Phase III: Research Questions Development

Once our Partnership and CAB were established, we began the process of exploring potential research questions. Because we were only able to find very few relevant existing research studies related to ADV among rural African American adolescents, we decided that our initial research studies needed to focus on understanding adolescents' knowledge, perceptions, beliefs, and skills regarding ADV. Thus, our collective research questions were: (1) What knowledge, perceptions, and beliefs do older, rural, African American adolescents hold about dating violence? (2) What are the perceived implications for mental and sexual health? (3) What knowledge, perceptions, and beliefs do younger rural, African American adolescents hold about ADV? and (4) What can be done from a multi-level/social-ecological perspective to address and prevent it? The nature of our research questions led to the adoption of qualitative methods, which will be described in the next section.

Project LOVE Phase IV: Methods

The research subcommittee was primarily responsible for phase four. However, additional CAB members offered their support as necessary. This phase includes recruitment, data collection and data analysis. A description of each follows.

Recruitment. In regards to recruitment, we decided to use flyers, radio broadcasts, and in-person recruitment. Flyers were posted at beauty salons, barbershops, and community-based organizations and agencies. Scripts were designed for local radio stations. Finally, CAB members also utilized in-person recruitment throughout local communities and neighborhoods. These recruitment efforts were successful in recruiting necessary research participants.

Data Collection. As previously mentioned, our CAB agreed that qualitative methods were appropriate to answer our research questions. As such, among the multiple data collection methods, we discussed and agreed to conduct semi-structured individual interviews and focus groups. This data collection method would enable the collection of in-depth responses and the opportunity to probe and ask additional questions deemed necessary. We also agreed that the PI, CAB members, and trained community-based facilitators would be appropriate data collectors.

Data Analysis. We used the grounded theory method (Glaser & Strauss, 1967; Strauss & Corbin, 1998) to analyze our data. The research subcommittee was responsible for all data analysis activities. The subcommittee members attended a data analysis training, which covered grounded theory (open, axial, and selective coding), qualitative research, transcript review, and the specifics related to the Project LOVE data analysis process. Once the data was analyzed, we began the process of dissemination.

Project LOVE Phase V: Dissemination

The CBPR process involves collaborative dissemination of research findings (*McGranaghan & Kauper-Brown, 2006*). As such, Project LOVE findings have consistently been collaboratively disseminated in multiple publications and venues. Each dissemination effort has included participation from at least two CAB members: one academic and one community-based member. We have primarily utilized three dissemination methods: Presentations, Publications, and Community Forums. We have presented our findings locally/regionally, nationally, and internationally. We have collaboratively published our findings in peer reviewed journals and books. We are currently in the process of planning a community forum that will enable us to share Project LOVE findings with the local community. Our *Dissemination Committee* will take the lead on this dissemination strategy. These dissemination activities have not only given us the opportunity to share our findings with both lay and academic audiences, they have also played an instrumental role in building community capacity in the area of research dissemination. Both our academic and community members have acquired additional knowledge and skills that have enabled us to be competitive in the grant-writing process, which is an integral component of many of the community-based organizations of which our CAB members are executive directors and/or employed.

Project LOVE Phase VI: Sustainability

Our sustainability efforts are in place to ensure that Project LOVE activities are successfully carried out. Project LOVE is a partnership designed to ensure that adolescents have the knowledge and skills necessary to build healthy dating relationships, recognize warning signs of unhealthy relationships, and know how to seek help, if necessary. As such, we believe that there are two critical sustainability components: Commitment and Funding. We chose to include commitment because the initial phases of our research were carried out on a volunteer basis and often with minimal external funding. Thus, our commitment to the goals of Project LOVE was a critical component to its success in the earlier stages and currently remains a critical component. Without commitment, we would not have been able to attain our level of success to date. Although we acknowledge and understand that funding is important, we believe that funding without commitment diminishes the overall quality and sustainability of research conducted using the CBPR approach.

Funding is the second critical sustainability component. Over the past several years, we have collaboratively written and applied for multiple research grants. Our efforts have resulted in receiving funding in the form of both internal institutional grants and an external NIH grant. These funding awards have enabled us to continue to pursue our research. Our most recent NIH grant will provide five years of support that will enable us to design and pilot test an ADV prevention intervention designed specifically for rural, African American adolescents.

Lessons Learned

The Project LOVE partnership has witnessed many successes over the past several years. The CBPR process has enriched our partnership and relationships with one another as well as our overall research program. A critical reflection of our partnership and the six phases described above highlight the following lessons learned:

1. When designing collaborative partnerships and research programs, it is important to engage the community at the

very beginning. Prolonged engagement is also a critical component of the process, as it can ensure that appropriate, effective, and thorough needs assessments are conducted. A thorough understanding of the communities in which one wishes to partner is crucial to research success and ample time must be spent gathering relevant community knowledge in multiple forms. Investment in and a commitment to the community coupled with building community capacity are essential.

2. Partnership development is a critical component to collaborative research. Transparency among partners is a valuable component to success and minimizes disagreements while simultaneously building trust among partners. Consistent efforts (i.e., regular meetings, trainings, retreats, evaluations, etc.) should be made to strengthen research partnerships and partners must remember to embrace flexibility in order to communicate respect for different value systems and/or paradigms.

3. Efforts should be made to collaboratively disseminate research in both academic and lay publications and venues.

4. The sustainability of a partnership and research program requires more than funding alone. A true commitment on the part of the partners must be coupled with multiple funding sources.

5. When engaging in collaborative research partnerships, it is important to remember the following quote, "People don't care how much you know, until they know how much you care!" (Theodore Roosevelt)

Project III: Our Bodies, God's Temples (OBGT) (P.I. Dr. Dawnavan Davis in collaboration with the OBGT Community Advisory Board)

Significance of OBGT

One of three children in the U.S. is obese or overweight, with African American (AA) youth disproportionately affected (Ogden, Carroll, Curtin, Lamb & Flegal, 2010; Ogden, Carroll, & Flegal, 2008). Obesity and overweight has been associated with a cadre of physical and psychological co-morbidities such as poor body image (Barlow, Dietz, Klish & Towbridge, 2002). The AA church plays a pivotal role in the lives of many AA families, and can serve as a powerful environment for health education and promotion efforts (Levin, Chatters, Ellison & Taylor, 1996; Chaves & Higgins, 1992; Lincoln & Mamiya, 1990). Specifically, AA churches serve a variety of functions including religious, social, and organizational, (Du Bois, 1903) and provides a setting conducive to addressing increased weight among AA youth and families. The overarching goals of OBGT were twofold: 1) engage in a collaborative, participatory formative research process to inform the development of a culturally-sensitive faith-based behavioral obesity intervention for African American youth and families; and 2) conduct a pilot feasibility test of a faith-based diet, physical activity, and body image behavioral intervention for AA youth and their families in churches for the purpose of intervention refinement. To accomplish these goals, a community-based participatory research (CBPR) approach was employed between academic and AA church partners to inform the development and conduction of the OBGT program.

Developing and Evaluating the Partnership

The OBGT program involved developing and sustaining equitable research academic-community partnerships with several AA churches and universities, and involved three critical steps: 1) multi-modal identification of key academic and community stakeholders and organizations; 2) ongoing visibility strategies; and 3) community participation, all of which were essential to better understand the current landscape related to church-based health priorities and interventions, and for initiation of the OBGT partnership development process. First, identification of key individuals and organizations of the AA faith community was achieved by three main approaches: website exploration, literature reviews, and formal and informal in-person interactions with internal and external academic and community individuals and organizations. Second, visibility activities entailed active and ongoing participation in church activities related and unrelated to health. Attending community-wide efforts led by organizations with common interests in the areas of obesity prevention and faith-based programming was critical, while participating in numerous church events and meetings allowed for initial engagement with a broad consistency of stakeholders. Understanding existing relationship and initiatives, relationship dynamics, and the engagement in mutual exploration by potential academic and community partners regarding the desire to enter a collaborative relationship; complementary and competing goals; assets; and partnership expectations among all parties was essential. Such strategies were an important part of the initial bi-directional relationship and trust building process, as well as the final determination to enter into a partnership. Based on the aforementioned strategies, a resultant 15-member community advisory board, comprised of academic and church partners, local community-based organizations, funding agencies, and AA youth and families, was formed. Over a two-year period, this entity developed a memorandum of understanding that clearly outlined the group's: 1) guiding principles; 2) nature/terms of partnership; 3) mission, goals, objectives; 4) operating norms, procedures, policies; 5) decision-making process; 6) communication approaches; and 7) resources to support partnership. Creation of the memorandum of understanding provided the necessary infrastructure to support the OBGT intervention development and execution objectives.

The PRECEDE-PROCEED Model

The PRECEDE-PROCEED Model (Green, 1992; Green & Kreuter, 1999) guided OBGT intervention development and implementation. This model provides a comprehensive structure for assessing health needs and for designing, implementing, and evaluating health-related programs and interventions to meet those needs. PRECEDE (*P*redisposing, *R*einforcing, and *E*nabling *C*onstructs in *E*ducational *D*iagnosis and *E*valuation) outlines the steps of the planning process to assist in the development of targeted and focused public health programs. PROCEED (*P*olicy, *R*egulatory, and *O*rganizational *C*onstructs in *E*ducational and *E*nvironmental *D*evelopment) guides the implementation and evaluation of the programs designed using PRECEDE. PRECEDE consists of five phases. Phase one involves determining the quality of life or social problems and needs of a given population. Phase two consists of identifying the health determinants of these problems and needs. Phase three involves analyzing the behavioral and environmental determinants of the health problems. In phase four, the factors that predispose, reinforce, and enable the behaviors and lifestyles are identified. Phase five involves ascertaining which health promotion, health education and/or policy-related interventions would best be suited to encourage the desired changes in the behaviors or environments and in the factors that support those behaviors and environments. PROCEED is composed of four additional phases. In phase six, the interventions identified in phase five are implemented. Phase seven entails process evaluation of those interventions. Phase eight involves evaluating the impact of the interventions on the factors supporting behavior and on behavior itself. The ninth and last phase comprises outcome evaluation—that is, determining the ultimate effects of the interventions on the health and quality of life of the population.

The PRECEDE and PROCEED phases function in a continuous, iterative cycle. Information gathered in PRECEDE guides the development of program goals and objectives in the implementation phase of PROCEED. This same information also provides the criteria against which the success of the program is measured in the evaluation phase of PROCEED. In turn, the data gathered in the implementation and evaluation phases of PROCEED clarify the relationships examined in PRECEDE between the health or quality-of-life outcomes, the behaviors and environments that influence them, and the factors that lead to the desired behavioral and environmental changes. These data also suggest how programs may be modified to more closely reach their goals and targets.

Developing the Intervention

Using the phases of the PRECEDE-PROCEED Model and a CBPR approach, the OBGT community advisory board and academic partners developed and implemented the OBGT program. The following presents the application of the PRECEDE-PROCEED model in OBGT:

Phase 1—Social Assessment: What are the needs and strengths of the African American Church Community?

OBGT community advisory board and academic partners conducted a comprehensive social analysis through informal and formal meetings as well as community and university event attendance and participation. Several factors were discovered that supported forming an academic-church community health-related collaboration. First was a mutual desire to enter a partnership and to collectively address the most salient health issues facing AA youth and families. Second, priority populations indentified by all stakeholders included AAs, youth, families, and AA church communities. Third, chronic disease prevention was the primary area of interest, with obesity in youth, families, and communities identified as the top health condition of concern. Lastly, programmatic orientation of the intended work should be evidence-based, asset-focused, integrative/faith-based, and contextually relevant to the AA church environment.

Phases 2, 3, & 4—Epidemiologic and Ecological Assessments: Understanding the Determinants of Obesity and the Overweight

Through the course of a yearlong process, the OBGT community advisory board and academic partners conducted epidemiologic and ecological analyses using qualitative focus groups and key informant interviews (led by trained community partners); literature reviews; and publicly accessible data sources. These strategies were employed to examine the cultural, environmental, community, and individual factors contributing to obesity in the targeted populations. Several factors such as cultural and social norms regarding food, weight, and body perception; lack of access to healthy dietary options in communities and at home; lack of neighborhood parks and areas of recreation; discontinuation of physical education instruction in schools; and the increased availability of fast-food restaurants in communities emerged as some of the most pressing contributing factors to obesity among youth and families. In addition, violence, unemployment, and lack of health insurance were some of other social and environmental determinants of obesity among AAs, children and adolescents and their families, and among church congregants, echoing local and national data. Conversely, numerous assets of AA churches and the potential role of these institutions in obesity prevention and treatment were identified: 1) multi-faceted role of churches for AA families presently and historically; 2) church mission aligning with community health and wellness; 3) strong and well-respected leadership in churches; and 4) established, well-defined structures of communication and dissemination. The aforementioned characteristics, present an environment conducive to obesity-related health promotion and education efforts targeting AA youth and families.

Phase 5:—Ascertaining Multi-level Obesity Interventions

Based on the formative qualitative work conducted by the advisory board, analysis of existing epidemiologic data sources, and the scientific literature review of published multi-level (individual, community, environment, and policy) obesity studies, the community advisory board decided to focus on the development of a culturally-tailored obesity intervention for AA youth, a population disproportionately burdened, within the context of the family system. Such an intervention would focus on behavior change and modification, and build upon existing theories such as Bandura's Social Learning Theory (Bandura, 1977) and Health Belief Model (Rosenstock, Strecher & Becker, 1988) within the broader framework of the Socio-ecological model (McElroy, Bibeau, Steckler & Glanz, 1988). In addition, this program would be based upon published evidence about behavioral obesity program models, and be tailored to the AA church education environment (i.e., Church Sunday School). Behavioral targets would include improved diet, physical activity, and body image—known contributors and consequences to obesity, respectively.

Development of the OBGT Intervention. Focus groups were conducted and surveys administered to AA youth, families, and church leaders across several AA churches. The main goal of the information gathering activities was to explore the current dietary and physical activity behaviors and body image perceptions in these groups. Additional information was gathered from families about topics related to obesity that were of greatest interest to be included in the OBGT program, and key facilitators and barriers to participating in a church-based behavioral obesity intervention. Church leaders provided information about the central role of churches in health intervention work and the importance of the intersection of faith and health messages around the behavioral intervention targets: moving beyond faith-placed to faith-based initiatives. The information collected above was used to develop the OBGT obesity intervention program.

Community and academic partners worked extensively to develop a 12-week behavioral obesity program comprised of five nutrition, three physical activity, three body image lessons, and one concluding session. Session topics were based on Phase 5. For integrative purposes, all lessons were developed to be implemented in the church Sunday school environment, designed to be led by Sunday school teachers, and written to contain both faith and health messaging. Lesson components included a teacher's guide; children lesson that contained didactic and interactive activities; food sampling; a physical activity portion; family session-specific homework activity; and a parent session overview. The duration of each of the 12 lessons was 90 minutes.

Phase 6—Implementation of OBGT

The 12-week OBGT program was pilot tested in a sample of 32 youth and families in one AA church to assess feasibility: attendance, session fidelity, program satisfaction, and impact on program primary outcome variables: diet, physical activity, and body-image knowledge and behaviors, and the exploratory outcome, weight. Diet, physical activity, body image and weight variables were measured at two time points: pre and post 12-week intervention to examine the influence of the OBGT program on obesity-related factors, while feasibility variables were assessed weekly and measured by attendance logs, session observation checklists, and evaluation surveys. The main objective of the OBGT pilot program was to gather preliminary information for program refinement and future large-scale replication.

Phases 7, 8, 9—Evaluation of OBGT: Partnership and Feasibility, Satisfaction and Behavioral Outcomes. *Evaluating the Partnership*

Essential to the sustainability of the OBGT partnership was the development of an evaluation plan to measure the short-term and long-term progress of the OBGT collaboration. To this end, since its inception, OBGT partners have engaged in quarterly evaluations that have included completing self-report surveys and participating in facilitated group discussions among partnership members. Quarterly evaluations are used to examine overall satisfaction of the partnership; achievement of partnership activities, goals and objectives; and to evaluate partnership accountability structures. Average positive satisfaction partnership ratings have ranged from 87-96% across the above partnership constructs. *Feasibility.* Weekly average attendance rate of families (63%) across the 12-week program, high session fidelity, and high degree of program satisfaction by children (87%); families (93%) and church Sunday School teachers (88%) provided promising preliminary findings regarding the feasibility of the OBGT program. Significant increase in knowledge related to program behavioral targets have been found, with improvements in self-report diet and physical activity behaviors witnessed. However as expected, given sample size limitations, the OBGT program did produce significant differences in weight among youth or family participants. Finally, church leaders continue to provide ongoing feedback to the OBGT community advisory board and academic collaborators about session delivery and faith-related program content, and have worked extensively with these groups to refine and further tailor the OBGT program for future replication and adaptation.

Conclusion

Research based on collaborative inquiry that purposively and systematically integrates community members into the research process has been identified as an important approach by which to address documented health disparities, particularly among communities of color. CBPR represents the ultimate example of community collaborative research and if used appropriately, the model increases the probability that research and resulting interventions can meet the particular needs of the target population (Viswanathan et al., 2004).

In this chapter, we discussed three community collaborative research projects designed to address issues that represent significant public health concerns among African American youth; HIV, adolescent dating violence and obesity. As evident in the program descriptions, substantial community involvement was essential to the success of each program. Although the projects represented different stages of the *Community Involvement Continuum* (Winer & Ray, 2000), there were a few fundamental principles that were integral to all of the programs, which can serve as a guide for future community collaborative research endeavors. These included principles of mutuality and equality among all partners, an open and transparent process, and an emphasis on culturally appropriate intervention and research strategies.

Mutuality and equity serve to foster ownership and empowerment among all team members. The three projects described in this chapter discussed the ways in which mutuality and equity were established using several strategies which included, 1) developing a shared mission among community and research partners, 2) ensuring shared power through mutual decision-making, and 3) fostering capacity building through learning exchanges that capitalize on the strengths of each partner. Project PIs also described the importance of ensuring group participation in all phases of research and program implementation. This not only helped to support the principles of mutuality and equity, but including partners in all aspects of the project also helped to foster an open and transparent process, the second fundamental principle of community collaboration that was shared by the three projects described in this chapter.

Each project described the importance of an open and transparent process in which experiences, resources, and a collective vision of research goals and objectives were shared, trust and open communication were fostered, and the roles and expectations of partner were clearly understood and documented. This often took place as each project established its Community Advisory Board (CAB). The operation of the CAB was of critical importance to the success of each of the projects described. Shared strategies that seemed to contribute to the success of each CAB included regular committee meetings, a feedback loop to foster efficient communication among the partners, and a plan for program dissemination and sustainability.

By following some of the fundamental principles of collaborative research and using several key strategies described above, each of this projects were successful in ensuring that the research and intervention methods used were community informed and culturally appropriate. Research suggests that programs, which are tailored to the specific needs and culture of its population, are more effective in addressing project outcomes (Wingood & DiClemente, 2000). Demonstrated indications of success for the three projects described above included, signs of community ownership, project sustainability beyond the funding period, preliminary results indicating program effectiveness, additional institutional and federal funding, and evidence of partnership satisfaction. It is hoped that the successes and challenges described by these three projects will provide a blueprint to assist other scholars with the development of effective community collaborative efforts.

References

Bandura, A. (1997). *Social Learning Theory*. Englewood Cliffs, NJ: Prentice Hall.

Barlow, S.E., Dietz, W.H., Klish, W.J., & Towbridge, F.L. (2002). Medical evaluation of overweight children and adolescents: Reports from pediatricians, pediatric nurse practitioners and registered dietitians. *Pediatrics, 110*, 222-28.

Braithwaite, R. L., Bianchi, C., & Taylor, S. E. (1994). Ethnographic approach to community organization and health empowerment. *Health Education Quarterly, 21*(3), 407-416.

CDC ATSDR, & Committee on Community Engagement (1997). *Principles of community engagement*. Atlanta, Ga.: Center for Disease Control and Prevention.

Centers for Disease Control and Prevention, & National Center for Injury Prevention and Control (2008). *Understanding teen dating violence fact sheet* Retrieved October 25, 2009, from http://www.cdc.gov/violenceprevention/pdf/DatingAbuseFactSheet-a.pdf.

Chaves, M., & Higgins, L.M. (1992). Comparing the community involvement of Black and White congregations. *Journal for the Scientific Study of Religion, 31*, 425-440.

DiClemente, R., Crosby, R., & Wingood, G. M. (2005). Community HIV prevention interventions: Theoretical and methodological considerations. In E. J. Trickett & W. Pequegnat (Eds.), *Community interventions and AIDS.* New York: Oxford University Press.

Du Bois, W.E.B. (1903) *The Negro church in America.* Atlanta, GA: Atlanta University Press.

Flicker, S. (2008). Who benefits from community-based participatory research? A case study of the Positive Youth Project. *Health Education & Behavior, 35*(1), 70-86.

Florin, P., & Wandersman, A. (1990). An introduction to citizen participation, voluntary organizations, and community-development: Insights for empowerment through research. *American Journal of Community Psychology, 18*(1), 41-54.

Glaser, B. G., & Strauss, A. L. (1967). *The discovery of grounded theory.* Chicago: Aldine.

Goodman, R. M., & Steckler, A. B. (1987-1988). The life and death of a health promotion program: An institutionalization case study. *International Quarterly of Community Health Education, 8*(1), 5-21.

Gray, B. (1989). *Collaborating-finding common ground for multiparty problems.* San Francisco, CA: Jossey-Bass.

Gray, B. (1996). Cross-sectoral partners: Collaborative alliances among business, government, and communities. In C. Huxham (Ed). *Creating collaborative advantage.* Thousand Oaks, CA: Sage Publications, 57-79.

Green, L. W. (1992). Prevention and Health Education. In J.M. Last and R. B. Wallace (Eds.), *Public health and preventive medicine,* 13th edition, Norwalk, CT: Appleton & Lange.

Green, L. W., & Kreuter, M. W. (1999). *Health promotion planning: An educational and ecological approach,* 3rd edition. Mountain View, CA: Mayfield.

Hanson, P. (1988-89). Citizen involvement in community health promotion: A role application of CDC's PATCH model. *International Quarterly of Community Health Education, 9*(3), 177-186.

Ingram, B. L., Flannery, D., Elkavich, A., & Rotheram-Borus, M. J. (2008). Common processes in evidence-based adolescent HIV prevention programs. *AIDS and Behavior, 12*(3), 374-383.

Institute of Medicine (1988). *The future of public health*. Washington, D.C.: National Academy Press.

Israel, B. A. (2000). Community-based participatory research: Principles, rationale and policy recommendations. In *Successful models of community-based participatory research*, pp. 16-22, March 2000, Washington, D.C.

Israel, B., Eng, E., Schulz, A. J., & Parker, E. A. (2005). Introduction to methods in community-based participatory research for health. In B. Israel, E. Eng, A. J. Schulz & E. A. Parker (Eds.), *Methods in community-based participatory research for health* (pp. 3-26). San Francisco (CA): Jossey-Bass.

Israel, B. A., Eng, E., Schulz, A. J., & Parker, E. A. (Eds.). (2005). *Methods in community-based participatory research for health*. San Francisco (CA): Jossey-Bass.

Israel, B. A., Parker, E. A., Rowe, Z., Salvatore, A., Minkler, M., Lopez, J., et al. (2005). Community-based participatory research: Lessons learned from the Centers for Children's Environmental Health and Disease Prevention Research. *Environmental Health Perspective, 113*(10), 1463-1471.

Israel, B. A., Schulz, A. J., Parker, E. A., & Becker, A. B. (1998). Review of community-based research: Assessing partnership approaches to improve public health. *Annual Review of Public Health, 19*, 173-202.

Leung, M. W., Yen, I. H., & Minkler, M. (2004). Community based participatory research: a promising approach for increasing epidemiology's relevance in the 21st century. [see comment]. *International Journal of Epidemiology, 33*(3), 499-506.

Levin, J.S., Chatters, L.M., Ellison, C.G., & Taylor, R.J. (1996). Religious involvement, health outcomes, and public health practice. *Current Issues in Public Health, 2*, 220-225.

Lincoln, C.E., & Mamiya, L.H. (1990). *The Black church in the African American experience*. Durham, NC: Duke University Press.

McElroy, K.R., Bibeau, D., Steckler, A., & Glanz, K. (1988). An ecological perspective on health promotion programs. *Health Education Quarterly, 15*, 351-377.

McGranaham, R. & Kauper-Brown, J. (2006). Unit 6: Disseminating the results of CBPR in the Examining Community-Institutional Partnerships for Prevention Research Group. *Developing and sustaining community-based participatory research partnerships: A skill-building curriculum.* www.cbprcurriculum.info.

Minkler, M. & Wallerstein, N. (2002). *Community-based participatory research for health.* San Francisco, CA: Jossey-Bass.

Minkler, M., Wallerstein, N., & Hall, B. (2008). *Community-based participatory research for health,* 2nd edition. San Francisco, CA: Jossey-Bass.

O'Fallon, L. R., & Dearry, A. (2002). Community-based participatory research as a tool to advance environmental health sciences. *Environmental Health Perspective, 110 Suppl 2,* 155-159.

Ogden, C.L., Carroll, M.D., Curtin, L.R., Lamb, M.M., & Flegal, K.M. (2010). Prevalence of high body mass index in US children and adolescents, 2007-2008. *JAMA, 303*(3), 242-249.

Ogden, C.L., Carroll, M.D., & Flegal, K.M. (2008). High body mass index for age among US children and adolescents, 2003-2006. *JAMA, 299,* 2401-2405.

Putnam, R. D. (1995). Bowling alone: America's declining social capital. *Journal of Democracy, 6*(1), 65-78.

Ray, K. (2004). *The nimble collaboration.* Saint Paul, MN: Amherst H. Wilder Foundation.

Rosenstock, I.M., Strecher, V.J., & Becker, M.H. (1998) Social learning theory and the health belief model. *Health Education Quarterly, 15,* 175-183.

Russell, N., Igras, S., Johri, N, Kuoh, H, Paving, M, & Wickstrom, J. (2008). The active community engagement continuum. *ACQUIRE Project Working Paper.* New York: USAID.

Scott, C.M., Thurston, W.E. (1997). A framework for the development of community health agency partnerships. *Canadian Journal of Public health, 88*(6), 416-420.

Scott-Taplin, C.M. (1993). *The development of partnerships among community agencies working with vulnerable populations.* University of Calvary, AB.

Seifer, S., & Maurana, C. (2000). Developing and sustaining community campus partnerships: Putting principles into practice. *Partnership Perspectives, 1*(2), 7-11.

Shaefer, J., & Bronheim, S. (2007). Community engagement brings credibility to risk reduction. *Promising Practices Series.*

Spencer, G. A., & Bryant, S. A. (2000). Dating violence: A comparison of rural, suburban, and urban teens. *Journal of Adolescent Health, 27*(5), 302-305.

Strauss, A., & Corbin, J. (1998). *Basics of qualitative research: Techniques and procedures for developing grounded theory* (2nd ed.). Thousand Oaks, CA: Sage.

Summit Health Institute for Research and Education (2004). *Building Coalitions among Communities of Color: A Multicultural Approach.* State Partnership Initiative, Office of Minority Health, Office of Public Health and Science, Department of Health and Human Services: Rockville, MD.

Thompson, B., & Kinne, S. (1990). Social change theory: Applications to community health. In N. Bracht (Ed.), *Health promotion at the community level.* Newbury Park, CA: Sage Publications.

Viswanathan, M., Ammerman, A., Eng, E., Gartlehner, G., Lohr, K., & Griffith, D. (2004). *Community-based participatory research: Assessing the evidence.* Summary, Evidence Report/Technology Assessment No. 99 (Prepared by RTI-University of North Carolina Evidence-based Practice Center under Contract No. 290-02-0016). AHRQ Publication 04-E022-1. Rockville, MD: Agency for Healthcare Research and Quality.

Weijer, C. (2000). Benefit-sharing and other protections for communities in genetic research. *Clinical Genetics, 58*(5), 367-368.

Winer, M & Ray, K. (1995). *Collaboration handbook: Creating, sustaining, and enjoying the journey.* Saint Paul, MN: Amherst H. Wilder Foundation.

Winer, M. & Ray, K. (2000). *Collaboration handbook.* Saint Paul, MN: Amherst H. Wilder Foundation.

Wingood, G.M. & DiClemente, R.J. (2000). Application of the theory of gender and power to examine HIV—related exposures, risk factors, and effective interventions for women. *Health Education & Behavior, 27(*5), 539-565.

Zimmerman, M. (2000). Empowerment theory. In J. Rappaport & E. Seidman (Eds.), *Handbook of community psychology*. New York: Kluwer Academic/ Plenum, pp. 43-64.

CHAPTER ELEVEN

Faith Based Approaches in the Delivery of Effective Health Care for Emerging Populations

Ernestine A.W. Duncan
Norfolk State
University

Karen Y. Holmes
Norfolk State
University

William Brokaw
Norfolk State
University

Abstract

This chapter addresses the need and rationale for faith based approaches in the delivery of health care for emerging populations. The majority of Americans indicate that religion plays a significant role in their lives. Among many minorities, the church is an important institution with strong ties to the community. Religious institutions and worship services function as major channels between communities and the health system. Given the unique role of faith-based institutions as trusted entities and their facilitation of social and health services, programs have been of increasing interest to policymakers, researchers and practitioners. Effective partnerships between religious institutions and health care organizations are emphasized by identifying programs that address health concerns with disproportionate representation among emerging populations. The chapter concludes with the implications of effective partnerships and future directions in the area of faith based approaches.

Introduction

Religious institutions and faith-based organizations have long been at the forefront in the delivery of social and health related services to the poor and underserved (Modesto, Weaver, Flannelly, 2006; Flannelly, Stern, Costa, Weaver, and Koenig, 2006). Viewed by many as vital and trusted community resources, these institutions are garnering increasing interest from researchers, practitioners, and policy makers who recognize them as logical settings for conducting community-based research and implementing health-related outreach and intervention programs for those in need (Chatters, Levin & Ellison, 1998; Chatters, 2000, Daniels,

Juarbe, Moreno-John & Perez-Stable, 2007). This view is especially relevant when we consider minority populations. For African Americans, the Black church is looked to for much more than worship and spiritual growth, but often serves as the community's key social, economic and political center (Campbell, Hudson, Resnicow, Blakeney, Paxton & Baskin, 2007). Additionally, research suggests that 61% of African Americans attend religious activities at least once per month, compared to 47% of Caucasians (Chaves 1993). The growing Hispanic population continues to transform the nation's religious landscape with an estimated 68% identifying as Catholic (Pew Hispanic Center, 2009). Similarly, there is a steady increase of Native American church membership among diverse North American tribes (Fikes, 1996). Additionally, a growing cultural diversity within the Asian American population contributes to an expanding diversity in multi-ethnic churches (Ghorpade, Lackritz, & Singh, 2006). It is clear that religion, and religious institutions play a significant role in the lives of many, and serve as important partners in the delivery of health-related interventions and services. However, what role do these organizations play in the delivery of health-related programs and initiative to minority populations? Furthermore, what is the effectiveness of these programs with respect to health-related outcomes in these populations?

This chapter considers the rationale for faith-based approaches to the delivery of health-related services to emerging populations and their effectiveness in implementing effective health-related initiatives in minority communities. We begin with a discussion of the role of religion in the lives of African Americans, Hispanic, Asians and Native Americans, and religion's impact on the physical and mental health of these groups. We consider the role that religious and faith-based organizations play in the delivery of health related programs and initiatives. Several effective partnerships between religious institutions and health care organizations that implement initiatives to address health concerns such as HIV/AIDS, substance abuse, cancer, obesity, diabetes and mental health are examined with respect to the African American population. The chapter concludes with a discussion of the implications of effective partnerships for the delivery of effective health care in the African American community, and similar minority communities, for community-based health initiatives. Consideration is presented with respect to possible future directions for the faith-based approach to the delivery of health care for historically underserved populations such as the African American community.

The Importance of Religion among Ethnic Groups

The Pew Forum on Religion & Public Life (2008) indicates that a substantial majority of people in the U.S. consider themselves religious. In this survey, 83% of the general population reported that they were affiliated with some form of organized religion, and another 6% said they were religious but unaffiliated with a particular religion. Further, 78% of the general population self-identified as Christian, whether Protestant or Catholic. As these statistics indicate, religion is an important part in the lives of most Americans. Evidence suggests that some ethnic groups in the U.S. show distinctive patterns of religiosity, which will be reviewed below.

African Americans

There is evidence to indicate that African Americans have higher levels of religiosity than other ethnic groups (Pew Forum, 2008). Of the African Americans surveyed, 85% described themselves as Christians, 2% as members of another organized religion, and 8% as religious but not affiliated with an organized religion (Pew Forum, 2008).

While African Americans tend to be religious, there are differences in the manner in which their religiosity is expressed. Gorpade et al. (2006) found that African Americans are more intrinsically religious (living their religion as opposed to attending church primarily for cultural or social reasons). Additionally, Taylor, Chatters, Jayakody, and Levin (1996) found that African Americans showed higher levels of religious behavior than Whites, both public (e.g. attending services) and private (e.g. prayer). A study on mid-life women of various ethnicities showed that African Americans had higher levels of religious involvement than Whites (Fitchett, Murphy, Kravitz, Everson-Rose, Krause, & Powell, 2007). However, Hunt and Hunt (2001) found that while African Americans were more likely than Whites to attend church intermittently (once a month), all were equally likely to attend weekly. Their results also indicated that region location (e.g. the rural South) was a better predictor of church attendance than ethnicity (Hunt & Hunt, 2001). Brodsky (2000) found that African American single mothers varied widely in their attitudes toward organized religion. These studies demonstrate that the stereotypical view of African Americans having a higher degree of religiosity and a distinctive manner of practicing religion might be an oversimplification.

Hispanic Americans

Demographic religious data among Hispanics is almost identical to that of African Americans (Pew Forum, 2008). One significant difference is that more Hispanic Christians reported practicing Catholicism, whereas more African American Christians report being members of a Protestant denomination. Hispanic individuals also demonstrated equal levels of intrinsic religious orientation as African Americans (Ghorpade, Lackritz, & Singh, 2006). Evidence suggests that higher levels of religious involvement among Hispanics are negatively correlated with acculturation into the majority culture (Ghorpade et al., 2006; Cavalcanti & Schleef, 2005).

Asian Americans

Among Asian Americans, 45% describe themselves as Christian, 30% as members of another world religion, and 8% as religious but unaffiliated with an organized religion (Pew Forum, 2008). Asian Americans also showed the highest level of secularism of any other ethnic group in the United States (Pew Forum, 2008). Asian Americans have scored lower on intrinsic religious orientation than African Americans and Hispanics (Ghorpade et al., 2006). Chinese—and Japanese-American mid-life women show similar levels of religious behavior as Whites (and less than African American and Hispanic women), except that White women pray more frequently (Fitchett et al., 2007).

Native Americans

There is a dearth of statistical information on Native American religious practices. The Pew Forum (2008) includes Native Americans in the "Other Ethnicities" category, so no data specific to Native Americans is given. Garroutte et al. (2009) surveyed religious differences between Native Americans from the Southwest and from the Northern Plains. Roughly 95% of both groups rated religion as being very or somewhat important to them (Garroutte et al., 2009). A greater percentage of Native Americans practicing aboriginal religion describe religion as "very important" compared to Native Americans belonging to the Native American Church or practicing Christianity (Garroutte, Beals, Keane, Kaufman, Spicer, Henderson, Henderson, Mitchell, & Manson, 2009).

In all ethnic groups in the United States, a majority of people actively practice some form of organized religion. As such, churches serve as a logical and effective institution to provide preventative education and services in the health care field.

Impact of Religion on Health

Empirical evidence suggests that religion, specifically regular church attendance, is positively correlated with health. Tully et al (2006) found that religious observance was associated with a lower risk of meningococcal infection among adolescents. Women who did not attend church regularly were seven times more likely to report having four or more risk factors for breast cancer than those who attended more than once per week (Gillum & Williams, 2009). Cline and Ferraro (2006) found that church attendance was negatively correlated with obesity among women.

Religion has also been negatively correlated with risk of mortality. A nine-year longitudinal study found that people who never attend religious services have a 1.87 times higher risk of dying compared to people who attend religious services (Hummer, Rogers, Nam, & Ellison, 1999). Similarly, Musick, House, and Williams (2004) found that attending religious services once a month or more results in a 30-35% lower risk of death over a 7.5 year follow up period. Dupre, Franzese, and Parrado (2006) found a strong negative correlation between church attendance and mortality.

Debate exists regarding exactly which aspects of religion and religious attendance are associated with positive health outcomes. In examining whether health practices, social support, psychosocial resources, and belief structures in religious people were correlated with positive health, George, Ellison, and Larson (2002) found inconclusive results.

Religion and Mental Health

In a meta-analysis, Chatters (2000) found that religion reduces risk of depression, substance abuse, delinquent behavior, suicide, and psychological distress, while also enhancing well-being and overall adjustment. Harold Koenig (2009) has examined a multitude of experiments studying the link between religion and mental health. Koenig and his colleagues found over 100 studies investigating the link between religion and depression (Koenig, McCullough, & Larson, 2001, as cited in Koenig, 2009). Roughly 2/3 of these studies found lower rates of depression among the more religious, while only four of them found higher rates among the more religious. Additionally, Koenig found 68 studies examining the link between religion and suicide (Koenig, McCullough, & Larson, 2001, as cited in Koenig, 2009). Fifty-seven of those studies reported fewer suicides and more negative attitudes toward suicide among the more religious participants. Koenig reviewed 69 observational studies which considered the relationship between religious involvement and anxiety (Koenig, McCullough, & Larson, 2001, as cited in Koenig, 2009). Of those, 35 found significantly less anxiety among the religious, 24 found no association, while only 10 reported greater anxiety among the religious participants. Of the 138 studies of substance abuse and religion that Koenig reviewed, 90% of them found significantly less substance use and abuse among the more religious (Koenig, McCullough, & Larson, 2001, as cited in Koenig, 2009). However, ten studies examining the link between psychoticism and religious involvement produced mixed results (Koenig, McCullough, & Larson, 2001, as cited in Koenig, 2009).

While the explanations for the apparent protective effect of religion on health remain open for debate, there is strong evidence that religion is indeed correlated with better mental health, better physical health, and a lower risk of mortality.

The Role of Religious Institutions in the Effective Delivery of Effective Health Care

Spirituality and religious involvement are vital to the lives of many Americans. In fact, most Americans are affiliated with a particular religious denomination and attend organized worship services (Kosmin, Mayer, & Keysar, 2006). Research, thus supports the importance of churches and other religious institutions as an important community resource and a key setting for initiating health promotion programs (Campbell, Hudson, Resnicow, Blakeney, Paxton & Baskin, 2006).

Places of worship have a legacy of providing for the physical as well as spiritual needs of its members (Nightingale, 1860; Ransdell, 1995). This "whole-person" view of delivering health care offers insight into the positive relationship between religion and spirituality and health (Peterson, Atwood & Yates, 2002); once more, suggesting that places of worship are ideal institutions for establishing health promotion initiatives (Peterson, Atwood & Yates, 2002).

Religious institutions are attractive venues for the initiation of health promotion programs as these institutions are trusted and highly esteemed, offering well establish social support networks that are reinforced by relatively stable memberships (Thomas, Quinn, Billingsley, & Caldewell, 1994). Additionally, religious institutions are likely to offer ministries that focus on the physical and psychological well-being of the member, making the incorporation of health promotion initiatives that much more appealing (Campbell, Hudson, Resnicow, Blakeney, Paxton & Baskin, 2006).

Research clearly suggests the importance of religion and religious institutions in the lives of Americans, but by far the most expansive literature, highlights the importance of the Black church to the African American community. In light of this, the following sections describe the significance of the Black church to the African

American community; and its role in the delivery of effective health-related programs and initiatives.

The Role of the Black Church in Delivering Effective Health Care

Without question, the Black church occupies a multifaceted role in the lives of many African Americans (Frazier, 1974, Taylor, Thornton, & Chatters, 1987; Lincoln & Mamiya, 1990; Chaves and Higgins, 1992; Taylor, Ellison, Chatters, Levin & Lincoln, 2000; Aaron, Levine, & Burstin, 2003), not only are they looked to for spiritual guidance, but are also viewed as the central social institution for the African American community (Chatters, Levin, & Ellison, 1998), serving as a meeting place, social hall, school, community center and in many cases, the principal source of social and economic support for many in the African American community (Levin, 1984; Billingsley, & Caldwell, 1991; Chaves and Higgins, 1992). Caldwell and her colleagues (1995) in a study of 635 Northern Black churches found that the overwhelming majority of them viewed the provision of social services as a vital part of their overall mission. As such, many Black churches provide social and educational programs such as health promotion, nutrition and exercise programs (Thomas, Quinn, Billingsley & Caldwell, 1994; Yanek, Becker, Moy, Gittelsohn, & Koffman, 2001; Peterson, Atwood & Yates, 2002), cancer screening (Markens, Fox, Taub, & Gilbert, 2002), and mental health services (Tobin, Anderson-Ray, Ellor, & Ehrepreis, 1985), programs for seniors (Caldwell et al., 1995).

It is clear, that for many African Americans, the Black church is more than a place of worship, but a community institution that provides support, guidance and healing for the African American community. Given its historical legacy and traditions, the Black church is an ideal setting in which to offer health-related programs and activities (Markens, Fox, Taube & Colbert, 2002).

The African American Pastor as Mental Health Practitioner

The pastor of the Black Church shares an equally esteemed position in the lives of many African Americans. Pastors represent an important source of support for the African American community and for many the first person of contact when experiencing personal and psychological distress (Neighbors, Musick & Williams, 1998; Taylor, Ellison, Chatters, Levin & Lincoln, 2000).

Though limited, research offers some insight into the role Black clergy play in meeting the personal and mental health needs of African Americans (Taylor et al, 2000). Findings from the National Comorbidity Survey (NCS) and the National Survey of Black Americans (NSBA) reveal that African Americans with serious mental health problems under utilize traditional mental health resources, often relying on the Black Church, and specifically, the Black clergy to meet their mental health needs (Neighbors, 1991; Williams, Griffith, Young, Collins & Dodson, 1999; Taylor, Ellison, Chatters, Levin & Lincoln, 2000).

Black clergy are often called upon to provide counseling to individuals suffering from a wide range of personal problems such as alcohol and substance abuse and marital and family conflict. In many instances they are called upon to address serious mental health problems (Neighbors, Musick & Williams, 1998). Despite the vital services that Black clergy provide to African Americans with serious personal and mental health problems, in many cases clergy lack the expertise to assess the severity of mental health problems and often interpret these problems within the context of their religious training (Larson, 1968; Hong & Wiehe, 1974). Research by Mollica, Streets, Boscarino & Redlich (1986) indicates that Black clergy make few referrals to mental health facilities. Subsequent research found that clergy who did refer their troubled congregants for mental health services were often younger, had more education and training, and espouse a more liberal theological philosophy (Gotlieb & Olfson, 1987; Williams, Griffith, Young, Collins & Dodson, 1999; Neighbors, Musick, & Williams; Taylor, et al 2000).

The pattern of results raises questions about the ability and many cases the willingness of Black clergy to provide counseling to and referral services for individuals with severe personal and mental health challenges. Yet, in spite of these concerns, many African Americans will continue to call upon their pastors for help and support when facing personal and mental health challenges.

Faith-Based Initiatives and Their Effectiveness

In light of religion's prominence in the lives of African Americans, it is no surprise that many turn to the church and other faith-based organizations for their emotional, physical and mental health needs. There is an expansive multidisciplinary literature describing the health-related programs and activities initiated faith-based organization (REF). This literature describes the collaboration between faith-based organizations and health promotion programs to provide effective health-related preventative education programs in areas such as cancer prevention and awareness (e.g. breast, prostate and cervical cancers, (Davis, Bustamante, Brown, 1994; Earp & Flax, 1999; Duan, Fox, Derose, & Carson, 2000), diabetes (McNabb, Quinn, Kerver, Cook & Karrison, 1997), hypertension and blood pressure control (Smith, Merrit, & Patel, 1997) diet, nutrition and weight loss (Kumanyika, & Charleston, 1992, Barnhart, Mossavar-Rahmani, Nelson, Raiford & Wylie-Rosett, 1998), smoking cessation (Shorling, Roach, Siegel, Baturka, Guterbock, & Stewart, 1997) among others.

However, a comprehensive literature review by Dehaven and his colleague (2004) reveals few studies that evaluate the scientific effectiveness of these programs. The programs that have been empirically studied show promise in decreasing ethnic disparities in adult vaccination rates (Daniels, Juarbe, Moreno-John & Perez-Stable, 2007) reductions in hypertension and hypertension hospitalization and morality (Levine et al, 1992) and decreases in body mass index through participation in a faith-based weight loss intervention program (Fitzgibbons, Stolley, Granshow, Schiffer, Wells, Simons, & Dyer, 2005).

Health Care and Faith-Based Partnerships

Faith based institutions have a long history of independently and collaboratively hosting health promotion programs to address chronic medical and mental health problems (Thomas, Quinn, Billingsley, & Caldwell, 1994; McNabb, Quinn, Kerver, Cook, & Harrison, 1997; Jensen, Flynn, Cozza, & Karabin, 2008). There is evidence that faith based programs can improve health outcomes (DeHaven, Hunter, Wilder, Walton, & Berry, 2004). While most programs focus on primary prevention, there are a significant number of programs that address specific health concerns. These concerns are consistent with those medical conditions that are most disproportionate in people of color. There are programs to address diabetes, cancer, HIV/AIDS, and substance abuse/mental health.

Representative programs and activities include church based health centers (Westburg, 1973), church based health promotion/disease prevention interventions (Hatch & Jackson, 1981; Hatch, Callan, Eng, & Jackson, 1984) and health policy initiatives (Hatch & Jackson, 1981; Hatch et al., 1984). Partnerships between public health and faith based organizations are more readily identified within the African American communities (Lewis, 1984; Lewis, 1986). However, health programs within a wide array of faith based settings are gaining broad based support from representatives of religious institutions and public health professionals (Evans, 1995; McLean & Chappel, 1992).

Evidence indicates that faith based institutions tend to have varied levels of involvement for health programs. "Faith placed" refers to those programs where health professionals utilize churches to test interventions. "Faith based" is the level of involvement where the health related program is a part of the church's health ministry. Programs are referred to as "collaborative when they combine faith placed and faith based features (DeHaven et al., 2004). In regard to outcome measures, it is significant to note that faith placed programs tend to report outcome data significantly more than the faith based or collaborative programs. Consequently, it has been recommended that there be an increase in the collaboration between faith based institutions and health professionals for the purposes of evaluating health activities. Disproportionately more is known about the effectiveness of faith placed programs (DeHaven et al., 2004).

Partnerships and Diabetes

African Americans are twice as likely to be diagnosed with diabetes as non-Hispanic whites. In addition, they are more likely to suffer complications from diabetes, such as end-stage renal disease and lower extremity amputations. African American adults are twice as likely than non-Hispanic white adults to have been diagnosed with diabetes by a physician. In 2006, African American men were 2.2 times as likely to start treatment for end-stage renal disease related to diabetes, as compared to non-Hispanic white men. Furthermore, in 2006, diabetic African Americans were 1.5 times as likely as diabetic Whites to be hospitalized. According to the Office of Minority Health, African Americans were 2.3 times as likely as non-Hispanic Whites to die from diabetes (Office of Minority Health, 2006). A major contributing factor for Type 2 diabetes is obesity. African American women have the highest rates of being overweight or <u>obese</u> compared to other groups in the U.S. About four out of five African American women are overweight or obese. In 2007, African Americans were 1.4 times as likely to be obese as Non—Hispanic Whites. From 2003-2006, African American women were 70% more likely to be obese than Non-Hispanic White women (Office of Minority Health, 2010).

Project DIRECT. Since 1994, Project Diabetes Interventions Reaching and Educating Communities Together (DIRECT), a community based intervention has served as a demonstration project to identify culturally sensitive and efficacious approaches to reduce Type 2 diabetes. This program was implemented to increase awareness among African American residents of North Carolina. The importance of compliance with recommended guidelines for activity/exercise, nutrition/diet and diabetes self management was the focus of this intervention. Community partnerships included churches, businesses, health care providers and colleges. Project Direct conducted focus groups and discussions with key stakeholders in the community about outreach and ways to collaborate among agencies. Similarly, the project staff informed medical providers about the scientific literature on the value of provider education for patients. The project reported that providers were then perceived to be more caring, motivated and willing to do things proven beneficial to patient education. Additionally, through interviews with patients living with diabetes, Project DIRECT gained insight about the local beliefs and actions. This in turn enabled the project to better focus outreach and education (Reid, Hatch & Parrish, 2003).

To assess the usefulness of three sources (faith-based organizations [FBOs], health system and community) for recruitment of African Americans with type 2 diabetes to a randomized controlled trial (RCT) design. African Americans with type 2 diabetes were recruited to a diabetes self-management program at four faith based organization sites. The findings suggest that African American adults with diabetes can be successfully recruited and retained in a racially targeted RCT conducted in FBOs. Key elements to consider are the use of a multifaceted approach for participant recruitment particularly the benefit of health system physician involvement in recruitment since the highest yield was achieved through health system providers and importance of site location for retention.

REACH 2010. The REACH 2010 Charleston and Georgetown Diabetes Coalition (the Coalition) is a diverse community-campus partnership that was formed in 1999 in response to the CDC REACH 2010 proposal to develop and implement a plan for reducing racial disparities in health status. The Coalition was formed with leadership from local communities, the South Carolina Department of Health and Environmental Control Diabetes Prevention and Control Program, and the Outreach Council of the Diabetes Initiative of South Carolina. The 28 Coalition partner organizations are diverse and include people with diabetes, volunteer and faith-based organizations, health care and academic institutions, local libraries, Greek sorority organizations, professional associations, local media groups, and government and business organizations. Before the Coalition was formed, most of the Coalition partners had worked together on numerous occasions to provide diabetes care, education, or outreach, but they had not been formally linked to one another with the common focus of identifying and reducing disparities for AAs diagnosed with diabetes.

After 24 months of program implementation, disparities were not observed for African Americans with diagnosed diabetes when compared to whites and others for annual A1C testing; an annual dilated eye examination or referral for an examination; an annual lipid profile; annual kidney testing; and blood pressure control. No significant changes for African Americans were observed for clinical diabetes education, nutrition education or both, and A1C control over the two year period (Jenkins, McNary, Carlson, King, Hossler, Magwood, Zheng, et al., 2004).

Partnerships and Cancer

Cancer is the second leading cause of death for most racial and ethnic minorities in the United States. For Asians and Pacific Islanders, it is the number one killer. In 2006, 63,082 African Americans, 26,633 Hispanics, 11,784 Asians and Pacific Islanders and 2,447 American Indians died of the disease. Cancer impacts African Americans particularly hard. African American men are over twice as likely to die from prostate cancer than Whites. While breast cancer is diagnosed 10% less frequently in African American women than White women, African American women are 36% more likely to die from the disease. In other minority communities, cancer is also taking a disproportionate toll. Among Hispanics, women are 1.8 times more likely to be diagnosed with cervical cancer than non-Hispanic White women. Asian and Pacific Islander women are twice as likely to be diagnosed with stomach cancer as non-Hispanic White women. Asian American men suffer from stomach cancer twice as often as non-Hispanic White men. Similarly, both American Indian/Native American men and women are twice as likely to develop and die from stomach cancer and liver cancer (Office of Minority Health, 2010).

Breast cancer is the second most common cause of cancer death among African American women (American Cancer Society, 2005) and the leading cause of cancer death among Latinas (American Cancer Society, 2003). While White women have the highest incidence of breast cancer, African American and Latina women are disproportionately more likely to die from it (Reid, Hatch, & Parrish, 2003). The higher breast cancer mortality rate for these women is partially related to the fact that a larger percentage is diagnosed later, at a less treatable stage (American Cancer Society, 2005; Phillips, 1995). Although the effectiveness of regular mammography screening is well established in various research studies (Eddy, 1989; Smart, Hendrick, & Rutledge, 1995; Eastman, 1997; Stockdale, Last, Tucker, & Thomas, 1988), underutilization of mammography screening prevents the realization of its full effectiveness. Barriers to regular mammography use remain for some groups of women; in particular, minority women and those of low socioeconomic status often lack access to regular care or tend to rely on emergency rooms for primary care (Mandelblatt, Freeman, Winczewski, Cagney,

Williams, Trowers, et al., 1997). Additionally, lack of knowledge and lack of physician recommendation are important contributing factors for not obtaining regular mammography screening (Fox, Siu, & Stein, 1994). While some strategies, primarily physician based, have been somewhat successful at increasing mammography use during the intervention period, evidence suggests that the effect is not sustained after the intervention period is over. It is for this reason that many researchers have recommended that interventions emphasize community based strategies that target underserved populations (Mandelblatt & Kanetsky, 1995).

Bells for Remembrance. Medicare Quality Improvement Organizations partner with religious organizations to reduce racial and ethnic disparities in the quality of healthcare. One such partnership is with the Georgia Medical Care Foundation which has recruited more than 500 partner organizations to increase awareness of the importance of early detection and to encourage women to get annual mammograms. These efforts have increased the state's breast cancer screening rate from 52.4% to 57.4% This project helps participating churches enhance their relationships what local health care providers and breast cancer support services. Additionally, the project helps churches to improve their knowledge of breast cancer so that they can serve as a resource for their congregations (American Health Quality Association, 2010).

The WIT Project. Witnessing In Tennessee (WIT) is referred to as "Saving Grace" by the African American female participants who experienced early detection of breast cancer and subsequent treatment. WIT was tailored after the Witness Project which was implemented to provide participants with the knowledge and skills necessary to increase screening practices among African American women (Erwin, Spatz, Scotts, Hollenberg, & Deloney, 1996). More specifically, WIT was developed to increase breast self-examination, clinical breast examination and mammography use for African American women in East Tennessee (Belin, Washington, & Greene, 2006). Women participating in this project were active members of their churches and facilitators were peer educators who were breast cancer survivors. The facilitators taught other women the importance of early detection by "witnessing" or talking about their cancer experience. The protocol for this program included increasing cancer screening, education and follow-up for hard to reach populations. The WIT Project increased women's performance of breast self-examination, increased their receipt of clinical breast examinations, and improved their knowledge and attitudes related to breast cancer and screening. Furthermore, the effectiveness of this project led to the model being adapted to prevent prostate cancer (Belin, Washington, & Greene, 2006).

Data indicate that there is an 85% greater likelihood of African American men being diagnosed with prostate cancer and a 114% great likelihood of African American men dying from prostate cancer than White men. A program designed to increase knowledge and self-efficacy for men was offered in African American churches in a major Midwestern city. Modeling was provided by trained lay educators who were African American men previously diagnosed and treated for prostate cancer. Results indicate that after completing the church based intervention, participants had significantly improved knowledge and self efficacy related to prostate cancer screening (Boehm, Schlenk, Funnell, Parzuchowski, & Powell, 1995).

Partnerships and Cardiovascular Health

Cardiovascular disease (CVD) is the No. 1 killer in America. In 2004, about 871,000 adults in the United States died of CVD, accounting for about 36 percent of all deaths. (American Heart Organization, 2011). A sedentary lifestyle has been associated with CVD. The relative risk of coronary heart disease associated with physical inactivity ranges from 1.5 to 2.4, an increase in risk comparable with that observed for high cholesterol, high blood pressure and cigarette smoking. People with lower incomes and less than a 12th grade education are more likely to be physically inactive (American Heart Organization, 2011). According to the 2004 National Health Interview Survey, the following have a physically inactive lifestyle:

- Among non-Hispanic whites, 18.4 percent of men and 21.6 percent of women

- Among non-Hispanic blacks, 27 percent of men and 33.9 percent of women
- Among Hispanics, 32.5 percent of men and 39.6 percent of women
- Among Asian/Pacific Islanders, 20.4 percent of men and 24.0 percent of women

Project JOY. The impact on cardiovascular risk profiles of African American women ages 40 years and older after one year of participation in one of three church-based nutrition and physical activity strategies: a standard behavioral group intervention, the standard intervention supplemented with spiritual strategies, or self-help strategies was tested. Women were screened at baseline and after one year of participation. A total of 529 women from 16 churches enrolled. Intervention participants exhibited significant improvements in body weight, waist circumference, systolic blood pressure, dietary energy, dietary total fat, and sodium intake. The self-help group did not. In the active intervention group, women in the top decile for weight loss at one year had even larger, clinically meaningful changes in risk outcomes. Intervention participants achieved clinically important improvements in cardiovascular disease risk profiles one year after program initiation, which did not occur in the self-help group. Findings indicate that church-based interventions can significantly benefit the cardiovascular health of African American women (Barnhart, Mossavar-Rahmani, Nelson, Raiford, & Wylie-Rosett, 1998; Campbell, Hudson, Resnicow, Blakeney, Paxton, & Baskin, 2007).

Partnerships and HIV/AIDS

HIV/AIDS has had a devastating impact on minorities in the United States. Racial and ethnic minorities accounted for almost 71 percent of the newly diagnosed cases of HIV and AIDS in 2008. In 2008, 73 percent of babies born with HIV/AIDS belong to minority groups. In the African American community, HIV/AIDS has become an epidemic. African Americans accounted for 52% of all HIV/AIDS cases diagnosed in 2008. African American men are more than nine times more likely to die of AIDS than non-Hispanic White men. AIDS is the third leading cause of death in African American women aged 35-44 and the third leading cause of death in African American men, aged 35-44, in 2007.

HIV/AIDS is spreading at a rapid rate in the Hispanic community. Hispanics accounted for 19 percent of AIDS cases in 2008, despite making up only 15 percent of the U.S. population. Hispanics are 2.8 times more likely to be diagnosed with AIDS than Whites. Hispanic males were also 2.5 times more likely to die of AIDS than their non-Hispanic White counterparts in 2006. Though the numbers are small, American Indians are also impacted disproportionately by HIV/AIDS. American Indians are 1.6 times more likely to have AIDS than Whites. For Asians and Pacific Islanders, HIV/AIDS is the seventh leading cause of death in men aged 25 to 34. Native Hawaiians/Pacific Islanders are almost 3 times as likely to be diagnosed with HIV/AIDS as the White population (Office of Minority Health, 2010).

Project F.A.I.T.H. To reduce the stigma of human immunodeficiency virus (HIV), Project F.A.I.T.H. (Fostering AIDS Initiatives that Heal) was established in (HIV) among African American faith-based organizations in South Carolina. During its first year, Project F.A.I.T.H. funded 22 churches to provide HIV-related programs and services to their congregations and surrounding communities. During 2007, 20 Project F.A.I.T.H. churches conducted cross—sectional surveys with 1,445 parishioners, 61 pastors, and 109 care team members measuring their HIV-related knowledge and stigmatizing attitudes. Project F.A.I.T.H. found that while most parishioners were very knowledgeable about HIV transmission via unprotected sex and needle sharing during injection drug use, they were less knowledgeable about transmission via casual contact, mosquitoes, donating blood, and an HIV test. Overall, HIV-related stigma was low at Project F.A.I.T.H. churches. However, males and older parishioners aged 65 years and older were significantly less knowledgeable and had greater HIV-related stigma than females and younger parishioners. Additionally, it was found that pastors and care team members at Project F.A.I.T.H. churches were significantly more knowledgeable and harbored significantly less stigma than their parishioners (Lindley, Coleman, Gadddist & White, 2010).

Partnerships and Substance Abuse/Mental Health

Alcohol and other drug use have been reported as serious concerns among Americans, but are disproportionately seen in racial and ethnic groups. This is particularly true for American Indian populations (Beauvais et al., 1989). Research indicates there is more substance use among

American Indians than most, if not all, ethnic minority groups in the United States (Office for

Substance Abuse Prevention, 1990). The high prevalence of American Indian substance abuse cuts across a wide range, affects both genders, and nourishes the cycle of poverty and disease (Robbins, 1994). American Indian youth begin using cigarettes and alcohol at an earlier age than their white counterparts (Young 1988), and they are more likely to try marijuana at an earlier age than do white youth (Office for Substance Abuse Prevention 1990). Past-month prevalence data show that American Indian/Alaskan Native youth use marijuana, cocaine, cigarettes, and alcohol at two or more times the ratio of white, black, or Hispanic youth. By age 12, lifetime rates of use of alcohol, tobacco, marijuana, and other drugs among American Indians exceed the rates for other groups (Federman et al., 1997).

African American high school seniors consistently have lower rates of licit and illicit substance use compared with whites. This finding also is true among African American youth in lower grades, where lower rates of dropout have occurred. Despite these findings, illicit drugs are a major problem in the African American community (Johnston et al., 1995). One reason for this is African Americans who use alcohol and other drugs experience higher rates of drug-related health problems than do users from other ethnic groups (Herd, 1989). Another reason is drug abuse is among a variety of long-standing factors believed to cause criminal behavior in African American communities.

It is important to note that data in surveys such as the Monitoring the Future Study (MTF), the Drug Abuse Warning Network (DAWN), and the Arrestee Drug Abuse Monitoring Program (ADAM) (formerly known as the Drug Use Forecasting System) are taken from samples in which African Americans typically are underrepresented. Consequently, the findings may not accurately reflect the true extent of the drug use problem in this population (Primm, 1987).

Studies on the prevalence of drug use among Hispanics indicate it is alarmingly high among adolescents and, because a large proportion of the Hispanic population is young, a larger proportion of Hispanics may be at increased risk for drug use (Johnston et al., 1991). Stresses associated with poor economic conditions, combined with low educational rates, a high degree of drug availability, and the impact of racism on self-esteem make Hispanics particularly vulnerable to alcohol and other drug use and abuse (Delgado, 1995). Data on current drug use from the 1997 MTF Survey indicate Hispanic high school seniors have the highest rates of use for cocaine, crack, other cocaine, and heroin (Johnston et al. 1997).

Victory Fellowship. Victory Fellowship is a 90-day faith-based substance abuse treatment program for men and women. The ministry was founded in 1972 and is based in San Antonio, Texas. There are 65 Fellowships in Texas, the Southwest United States, and Central and South America. The ministry serves approximately 150 to 200 men per year and the home currently houses 21 men, nearly all of whom are considered in poverty. They vary in race/ethnicity, although many are Hispanic. The program consists of an intake assessment, non-medical detoxification and 90 days of treatment that consists largely of daily worship services, prayer, Bible studies and large group, small group and one-on-one meetings with program counselors. Perhaps the most recognized faith-based substance abuse intervention based on the moral model is Teen Challenge. Teen Challenge seeks to treat substance abuse by promoting spiritual well being. People in the program are encouraged to connect with their inner selves, God and others, and to view addiction as a moral problem that can be cured through a relationship with Jesus Christ

Conclusion

Research clearly suggests the importance of religion and religious institutions in the lives of Americans. This chapter addresses the need and rationale for faith based approaches in the delivery of health care for minority populations. A substantial majority of people in the U.S. consider themselves religious and data supports the importance of churches and other religious institutions as an important community resource. Religious institutions are likely to offer ministries that focus on the physical and psychological well-being its members, making these institutions, uniquely suited for the incorporation of health promotion initiatives. Faith based institutions have a long history of independently and collaboratively hosting health promotion programs to address chronic medical and mental health problems and there is evidence that faith based programs can improve health outcomes. While most programs focus on primary prevention, there are a significant number of programs that address specific health concerns. There are programs to address diabetes, cancer, HIV/ AIDS, and substance abuse/mental health and all show promising results in educating and effecting behavior change in the populations served. The most expansive literature highlights the importance of the Black church to the African American community. Similarly, a preponderance of research investigates the effects of faith based approaches with African American communities. Additional research is warranted to assess the effectiveness of faith based approaches with other diverse populations.

References

American Cancer Society. (2003). Cancer Facts and Figures. http:// www.cancer.org/research/cancerfactsfigures/index.   Retrieved November 3, 2012.

American Cancer Society. (2005). Cancer Facts and Figures. http:// www.cancer.org/research/cancerfactsfigures/index.   Retrieved November 3, 2012.

American Health Quality Association (2010). http://www.ahqa.org/ pub/inside/158_716_2487.CFM?CFID=161479250&CFTOK EN=14604022. Retrieved November 5, 2012.

American Heart Association (2011). http://www.google.com/searc h?sourceid=navclient&aq=&oq=american+Heart+Association &ie=UTF-&rlz=1T4ADBS_enUS327US442&q=american+he art+association&gs_l=hp.0.0l5.0.0.9.2481200.N5f6hMvfjGc. Retrieved February 1, 2011.

Barnhart, J. M., Mossavar-Rahmani, Y., Nelson, M., Raiford, Y., and Wylie-Rosett, J. (1998). Innovations in practice. An innovative, culturally-sensitive dietary intervention to increase fruit and vegetable intake among African-American women: a pilot study. *Topics in Clinical Nutrition, 13*(2), 63-71.

Beauvais, F., Oetting, E. R., Wolf, W., & Edwards, R. W. (1989). American Indian youth and drugs, 1976-1987: A continuing problem. *American Journal of Public Health, 79*, 634-636.

Belin, P.L., Washington, T.A., Greene, Y. (2006). Saving Grace: a breast cancer prevention program in the African American community. *Health Social Work*. Feb; *31*(1), 73-76.

Billinglsey, A., & Caldwell, C.H. (1991). The church, the family, and the school in the African American community. *Journal of Negro Education, 60*, 427-440.

Boehm, S., Coleman-Burns, P., Schlenk, E.A., Funnell, M.M., Parzuchowski, J., Powell, I.J. (1995). *Journal of Community Health Nursing. 12*(3), 161-169

Brodsky, A.E. (2000). The role of religion in the lives of resilient, urban, African American, single mothers. *Journal of Community Psychology, 28(2)*, 199-219.

Caldwell, C.H., Chatters, L.M., Billingsley, A., & Taylor, R.J. (1995). Church-based support programs for elderly black adults: congregational and clergy characteristics. In M.A. Kimble, S.H. McFadden, J.W. Ellor, & J. Seeber (Eds.), *Handbook on religion, spirituality, and aging.* Minneapolis: Augsburg Fortress.

Campbell, M.K., Hudson, M.A., Resnicow, K., Blakeney, N., Paxton, A., Baskin, M., (2007). Church-based health promotion interventions: evidence and lessons learned. *Annual Review of Public Health. 2007,* 213-34.

Cavalcanti, H.B., & Schleef, D. (2005). The case for secular assimilation? The Latino experience in Richmond, Virginia. *Journal for the Scientific Study of Religion, 44(4)*, 473-483.

Chatters, L.M. (2000). Religion and health: public health research and practice. *Annual Review of Public Health, 21*, 335-367.

Chatters, L.M., Levin, J.S., Ellison, C.G. (1998). Public health and health education in faith communities. *Health Education Behavior, 25(6)*, 689-699.

Chaves, M. (1993). Intraorganizational power and internal secularization in protestant denominations. *American Journal of Sociology*, *9*, 1-48.

Chaves, M. & L. M. Higgins. (1992). Comparing the community involvement of black and white congregations. *Journal for the Scientific Study of Religion, 31*, 425-40.

Cline, K.M.C., & Ferraro, K.F. (2006). Does religion increase the prevalence and incidence of obesity in adulthood? *Journal for the Scientific Study of Religion, 45(2)*, 269-281.

Daniels, N.A., Juarbe, T., Moreno-John, G., Pérez-Stable, E.J., (2007). Effectiveness of adult vaccination programs in faith-based organizations. *Ethnicity and Disease,* Winter, *17,* 15-22.

Davis, D. T., Bustamente, A., Brown, C. P. (1994). The urban church and cancer control: a source of social influence in minority communities. *Public Health Reports, 109 4*, 500-506.

Delgado, M. (1995). Community asset assessment and substance abuse prevention: A case study involving the Puerto Rican community. *Journal of Child and Adolescent Substance Abuse, 4(4)*, 57-78.

DeHaven, M.J., Hunter, I.B., Wilder, L., Walton, J.W., & Berry, J. (2004). Health programs in faith-based organizations: Are they effective? *American Journal of Public Health. Vol. 94*, 1030-1036.

Duan, N., Fox, S.A., Derose, K.P., & Carson, S. (2000). Maintaining mammography adherence through telephone counseling in a church-based trial. *American Journal of Public Health, Vol. 90(9)*, 1468-1471.

Dupre, M.E., Franzese, A.T., & Parrado, E.A. (2006). Religious attendance and mortality: Implications for the black-white mortality crossover. *Demography, 43(1)*, 141-164.

Earp, J.A. and Flax, V. (1999). What lay health advisors do: An evaluation of advisors' activities. *Cancer Practice, 7(1),* 16-21.

Eastman, P. (1997). NCI adopts new mammography screening guidelines for women. *Journal of the National Cancer Institute, 89*, 538-9.

Eddy, D.M. (1989). Screening for breast cancer. *Archives of Internal Medicine, 111*, 389-99.

Ellison, C.G., & Levin, J.S. (1998). The religion-health connection: Evidence, theory, and future directions. *Health Education & Behavior, Vol. 25(6)*, 700-720.

Erwin D.O., Spatz, T.S., Stotts, R.C., Hollenberg, J.A., Deloney, L.A. (1996). Increasing mammography and breast self-examination in African American women using the Witness Project model. *Journal of Cancer Education.* Winter, *11(4)*, 210-215.

Evans, C.A. (1996). Presidential address: Public health, vision and reality. *American Journal of Public Health. 6(4)*, 476-479.

Farris, K. (2006). The role of African-American pastors in mental health care. *Journal of Human Behavior in the Social Environment, 14(1/2)*, 159-182.

Federman, E.B.; Costello, E.J.; Angold, A.; Farmer, E.M.Z.; and Erkanli (1997). A development of substance use and psychiatric comorbidity in an epidemiologic study of White and American Indian young adolescents: The Great Smoky Mountains Study. *Drug and Alcohol Dependence, 44*, 69-78.

Felix-Aaron, K., Levine, D., & Burstin, H. (2003). African American church participation and health care practices. *Journal of General Internal Medicine, 18(11)*, 908-913.

Fikes, J. (1996). *A brief history of the Native American church. One nation under God.* Santa Fe, NM: Clear Light Publishers.

Fitchett, G., Murphy, P.E., Kravitz, H.M., Everson-Rose, S.A., Krause, N.M., Powell, L.H. (2007). Racial/ethnic differences in religious involvement in a multi-ethnic cohort of midlife women. *Journal for the Scientific Study of Religion, 46(1)*, 119-132.

Fitzgibbons, M.L., Stolley, M.R., Granschow, P., Schiffer, L., Wells, A., Simon, N., Dyer, A. (2005). Results of faith-based weight loss intervention for Black women. *Journal of the National Medical Association, 97(10)*, 1393-1402.

Flannelly, K. J.; Stern, R. S., Costa, K. G., Weaver, A. J., & Koenig, H. G. (2006). Rabbis and health: A half-century review of the mental and physical health care literature:1950-1999. *Pastoral Psychology, 54*, 545-554.

Fox, S.A., Siu, A.L., and Stein, J.A. (1994). The importance of physician communication on breast cancer screening of older women. *Archives of Internal Medicine, 154(26)*, 2058-2068.

Frazier, E. (1974). *The Negro church in America.* New York: Schocken.

Garroutte, E.M., Beals, J., Keane, E.M., Kaufman, C., Spicer. P., Henderson, J., Henderson, P.N., Mitchell, C.M., Manson, S.M. (2009). Religiosity and spiritual engagement in two American Indian populations. *Journal for the Scientific Study of Religion, 48(3),* 480-500.

George, L.K., Ellison, C.G., & Larson, D.B. (2002). Explaining the relationships between religious involvement and health. *Psychological Inquiry, 13(3),* 190-200.

Ghorpade, J., Lackritz, J.R., Singh, G. (2006). Intrinsic religious orientation among minorities in the United States: a research note. *The International Journal for the Psychology of Religion, 16(1)*, 51-62.

Gillum. F., & Williams, C. (2009). Associations between breast cancer risk factors and religiousness in American women in a national health survey. *Journal of Religion & Health, 48,* 178-188.

Gottlieb, J. F., & Olfson, M. (1987). Current referral practices of mental health care providers. *Hospital and Community Psychiatry, 38,* 1171-1181.

Hatch, J.W, & Jackson, C. (1981). North Carolina Baptist church program. *Urban Health*, May, 70-71.

Hatch, J.W., Callan. A.E., Eng, E, & Jackson, C. (1984). The general Baptist state convention health and human services project. *Contact, 77,* 1-7.

Herd, D. (1989). The epidemiology of drinking patterns and alcohol related problems among U.S. African Americans. In: *Alcohol Use among U.S. Ethnic Minorities.* Research Monograph 18. DHHS Pub. No. (ADM) 89-1435. Rockville, MD: National Institute on Alcohol Abuse and Alcoholism, 3-50.

Hong, B.A., & Wiehe, V.R. (1974). Referral patterns of the clergy. *Journal of Psychology and Theology, 2,* 291-297.

Hummer, R.A., Rogers, R.G., Nam, C.B., & Ellison, C.G. (1999). Religious involvement and U.S. adult mortality. *Demography, 36(2),* 273-285.

Hunt, L.L., & Hunt, M.O. (2001). Race, region, and religious involvement: a comparative study of Whites and African Americans. *Social Forces, 80(2)*, 605-631.

Jenkins, C., McNary, S., Carlson, B.A., King, M.G., Hossler, C.L., Magwood, G., Zheng, D., Hendrix, K., Beck, L.S., Linnen, F., Thomas, V., Powell, S., & Ma'at, I. (2004). Reducing disparities for African Americans with diabetes: progress made by the REACH 2010 Charleston and Georgetown Diabetes Coalition. *Public Health Repo*rt, *119(3)*, 322-30.

Jensen, C.A., Flynn, S., Cozza, M.A., Karabin, J. (2008). Including the ultimate: a spiritual focus treatment program in an inpatient psychiatric area of a hospital in partnership with a pastoral counseling center. *Journal of Pastoral Care, 52*, 339-348.

Johnston, L.D., & O'Malley, P.M. (1986). Why do the nation's students use drugs and alcohol? Self—reported reasons from nine national surveys. *Journal of Drug Issues* 16:29-66.

Johnston, L. D., O'Malley, P. M., & Bachman, J. G. (1995). National survey results on drug use from the Monitoring the Future study, 1975-1994. Volume I: Secondary school students. (NIH Publication No. 95-4026). Rockville, MD: National Institute on Drug Abuse.

Koenig, H.G. (2009). Research on religion, spirituality, and mental health: a review. *Canadian Journal of Psychiatry, 54(5)*, 283-291.

Koenig, H.G., McCullough, M.E., & Larson, D.B. (2001). *Handbook of religion and health*. New York: Oxford University Press.

Kosmin, B.A. & Keysar, A. (2006). *Religion in a free market: Religious and non-religious Americans: Who, what, why, where.* Ithaca, NY: Paramount Market Publishing.

Kumanyika, S. K., & Charleston, J. B. (1992). Lose Weight and Win: A church-based weight loss program for blood pressure control among Black women. *Patient Education and Counseling, 19(1),* 19-32.

Larson, R. F. (1968). The clergyman's role in the therapeutic process: Disagreement between clergymen and psychiatrists. *Psychiatry, 31,* 250-260.

Levin, J.S. (1984). The role of the Black church in community medicine. *Journal of the National Medical Association, 76(5)*, 477-483.

Levin, D.M., Becker, D.M, Bone, L.R., Stillman, F.A., Tuggle, M.B., Prentice, M., Carter, J. & Fillippeli, J.A. (1992). Partnership with minority populations: A community model of effectiveness in research. *Ethnicity & Disease, 2(3)*, 296-305.

Lewis, R.K. (2005). Using a Culturally Relevant Theory to Recruit African American Men for Prostate Cancer Screening. *Health Education & Behavior*, *32(4)*, 452-454.

Lincoln, C. & Mayima, L. (1990). *The Black church in the African-American experience*. Durham, NC: Duke University Press.

Mandelblatt J, Freeman H, Winczewski D, Cagney, K., Williams, S., Trowers, R., Tang, J., Gold, K., Lin, T.H. & Kerner, J. (1997). The costs and effects of cervical and breast cancer screening in a public hospital emergency room. The Cancer Control Center of Harlem. *American Journal of Public Health. 87(7)*, 1182-1189.

Mandelblatt J. & Kanetsky, P.A. (1995). Effectiveness of interventions to enhance physician screening for breast cancer. *The Journal of Family Practice. 40*, 162.

Markens, S., Fox, S.A., Taub, B., et al. (2002). Role of Black churches in health promotion programs: Lessons from the Los Angeles Mammography Promotion in Churches Program. *American Journal of Public Health*, *92*, 805-810.

McKee, D.D., & Chappel J.N. (1992). Spirituality and medical practice. *Journal of Family Practice, 35*, 201, 205-208,

McNabb, W.L., Quinn, M,T., Kerver. J., Cook, S., & Karrison, T. (1997). The PATHWAYS church-based weight loss program for urban African-American women at risk for diabetes. *Diabetes Care. Oct. 20*, 1518-1523.

Modesto, K., Weaver, A. & Flannelly, K. (2006). A systematic review of religious and spiritual research in social work. *Social Work and Christianity, 33(1)*, 77-89.

Mollica, R. R., Streets, F. J., Boscarino, J., & Redlich, F. C. (1986). A community study of formal pastoral counseling activities of the clergy. *American Journal of Psychiatry, 14*, 323-328.

Musick, M.A., House, J.S., & Williams, D.R. (2004). Attendance at religious services and mortality in a national sample. *Journal of Health and Social Behavior*, *45(2)*, 198-213.

Neighbors, H. W. (1991). Mental health. In J. S. Jackson (Ed.), *Life in black America* (pp. 221-237). Newbury Park, CA: Sage Publications.

Neighbors, H. W., Musick, M.A., & Williams, D.R. (1998). The African American minister as a source of help for serious personal crises: Bridges and barrier to mental health care? *Health Education & Behavior*, *25(6)*, 759-777.

Nightingale, F. (1990). *Notes on Nursing-1860. London: Harrison.* Office for Substance Abuse Prevention. http://uscodebeta.house.gov/view.xhtml?req=granuleid:USC-prelim-title42-section290bb-21&num=0&edition=prelim. Retrieved November 7, 2010.

Office of Minority Health. (2006). National Diabetes Surveillance System.   http://www.cdc.gov/diabetes/statistics/esrd/fig5.htm. Retrieved November 6, 2012.

Office of Minority Health. (2010). National Diabetes Surveillance System.   http://www.cdc.gov/diabetes/statistics/esrd/fig5.htm. Retrieved November 6, 2012.

Peterson, J., Atwood, J.R., & Yates, B. (2002). Key Elements for Church-Based Health Promotion Programs: Outcome-Based Literature Review. *Public Health Nursing, 19(6),* 401-411.

Pew Forum on Religion & Public Life (2008). *U.S. religious landscape survey.* Washington, DC: Pew Research Center. Retrieved from http://www.religions.pewforum.org/reports#.

Phillips, J., & Wilbur, J. (1995). Adherence to breast cancer screening guidelines among African American women of differing employment status. *Cancer Nursing: An International Journal for Cancer Care, 18(4),* 258-269.

Primm, B.J., Perez, L., Dennis, G.C., et al. (2006). Managing pain: The Challenge in Underserved Populations: Appropriate Use versus Abuse and Diversion. *Journal of the National Medical Association, 96,* 1152-61.

Randsdell, C. (1995). Church-based health promotion: An untapped resource for women 65 and older. *American Journal of Health Promotion, 9,* 333-336.

Reid, L., Hatch, L., Parrish, T., (2003). The role of a historically black university and the black church in community based health promotion initiatives: The Project DIRECT Experience. *The Journal of Public Health Management and Practice.* November Supplement. S70-73.

Robbins, M.L. Native American perspective. In: J.U. Gordon (eds.), *Managing multiculturalism in substance abuse services.* Thousand Oaks, CA: SAGE Publications, Inc., 1994. pp. 148-176.

Schorling, J.B., Roach, J., Sigel, M., Baturka, D.E., Guterbock, T.M., Stewart, H.L. (1997). A trial of church-based smoking cessation interventions for rural African-Americans. *Preventive Medicine, 26(1),* 92-101.

Smart, C.R., Hendrick, R.E., Rutledge JH III, et al. (1995). Benefit of mammography screening in women aged 40 to 49 years: current evidence from randomized controlled trials. *Cancer, 75,* 1619-1626.

Smith, E. D., Merritt, S. L., & Patel, M. K. (1997). Church-based education: An outreach program for African Americans with hypertension. *Ethnicity & Health, 2(3),* 243-53.

Stockdale, A. D., Last, P., Tucker, A. K. and Thomas, J. M. (1988), Screening for breast cancer: some clinical aspects. *British Journal of Surgery, 75,* 697-699. doi: 10.1002/bjs.1800750724.

Taylor, R.J., Chatters, L.M., Jayakody, R., & Levin, J.S. (1996). Black and White differences in religious participation: a multisample comparison. *Journal for the Scientific Study of Religion, 35(4),* 403-410.

Taylor, R.J., Ellison, C.G., Chatters, L.M., Levin, J.S. & Lincoln, K.D. (2000). Mental health services in faith communities: The Role of Clergy in Black Churches. *Social Work, Volume 45(1),* 73-87.

Taylor, R.J., Thornton, M.C., Chatters, L.M. (1987). Black Americans' perceptions of the sociohistorical role of the church. *Journal of Black Studies, 18(2),* 123-138.

The Texas Faith-Based Initiative at Five Years: Warning Signs as President Bush Expands Texas-style Program at National Level. http://www.tfn.org/site/DocServer/TFN_CC_REPORT-FINAL. pdf. Retrieved January 7, 2011.

Thomas, S.B., Quinn, S.C., Billingsley, A. & Caldwell, C. (1994). The characteristics of northern Black churches with community health outreach programs. *American Journal of Public Health, 84(4),* 575-579.

Tully, J., Viner, R.M., Coen, P.G., Stuart, J.M., Zambon, M., Peckham, G., Booth, C., Kaczmarski, E., & Booy, R. (2006). Risk and protective factors for meningococcal disease in adolescents: matched cohort study. *British Medical Journal. 332,* 445-450.

Westberg, G.F. (1973). Churches are joining the health care team. *Urban Health, 13(9),* 34-36.

Williams, D. R., Griffith, J. Young, C., Collins, C., & Dodson, J., (1999). Structure and provision of services in New Haven black churches. *Cultural Diversity and Ethnic Minority Psychology, 5,* 118-33.

Yanek, L.R., Becker, D.M., Moy, T.F., Gittelsohn, J. & Koffman, D.M. (2001). Project Joy: Faith based cardio vascular health promotion for African American women. Public Health Reports, *116* (Suppl. 1), 68-81.

Young, T. J. (1988). Substance use and abuse among Native Americans. *Clinical Psychology Review, 8,* 125-138.

Part IV

Future Directions: Challenges for the Twenty-First Century

CHAPTER TWELVE

Future Directions in Culturally Competent Health Care Delivery for Underserved Populations

Lula A. Beatty
American Psychological
Association

Dionne Jones
University of Maryland University
College

Abstract

Over the past forty years, a number of initiatives have been pursued with varying degrees of success to reduce health disparities among underserved populations. These initiatives include Healthy People (2010), the Secretary Task Force on Black and Minority Health (1985), the Institute of Medicine Report (2002), and the NIH Health Disparities Strategic Plan and Budget (2004-2008). This chapter highlights five challenges to achieving good health care for racial/ethnic minority and other underserved populations. The first challenge is to eliminate the social determinants and structural inequities associated with poor health and health care. The second challenge is to improve access, availability, and the quality of health care. Challenge number three is to vigilantly monitor, document and better understand health disparities and health needs of racial/ethnic and other underserved populations. Challenge number four is to work to better understand and implement cultural competency in all aspects of health care and research on health. The fifth challenge is to prepare the work force to deliver high quality health care.

Introduction

Reducing health disparities is a goal of the United States that has been deliberately pursued at the federal level since the late 1970's through initiatives such as Healthy People (2010) and various minority and health disparities efforts (e.g., the 1985 Report of the Secretary Task Force on Black and Minority Health, the NIH Health Disparities Strategic Plan and Budget (2004-2008). The impetus for these programs grew in large part from data that showed that good health and better health outcomes were not equally experienced by all U. S. population groups, that persistent gaps exist in the health status of racial and ethnic minorities in the US compared to their white counterparts (Fernandez, South-Paul, & Matheny, 2003), and that lack of health care and poorer quality health care were likely related to the disparities observed

In the late 1990s the U.S. Congress tasked the Institute of Medicine (IOM) to determine the cause of disparities in health care and make recommendations to eliminate them. The now landmark Institute of Medicine (IOM) Report (2002), *Unequal Treatment: Confronting Racial and Ethnic Disparities in Health Care*, found that racial and ethnic disparities in health care are associated with worse health outcomes; disparities occur in the context of broader historic and contemporary social and economic inequality, and there is evidence of persistent racial and ethnic discrimination in many sectors of society; and contributors to these disparities include health systems, healthcare providers' bias, stereotyping, prejudice, clinical uncertainty, utilization managers and patients themselves (Smedley, Stith, & Nelson, 2003). To effectively eliminate disparities in health care, the committee recommended changes in six areas: legal, regulatory and policy interventions; health systems interventions; patient education and empowerment; cross-cultural education in the health professions; data collection and monitoring; and research needs. Cultural awareness and competency are underlying factors evident in each area.

Other research has confirmed and further delineated the IOM findings and identified other contributing factors associated with poorer health outcomes for underserved populations. The World Health Organization (WHO) posits that poorer health outcomes are caused by social determinants of health, which includes those everyday life conditions and circumstances shaped by the distribution of money, power and resources at local, national and global levels. These social determinants of health are believed to be mostly responsible for health disparities through the creation of pervasive structural inequities manifested in such conditions as lower levels of education, lower socioeconomic status, inadequate and unsafe housing, racism and living in close proximity to environmental hazards (Commission on the Social Determinants of Health, 2008).

Work on health disparities has grown rapidly since the 1980s, but resulting efforts to eliminate health disparities have met with mixed and inconsistent success, at best (Adler & Rehkopf, 2008; LaViest, Gaskin & Richard, 2009; Dykes & White, 2009; Adler & Stewart, 2010). The Agency for Healthcare Research and Quality, the agency charged with monitoring the nation's progress on reducing health disparities, found that in 2011 50% of 250 health care index measures tracking access to care showed no improvement and 40% of the measures actually worsened (2012). Health disparities and the urgent need for better health care for underserved populations still exist as do many challenges. Major challenges blocking the elimination of health disparities and the achievement of good health care for racial/ethnic minority and other underserved populations are presented and briefly discussed.

Challenge 1. Eliminate the Social Determinants and Structural Inequities Associated with Poor Health and Health Care

Risk avoidance approaches with their foci on changing individual behavior have prevailed in efforts to reduce health disparities. As previously indicated, there is consensus that health and health care can best be achieved by addressing the social determinants and structural inequities predictive of good health and health care, although both approaches—individual and system level—are needed to effect long-term change. Changing the systems or environmental contexts in which healthcare is accessed or provided is necessary to reduce disparities and improve health for underserved population groups (Smedley & Syme, 2001). Concerns regarding the ability to meaningfully change large systems have been expressed, but if properly defined, structural factors such as availability/accessibility, social policies and cultural messages are amenable to change (Cohen, Scribner, and Farley, 2000).

Socio-economic status has long been found to be a strong predictor of health status (Marmot, Rose, Shipley & Hamilton, 1978), even acknowledging the confounding relationship between race and socioeconomic status for U.S. racial/ethnic minority populations, particularly African Americans (Adler & Rehkopf, 2008). For example, the unemployment rate among African

Americans was 15.7 percent in January 2011, higher than white men (8.0 percent), Hispanic men (11.9 percent), and adult women (7.9 percent). Note that this is likely a conservative low estimate for African Americans and perhaps other underrepresented groups given that unemployment rates do not include discouraged workers or people no longer looking for work. Eliminating poverty, improving educational attainment and increasing the employment rate and incomes of racial/ethnic minorities will improve health within poorer populations. Outlining the myriad actions and policies needed to achieve full economic, political and social parity for underserved populations is beyond the scope of this discussion, but its importance has to be acknowledged.

Challenge 2. Improve Access, Availability, and the Quality of Health Care. Access and Availability

In a review of the literature where over 100 suggested solutions for eliminating health disparities were identified, access was acknowledged as a major continuing issue (Dykes & White, 2009). Access to health care is most often available through employment-based insurance. Groups with higher unemployment, e.g., racial/ethnic minorities, are more likely to be uninsured in comparison to White Americans, with Hispanics and Blacks among the groups more likely to be uninsured (National Center for Health Statistics, 2010). A person was defined as uninsured if he or she did not have any private health insurance, Medicare, Medicaid, State Children's Health Insurance Program (SCHIP), state-sponsored or other government-sponsored health plan, or military plan. A person was also defined as uninsured if he or she had only Indian Health Service coverage or had only a private plan that paid for one type of service such as accidents or dental care. Consequences of being uninsured can be far-ranging. Uninsured persons have limited access to care and are not likely to have a regular source of care, thus they delay seeking care and often do not receive needed care. Moreover, lack of insurance has consequences for family health. If one family member is without health insurance, other members are affected as well (Institute of Medicine, 2002).

Providing health insurance to every American would address the major access barriers to health care. The Patient Protection and Affordable Care Act of 2010 initiated by President Obama and passed by Congress seeks to expand health coverage, control costs and improve the health care delivery system (Kaiser Family Foundation, 2010). It would, for example, allow coverage under Medicaid of persons under 65 with no dependent children who were not previously eligible for coverage, a group that includes many racial/ethnic minority individuals especially men. Andrulis, Siddiqui, Purtle, and Duchon (2010) analyzed the legislation to determine how it would advance health equity for racial/ethnic minority populations. They found provisions that would increase workforce diversity including investments in HBCUs and minority-serving institutions; support cultural competence education; support health disparities research; and initiate prevention efforts to address health disparities including campaigns on oral health and programs for American Indians/Alaska Natives. In addition, sections of the law addressed insurance coverage issues specific to health disparities including nondiscrimination in federal health programs, "plain language" requirements, incentive payments, and culturally/ linguistically appropriate claims appeals.

With the implementation of the Patient Protection and Affordable Care Act (Affordable Care Act), insurance plans will be more available to racial/ethnic minorities and provide them with continuing access to quality health care. Monitoring of health centers and ongoing research and quality assurance will ensure that goals are being met. Moreover, there should be more cultural diversity training for providers and culturally adapted patient education materials shown to be effective among providers in primary care settings (Paez, Allen, Carson & Cooper, 2008).

The Affordable Care Act was threatened with legal challenges, but the Supreme Court upheld the constitutionality of the legislation on June 28, 2012. With full funding from Congress, the law will improve access to health insurance for 32 million Americans, remove obstacles to care disproportionately experienced by racial/ ethnic minorities (Smedley, 2012) and there will be greater parity in access to mental health and substance use services (Practice Directorate, APA, 2012). African Americans are expected to benefit in significant ways from provisions in the law including the limits imposed on co-pay and out-of-pocket expenses, tax credits for Americans who cannot afford quality health insurance, and prohibitions on insurance denial based on pre-existing conditions (WhiteHouse.Gov, 2012). It is estimated that 17 million children with preexisting conditions can no longer be denied coverage and that 5.3 million Americans on Medicare will save about $600 on prescription drugs. Moreover, the Affordable Care Act has provided free preventive services to 2.4 million African American seniors and has insured approximately 410,000 African American young adults who would otherwise not have health insurance (BlackAmericaWeb. com, 2012).

It is too early to measure the full impact of the proposed reforms. But consider the impact of Social Security, a federal "New Deal" program of 1935 created to assist in the economic recovery from the great depression. Social Security has become a major source of income for African American elderly with 28 percent of elderly African American married couples and 54 percent of African American unmarried elderly persons relying on Social Security for 90 percent or more of their income in 2008 (Social Security, 2010). Similarly, Medicare, a federal program established in 1965 as an amendment to the Social Security Act, provides health insurance to all Americans 65 and over who have worked at least 10 years in a covered program or persons under 65 with certain disabilities.

Telemedicine, the provision of interactive health care through the use of modern technology and communication systems, is growing in use worldwide especially in developing countries and may be an effective way to make health care accessible and available to U. S. populations in rural and other underserved areas. A review of studies found that telemedicine had advantages in certain specialty areas such as teleradiology, telemental health, home telecare, some medical consultations, and certain costs (e.g., travel), but the authors noted that more good quality studies were needed before benefits could be definitively identified (Hailey, Roine & Ohinmaa, 2002). Other studies have found some level of patient acceptance of consumer health technology (Or & Karsh, 2009), no significant differences between usual care for diabetes and asynchronous and synchronous teleconsultation (Verhoeven, Tanja-Djiksra, Nijland, Eysenbach, & van Gemert-Pijnen, 2010), and the successful use of telemedicine and tele-educational programs to develop health care capacity in sub-Saharan Africa (Mars, 2010).

Quality of Care. Even when racial/ethnic minority individuals have insurance and are in the health care system, they are more likely to receive lower quality of care and encounter negative attitudes, bias, and stereotyping by providers, contributing to their under-utilization of needed care and services (Betancourt & Maina, 2004). More alarmingly, after controlling for income, age, insurance status, co-morbid conditions and symptom expression, disparities persisted. Barriers to care have been found at multiple levels including organizational (leadership/workforce), structural (processes of care), and clinical (provider-patient encounter) (Betancourt, Green, Carrillo, Ananeh-Firempong, 2003).

Racial/ethnic program participants in Medicare may not receive the same quality care as white participants. African Americans, for example, in comparison to whites enrolled in Medicare managed plans were less likely to receive recommended clinical care in four specific areas (e.g., diabetes related eye care, breast cancer screening) (Schneider, Zaslavsky, & Epstein, 2002). In a later study it was found that quality of care measures of clinical performance improved for both white and black Medicare patients between 1997 and 2003, but some racial disparities persisted (Trivedi, Zaslavsky, Schneider, & Ayanian, 2005). Gender and race effects have also been reported among Medicare patients being treated for diabetes with women more likely receiving HbA(1c) eye screening and white women receiving more of the performance measures related to the process of care. African Americans fared worse in process of care and intermediate health outcome measures (Chou, Brown, Jensen, Shih, Pawlson, & Scholle, 2007). Improvement of existing programs such as Medicare is addressed in the Health Care Reform Act (2011).

Health care systems can be improved to address disparities by collecting and reporting health care access and utilization data by patient's race/ethnicity; encouraging the use of evidence-based guidelines and quality improvement; supporting the use of language interpretation services in the clinical setting; providing appropriate education and training: increasing awareness of racial/ ethnic disparities in health care; increasing the proportion of underrepresented minorities in the health care workforce; and integrating cross-cultural education into the training of all health care professionals (Betancourt & Maina, 2004).

Challenge 3. Vigilantly Monitor, Document and Better Understand Health Disparities and Health Needs of Racial/ Ethnic and Other Underserved Populations

Health status and disparities are dynamic variables, subject to change and requiring continuous monitoring. Research must be in place to forecast, understand, prevent and treat emerging or changing health concerns. Research content and methodological concerns of particular significance to racial/ethnic minority and other underserved populations include the following:

Obesity. Obesity and poor dietary habits are established risk factors for a number of chronic diseases, e.g., diabetes, hypertension, and certain racial/ethnic minority populations, e.g., African Americans and Hispanics, have higher rates of obesity (CDC, 2009). As obesity rates continue to rise, there is concern that gains previously made in health and longevity may be lost. New cases of diabetes and hypertension resulting from obesity may outpace or reverse gains made in the prevention and treatment of those conditions. Understanding the rise in obesity in each population is necessary to develop culturally appropriate strategies. Neighborhoods with access to supermarkets have been found to have residents with healthier diets and lower rates of obesity. Residents in low-income and minority communities are more likely to have poorer access to supermarkets and healthy food and greater availability of fast—food (Larson, Story, & Nelson, 2009). Interestingly, one study found that wealthy black communities had fewer grocery stores within a five-minute travel distance than similar wealthy white communities (Helling and Sawicki, 2003). Limited transportation can aggravate access to healthier food as well as medical care. RE-AIM, (reach, effectiveness, adoption, implementation, maintenance), a framework used initially to evaluate the best interventions to change individual behaviors, has been shown to have promise as a means of evaluating built environmental strategies, e.g., farmer's market, safe and accessible streets, to prevent obesity through promoting healthful eating and active living (King, Glasgow, & Leeman-Castillo, 2010).

Focus on Specific Populations. Research and programs must focus on each population group, paying attention to each group's distinctive health status and needs, and, cultural, social, and historical experiences. For example, African Americans, historically and currently have the worst health profile among the racial/ethnic groups with health inequalities among African Americans amounting to more than $135.9 billion in excess direct medical costs between 2003 and 2006 (LaVeist, Gaskin & Richard, 2009). Thirteen percent (13%) of African Americans of all ages are reported being in fair or poor health. African American men have the shortest life span than men of any race or ethnicity in the US (65.0 years compared to 71.8 years for white men) and African American women have a lower life expectancy than white women (73.7 years for African American women vs. 78.7 years for white women) (National Center for Health Statistics, 2010). Moreover, the widest gap in mortality between African American and white men occur in the prime adult ages of 25-54 years (LaViest, 2005). The health status of African American men has been compared to men in 'Third World' countries noting, for example, that African American men have a shorter life expectancy than men in Iran, Columbia, and Sri Lanka (US Central Intelligence Agency, 2006).

Environmental Exposures. Racial/ethnic minority and poor people are more likely to experience disparities in exposure to environmental conditions that impact health, including for example, the higher prevalence of asthma in African American communities (Hill, Graham, & Divgi, 2011; Powell & Stewart, 2001). Environmental exposure may also be related to lung diseases, cancer and lupus. Three of the five major hazardous waste landfills are located in predominantly African American and Latino communities living disproportionately below the poverty line (Mohai & Bryant, 1992; Harding & Greer, 1993). Attention to environmental issues is growing. Clark Atlanta University established an environmental justice clearinghouse in 1994 that provides information and resources related to environmental justice, race and the environment, civil rights and human rights, facility siting, land use planning, brownfields, transportation equity, suburban sprawl and smart growth, energy, global climate change, and climate justice (www.CAU.edu).

Drug Use and Addiction. Historically there have been few significant differences in the overall use of alcohol, tobacco and illicit drugs by race/ethnicity. Moreover, across all groups, males have used drugs more than females and racial/ethnic minority women were less likely to use drugs than other groups, especially African American women who were more likely to be abstainers. That pattern has been changing in the last few years with girls' use mimicking that of boys (Cotto, Davis, Dowling, Elcano, Staton & Weiss, 2010). Recent findings, showed a significant increase in drug use among teens and certain groups of minority teens. Black/Non-Hispanic females, ages 12-17 years old, increased their drug use from 7.3 percent in 2008 to 10.4 percent in 2009, a statistically significant increase (CADCA, SAMHSA, 2010). Research is needed to monitor this changing drug use pattern, understand the reasons for this change and develop prevention programs to curtail use.

Drug use results in more severs social and medical consequences for racial/ethnic minority populations, that is equivalent risky behavior for Whites and racial/ethnic minority populations do not equal equivalent outcomes. African American drug users have significantly higher drug related incarceration rates (Iguchi, Bell, Ramchand & Fain, 2005). HIV/AIDS and other infections and health problems are disproportionately experienced by people of color (Young, Reviere & Ackah, 2004. Almost half of the people living with HIV infection (46%) in 2008 and an estimated 44% of all new HIV infections in 2009 were among Blacks. Between 2007 and 2010, Black women represented 62% of all women with HIV infection. Black women were infected with HIV at the rate of 15 times that of white women and over three times Hispanic/Latina women (CDC 2010). Although sexual contact is the most frequent route of HIV transmission, risky sexual behavior (i.e., no self-protective measures taken) is often related to drug use, e.g., drinking.

Ethnic differences in drug abuse treatment initiation and treatment retention have been reported. In comparison to white youth, Native American adolescents are less likely to return to treatment after intake and African American adolescents spend less time in treatment (Campbell, Weisner, & Sterling, 2006).

Chronic Stress. There is a relationship between exposure to chronic stress, poor health outcomes, and health disparities, which need to be better understood. Neighborhood stressors are associated with racial/ethnic differences in hypertension prevalence (Mujahid, et al, 2011; Spruill, 2010) and the stress resulting from a natural disaster, displacement by Hurricane Katrina, was found to impact the long-term mental health of survivors with the most impact experienced by females, the less-educated and African Americans (Picou & Hudson, 2010). Jackson, Knight and Rafferty (2010) found a positive association between number of unhealthy behaviors and number of chronic conditions among Blacks and concluded that persons living in chronically stressful environments are more likely to engage in unhealthy behaviors for their protective mental health effects. These unhealthy behaviors, unfortunately, in combination with negative environmental conditions are posited to contribute to disparities in morbidity and mortality. The relationship between stress and health, however, is not a direct one, but may be moderated by social support and coping (Kessler, Price, & Wortman, 1985). Lekan (2009) describes the Sojourner syndrome in African American women and the likely impact of persistent stress and active coping on health deterioration.

Actively Involve all Stakeholders in Research and Program Development. Engaging key, vested parties in research and program development and implementation can be critical to achieving the goals of health disparities research and programming. A review of published reports on the effectiveness of heart disease, substance abuse, violence and HIV prevention interventions with low income populations found that programs were able to reach diverse populations, but that most programs limited their effectiveness by not involving participants in planning, attempting to change underlying social causes, and tailoring programs for subpopulations (Freudenberg et al., 2000). Community-based participatory research (CBPR) models can facilitate access to and utilization of health care systems in a culturally competent way, primarily because CBPR emphasizes a partnership approach to problem identification and solution and addresses the whole range of activities needed to effect structural change including capacity development, research, and policy advocacy (Israel et al., 2010). When CBPR models are not appropriate for the research proposed some other form of community involvement, e.g., use of a community advisory committee, should be explored to ensure validity, significance and responsiveness.

Challenge 4. Work to Better Understand and Implement Cultural Competency in all Aspects of Health Care and Research on Health

Focus groups of African Americans, Asians, Hispanics, and Native Americans asked to identify barriers to healthcare and priorities for action identified among other concerns difficulty in making informed choices when selecting providers, poor service from medical office staff, provider communication and cultural competence barriers (Gaston-Johansson et al., 2007). Cultural competency in health care delivery is not limited to one-on-one interactions of the patient and the health care provider, but applies to every access and therapeutic point of contact between the patient and the health care agent or agency.

Cultural competency can be difficult to theoretically define and methodologically operationalize and measure given the wide range of definitions, variables, and iterations of expression across and within cultural groups and the dynamic evolution of culture. Common elements found in definitions of cultural competence include 1) valuing diversity; 2) having the capacity for cultural self-assessment; 3) being conscious of the dynamics inherent when cultures interact; 4) having institutionalized culture knowledge; and 5) having developed adaptations to service delivery reflecting an understanding of cultural diversity. (Cross, Bazron, Dennis, & Isaacs,1989). Cultural competence has also been defined as the demonstrated awareness and integration of three population-specific issues, namely, health-related beliefs and cultural values, disease incidence and prevalence, and treatment efficacy (Lavizzo-Mourey & Mackenzie, 1996). Eiser and Ellis (2007) propose that specific information about a cultural group is necessary for cultural competence. In the case of African Americans, they suggest that providers should know about slavery, Jim Crow discrimination, religious beliefs, and the Tuskegee syphilis study, for example. Using expert consensus, the National Minority AIDS Education and Training Center developed the "Be Safe Model," to assist healthcare providers in fostering a relationship of mutuality and health promotion. The model addresses six core elements which are barriers to health care, ethics in cultural competency, sensitivity of the provider, assessment appropriate to a cultural determination, facts related to ethnocentric physiologic differences, and encounters (McNeil, 2003). Thus, cultural competence in health care requires a provider to understand the importance of social and cultural influences on the health beliefs and behaviors of clients and deliver quality care that meets their social, cultural and linguistic needs.

Studies on the effectiveness of offering culturally competent care show promising results. Williamson and Harrison (2010) conducted a literature review of studies on how midwives provide culturally sensitive care in their practice. They identified two approaches: a cognitive approach which emphasized language and, concomitantly a static view of culture, and a social position approach that attempts to address culture in a wider, structural framework rather than on individual behaviors. They argue that the second approach will avoid stereotyping and encourage viewing the individual within the concept of cultural safety. A patient-based approach that utilized an ESFT (explanatory/social/fears/treatment) model in cross-cultural care led to better adherence (Betancourt, 2006) and positive patient-provider relationships as measured by patient's belief that the provider knew them "as a person" resulted in better outcomes in HIV patients, e.g., more likely to receive HAART, undetectable serum HIV RNA, fewer missed appointments, less drug use and higher reported quality-of-life for HIV patients (Beach, Keruly & Moore, 2006).

While racial/ethnic minority populations express less trust in health care providers, the range of trust held by individuals within populations varies. It is important to be cognizant of the factors that contribute to this variation. For example, in a telephone survey of African American women over 40 in Washington, DC, higher trust was associated with being over 65, primary care characteristics such as accessibility of the practice and coordination of specialty care, and greater use of prevention services (O'Malley, Sheppard, Schwartz, & Mandelblatt, 2004). Low income African American men and women receiving treatment for hypertension in comparing nurse practitioners, medical doctors, and clinic type reported no significant differences in mistrust by provider type, but trust was higher for patients seen by nurse practitioners (Benkert, Peters, Tate, & Dinardo, 2008). Patient and provider race concordance did not affect the findings.

Drevdahl, Canales and Dorcy (2008) note the lack of a strong empirical base showing a relationship between culturally competent interventions and the reduction of health disparities and suggest that the field may need to move beyond cultural competency. In a review of five interventions to improve cultural competence in healthcare systems (used variables such as providing bilingual providers, recruiting staff members who reflected the cultural diversity of the community served, use of culturally appropriate materials), effectiveness of the interventions could not be determined due to methodological incompatibility or rigor, e.g., no comparative studies, outcome measures of the review were not part of the study, (Anderson, Scrimshaw, Fullilove, Fielding, & Normand, 2003).

Challenge 5. Prepare the Work Force to
Deliver High Quality Health Care

Efforts must be expanded and strengthened to increase the recruitment and participation of racial/ethnic minority and other underserved communities in health care research and delivery. Betancourt et al. (2003) developed a framework of cultural competence interventions that include minority recruitment into the health professions, development of interpreter services and language-appropriate health educational materials, and provider education on cross-cultural issues and identified guidelines to measure cultural competence training on health care outcomes (Betancourt & Green, 2010). Historically Black Colleges and Universities (HBCUs) and minority serving institutions with their missions to improve the status of communities of color and their role in producing health care providers should continue to play an active leadership role in the development of health care professionals and increase their involvement in providing culturally competent training to others.

Concluding Remarks

Health disparities focuses on closing the gap, e.g., reducing excess deaths, between the most and least privileged groups in the

U. S. It is a useful pragmatic strategy to focus attention on inequities in health status and care, and it provides useful markers to evaluate success. It runs the risk, however, of not attending to certain conditions where disparities do not exist, but still may be significant areas of concern within communities. Communities must not lose sight of working to achieve optimal health for its citizens.

Communities will have to actively advocate for the systemic structural and policy changes needed to eliminate health disparities and provide excellent health care to everyone regardless of employment status, race/ethnicity, gender, or age. There must be a constant, well-informed chorus of voices advocating for health care access and quality for underserved communities, for research needed to form the knowledge base for program development and culturally competent health care, and for the training needed to ensure that all persons involved in the health care delivery system including consumers are well-informed.

Strong, creative leadership is needed to steadily advance the vision of establishing a culturally competent health care delivery system, construct feasible strategies, motivate and influence stakeholders, and train persons on cultural competency in health disparities, research and health care delivery. Racial/Ethnic minority institutions and organizations, with their experience and access to populations, have much to contribute to this effort.

References

Adler, N.E. & Rehkopf, D.H. (2008). U.S. disparities in health: Descriptions, causes, and mechanisms. *Annual Review of Public Health, 29*, 235-252.

Adler, N.E. & Stewart, J. (2010). Health disparities across the lifespan: Meaning, methods, and mechanisms. *Annals of the New York Academy of Sciences, 1186*, 5-23.

Agency for Healthcare Research and Quality. (April 20, 2012). Disparities report highlights health care challenges for racial and ethnic minorities. Underscores importance of Affordable Care Act efforts to improve health care quality and access. Retrieved August 7, 2012 from www.ahrq.gov/news/press/pr2012/qrdr11pr.htm.

Anderson, L.M., Scrimshaw, S.C., Fullilove, M.T., Fielding, J.E., Normand, J., Task Force on Community Preventive Services (2003). Culturally competent healthcare systems. A systematic review. *American Journal of Preventive Medicine, 24*(3 Supplement), 68-79.

Andrulis, D.P., Siddiqui, N.J., Purtle, J.P. & Duchon, L. (2010). Patient protection and affordable care act of 2010: advancing health equity for racially and ethnically diverse populations. Washington, DC: Joint Center for Political and Economic Studies.

Beach, M.C., Keruly, J. & Moore, R.D. (2006). Is the quality of the patient-provider relationship associated with better adherence and improved health outcomes for patients with HIV? *Journal of General Internal Medicine,* 21(6), 661-665.

Benkert, R., Peters, R., Tate, N. & Dinardo, E. (2008). Trust of nurse practitioners and Physicians assistants among African Americans with hypertension. *Journal of American Academic Nurse Practitioners, 20*(5), 273-280.

Betancourt, J.R. (2006). Cultural competency: Providing quality care to diverse populations. *Consulting Pharmacology, 21*(12), 988-995.

Betancourt, J.R., & Green, A.R. (2010). Commentary: Linking cultural competence training to improved health outcomes: perspectives from the field. *Academic Medicine, 85*(4), 583-585.

Betancourt, J.R., Green, AR, Carrillo, JE, & Ananch-Firempong,O. 2nd (2003). Defining cultural competence: a practical framework for addressing racial/ethnic disparities in health and health care. *Public Health Reports, 118*(4), 293-302.

Betancourt, J.R. & Maina. (2004). The Institute of Medicine Report "Unequal treatment": Implications for academic health centers. *Mt. Sinai Journal of Medicine, 71*(5), 314-321.

BlackAmericaWeb.com (June 29, 2012). What Black Americans can expect from the Affordable Care Act. Retrieved on 8/6/2012 from www.blackamericaweb.com/news/national-news. CADCA, SAMHSA. Nov. 17, 2010. Minority teens using drugs at higher rates.www.cadca.org. Retrieved Nov 18 2010.

Campbell, C.I., Weisner, C., & Sterling, S. (2006). Adolescents entering chemical dependency treatment in private managed care: ethnic differences in treatment initiation and retention. *Journal of Adolescent Health, 38*(4), 343-350.

Chou, A.F., Brown, A.F., Jensen, R.E., Shih, S., Pawlson, G. & Scholle, S.H. (2007). Gender and racial disparities in the management of diabetes mellitus among Medicare patients. *Women's Health Issues, 17*(3), 150-161.

Clark Atlanta University, Academics Environmental Justice Resource Center. Available at: www.cau.edu/Environmental_Justice_Resource_Center_ERIC. Accessed March 2, 2012.

Centers for Disease Control and Prevention. (2009). Differences in prevalence of obesity among Black, White, and Hispanic adults—United States, 2006-2008. *MMWR. 58*(27), 740-744.

Centers for Disease Control and Prevention. (2010). Diagnoses of HIV Infection and AIDS in the United States and Dependent Areas, 2009. *HIV Surveillance Report, Vol. 21.* Available at: www.cdc.gov/hiv/surveillance/resources/reports/2009report. Accessed March 26, 2012.

Cohen, D.A., Scribner, R.A., & Farley, T.A. (2000). A structural model of health behavior: A pragmatic approach to explain and influence health behaviors at the population level. *Preventive Medicine, 30*(2), 146-154.

Commission on the Social Determinants of Health. (2008). Closing the gap in a generation: Health equity through action on the social determinants of health. Final Report of the Commission on Social Determinants of Health. Geneva, World Health Organization.

Cotto, J. H., Davis, E., Dowling, G.J., Elcano, J. C., Staton, A. B. & Weiss, S. R. (2010). Gender effects on drug use, abuse, and dependence: A special analysis of results from the National Survey on Drug Use and Health. *Gender Medicine 7* (5), 402-413.

Cross, T., Bazron, B., Dennis, K., & Isaacs, M. *Towards a culturally competent system of care, Volume 1.* Washington, DC: Georgetown University Child Development Center, CASSP Technical Assistance Center, 1989.

Drevdahl, D.J., Canales, M.K., & Dorcy, K.S. (2008). Of goldfish tanks and moonlight tricks: can cultural competency ameliorate health disparities? *ANS Advances in Nursing Science, 31*(1), 13-27.

Dykes, D., & White, A. A. (2009). Getting to Equal: strategies to understand and eliminate general and orthopaedic healthcare disparities. *Clinical Orthopaedic Related Research, 467,* 2598-2605.

Eiser, A.R., & Ellis, G. (2007). Viewpoint: Cultural competence and the African American experience with health care: The case for specific content in cross-cultural education. *Academic Medicine, 82*(2), 176-183.

Fernandez, E.S., South-Paul, J.E. & Matheny, S.C. (2003). Mental health: Culture, race, and ethnicity: A supplement to mental health: A report of the Surgeon General.

Freudenberg, N., Silver, D., Carmona, J.M., Kass, D., Lancaster, B. & Speers, M. (2000). Health promotion in the city: A structured review of the literature on interventions to prevent heart disease, substance abuse, violence and HIV infection in US metropolitan areas, 1980-1995. *Journal of Urban Health, 77*(3), 443-457.

Gaston-Johansson, F., Hill-Briggs, F., Oguntomilade, L, Bradley, V., & Mason, P. (2007). Patient perspectives on disparities in healthcare from African-American, Asian, Hispanic, and Native American samples including a secondary analysis of the Institute of Medicine focus group data. *Journal of the National Black Nurses Association, 18*(2), 43-52.

Hailey, D., Roine, R., & Ohinmaa, A. (2002) Systematic review of evidence for the benefits of telemedicine. *Journal of Telemedicine and Telecare, 8*, Supplement 1, 1-30.

Harding, AK. & Greer, ML. The Health Impact of Hazardous Waste Sites on Minority Communities: Implications for Public Health and Environmental Health Professionals. *Journal of Environmental Health* Vol. 55; 1993, Retrieved Online at: www.questia.com/googleScholar.qst?docID=5002192383. Accessed January 13, 2011.

Helling, A. & Sawicki, D.S. (2003). Race and residential accessibility to shopping and services. *Housing Policy Debate, 14* (1,2), 69-101.

Hill, T.D., Graham, L.M. & Divgi, V. (2011). Racial disparities in pediatric asthma: a review of the literature. *Current Allergy and Asthma Report, 11* (1), 85-90.

Iguchi, M.Y., Bell, J., Ramchand, R.N. & Fain, T. (2005). How criminal system racial disparities may translate into health disparities. *Journal of Health Care for the Poor and Underserved, 16*(4 Suppl. B), 48-56.

Institute of Medicine. (2002). Health insurance is a family matter. (2002). Board on Health Care Services. Washington, DC: The National Academies Press.

Israel, B.A., Coombe, C.M., Cheezum, R.R., Schulz, A.J., McGranaghan, R.J., Lichtenstein, R., Reyes, A. G., Clement, J., & Burris, A. (2010). Community-based participatory research: a capacity-building approach for policy advocacy aimed at eliminating health disparities. *American Journal of Public Health, 100*(11), 2094-2102.

Jackson, J.S., Knight, K.M. & Rafferty, J.A. (2010). Race and unhealthy behaviors: chronic stress, the HPA axis, and physical and mental health disparities over the life course. *American Journal of Public Health, 100*(5), 933-939.

Kaiser Family Foundation. (2010). Health reform and communities of color: Implications for racial and ethnic health disparities. Available at www.kff.org.

Kessler, R.C., Price, R.H., & Wortman, C.B. (1985). Social factors in psychopathology: stress, social support, and coping processes. *Annual Review of Psychology, 36,* 531-572.

King, D., Glasgow, R.E., & Leeman-Castillo, B. (2010). Re-aiming RE-AIM: using the model to plan, implement, and evaluate the effects of environmental change approaches to enhancing population health. *American Journal of Public Health, 100*(11), 2076-2084.

Larson, N.I., Story, M.T., & Nelson, M.C. (2009). Neighborhood environments: disparities in access to healthy foods in the U.S. *Journal of Preventive Medicine, 36* (1), 74-81

Lekan, D. (2009). Sojourner syndrome and health disparities in African American women. *ANS Advances in Nursing Science, 32(*4), 307-321.

Lavizzo-Mourey, R., & Mackenzie, E.R. (1996). Cultural competence: Essential measurements of quality for managed care organizations. *Annals of Internal Medicine, 124*(10), 919-921.

LaVeist, T.A. (2005). Distentangling race and socioecomic status: A key to understanding health inequities. *Journal of Urban Health, 82*(2 Supplement 3), iii 26-34.

LaVeist, T.A., Gaskin, D.J., & Richard, P. (2009). The economic burden of health inequalities in the United States. *The Joint Center for Political and Economic Studies*, Washington, DC. Available at: www.jointcenter.org/publications.recent. publications/health.

Mars, M. (2010). Health capacity development through telemedicine in Africa. *Yearbook of Medical Informatics, 87*-93.

Marmot, M.G., Rose, G., Shipley, M. & Hamilton, P.J. (1978). Employment grade and coronary heart disease in British civil servants, *Journal of Epidemiology and Community Health, 32*(4), 244-249.

McNeil, J.I. (2003). A model for cultural competency in the HIV managements of African American patients. *Journal of the National Medical Association, 95*(2 Supplement 2), 3S-7S.

Mohai, P. & Bryant, B. Environmental Injustice: Weighing Race and Class as Factors in the Distribution of Environmental Hazards. 63 *U Colo L. Rev.*, 1992. 921; HeinOnline Law Journal Library, Available at: http://heinonline.org/HeinDocs/LawJournalLibrary. pdf. Accessed January 13, 2011.

Mujahid, M.S., Diez Roux, A.V., Cooper, R.C., Sea, S. & Williams, D.R. (2011). Neighborhood stressors and race/ethnic differences in hypertension prevalence (the multi-ethnic study of atherosclerosis). *American Journal of Hypertension, 24*(2) 187-193.

National Center for Health Statistics. Early Release of Selected Estimates Based on Data From the 2009 National Health Interview Survey, Table 1.3, Percent Persons without health insurance coverage at time of interview by race/ethnicity, June 2010.

National Center for Health Statistics, *National Vital Statistics Reports (NVSR)*, Deaths: Final Data for 2007, Vol. 58, No. 19, May 2010.

National Institutes of Health. *Health Disparities Strategic Plan and Budget, 2004-2008*, Bethesda, MD, 2009.

O'Malley, A.S., Sheppard, V.B., Schwartz, M., & Mandelblatt, J. (2004). The role of trust in use of preventive services among low-income African-American women. *Preventive Medicine, 38*(6), 777-785.

Or, C.K. & Karsh, B.T. (2009). A systematic review of patient acceptance of consumer health information technology. *Journal of American Medical Information Association, 16* (4), 550-570.

Paez, K.A., Allen, J.K., Carson, K.A., & Cooper, L.A. (2008). Provider and clinic cultural competence in a primary care setting. *Social Science and Medicine, 66*(5), 1204-1216.

Picou, J.S. & Hudson, K. (2010). Hurricane Katrina and mental health: a research note on Mississippi Gulf Coast residents. *Sociological Inquiry, 80* (3), 513-524.

Powell, D.L., & Stewart, V. (2001). Children: The unwitting target of environmental injustices. *Pediatric Clinics of North America, 48*(5), 1291-1305.

Practice Directorate, American Psychological Association. (July 16, 2012). Supreme Court upholds Affordable Care Act: what psychologists need to know. Practice Update. Retrieved on 8/8/2012 from www apapracticecentral.org/update2012/04-16/ affordable-care-act. Quality Affordable Health Care for All Americans (Patient Protection and Affordable Care Act), 42 U.S.C.A. § 18001 (West 2011).

Schneider, E.C., Zaslavsky, A.M., & Epstein, A.M. (2002). Racial disparities in the quality of care for enrollees in medicare managed care. *Journal of the American Medical Association, 287*(10), 1288-1294.

Social Security Administration. (2010). *Source of income for AA elderly*. Washington, DC: Government Printing Office.

Smedley, B. (June 28, 2012). Health care bill could reduce inequities. Opinion. Retrieved 8/8/2012. Retrieved from www. thegrio.com 2012/06/28.

Smedley, B.D., Stith, A.Y., & Nelson, A. R. (Eds.), 2003. *Unequal treatment: Confronting racial and ethnic disparities in health care*. Washington, DC: National Academy Press.

Smedley, B.D. & Syme, S.L. (2001). Promoting health: intervention strategies from social and behavioral research. *American Journal of Health Promotion, 15*(3), 149-166.

Spruill, T.M. (2010). Chronic psychosocial stress and hypertension. *Current Hypertension Reports, 12*(1), 10-16.

Trivedi, A.N., Zaslavsky, A.M., Schneider, E. C. & Ayanian, J.Z. (2005). Trends in the quality of care and racial disparities in Medicare managed care. *New England Journal of Medicine, 353*(7), 692-700.

U.S. Department of Health and Human Services. (2010). Office of Disease Prevention and Health Promotion. Healthy People 2020. Washington, DC. Available at www.healthypeople.gov. Accessed March 2, 2012.

U.S. Department of Health and Human Services. (1985). *Report of the Secretary's Task Force on Black and minority health.* Washington, DC: U.S. Government Printing Office.

US Central Intelligence Agency, 2006. The World Fact Book, 2005, Available from www.cia.gov.cia/publications Accessed January 20, 2013.

Verhoeven, F., Tanja-Dijksra, K., Nijland, N., Eysenbach, G., & van Gemert-Pijnen, L. (2010). Asynchronous and synchronous teleconsultation for diabetes care: A systematic literature review. *Journal of Diabetes Science and Technology, 4*(3), 666-684.

WhiteHouse.Gov. Health Reform for African Americans (2012). The affordable Care Act gives African Americans control over their own health care. Retrieved on 8/8/2012 from WhiteHouse. Gov/HealthReform.

Williamson, M. & Harrison, L. (2010). Providing culturally appropriate care: a literature review *International Journal of Nursing Studies, 47*(6), 761-769.

Young VD, Reviere R, Ackah Y. (2004). Behind Bars: An Examination of Race and Health Disparities in Prison. In: Livingston IL, ed. *Praeger handbook of Black American health: policies and issues behind disparities in health. Vol 11.* 2nd ed. Westport, CT: Praeger; 638-652.

INDEX

www.ingramcontent.com/pod-product-compliance
Lightning Source LLC
Chambersburg PA
CBHW031815170526
45157CB00001B/65